ATLAS OF
GASTROINTESTINAL
ENDOSCOPY

ATLAS OF
GASTROINTESTINAL
ENDOSCOPY

FRED E. SILVERSTEIN, M.D.

Professor of Medicine
Director of Gastrointestinal Endoscopy
University Hospital
University of Washington
Seattle, Washington

GUIDO N.J. TYTGAT, M.D., Ph.D.

Professor of Medicine and Gastroenterology
Chief, Division of Gastroenterology-Hepatology
Academic Medical Center
University of Amsterdam
Amsterdam, The Netherlands

Foreword by
KURT J. ISSELBACHER, M.D.

Mallinckrodt Professor of Medicine
Harvard Medical School
Physician and Chief
Gastrointestinal Unit
Massachusetts General Hospital
Boston, Massachusetts

W.B. Saunders Company   PHILADELPHIA • TORONTO

Gower Medical Publishing   NEW YORK • LONDON

Published in North America by:
W.B. Saunders Company
West Washington Square
Philadelphia, PA 19105

Distributed worldwide except North America and Japan by:
Churchill Livingstone
Medical Division of Longman Group Ltd
Robert Stevenson House
1-3 Baxter's Place, Leith Walk
Edinburgh EHI 3AF, UK

ISBN 0-03-012792-0 (W.B. Saunders)
ISBN 0-912143-06-1 (Gower)
ISBN 0443-03862-7 (Churchill Livingstone)

Library of Congress Cataloging-in-Publication Data
Silverstein, Fred E., 1942–
    Atlas of gastrointestinal endoscopy.

    Includes bibliographies and index.
    1. Endoscope and endoscopy--Atlases.
2. Gastrointestinal system--Diseases--Diagnosis--
Atlases. I. Tytgat, G. N. J. II. Title. [DNLM:
1. Endoscopy--atlases. 2. Gastrointestinal Diseases--
diagnosis--atlases. WI 17 S587a]
RC804.E6S536   1987   616.3'307'545   86–12089

Editor: Abe Krieger
Designers: Keith Stout, Jill Feltham, Jessica Stockholder
Illustrators: Alan Landau, Laura Pardi

Printed in Hong Kong by Mandarin Offset.

Foreword

As the reader will instantly appreciate, this is an impressive atlas and an important contribution to gastrointestinal endoscopy. Moreover, it provides a unique resource in the field of gastroenterology especially because the quality of the photography is so exceptional. The atlas reviews the appearance of normal anatomy, variations within normal limits, and provides examples of the endoscopic manifestations of nearly all gastrointestinal diseases. A brief yet sufficient text guides the reader through the sequence of photographs while line drawings aid in the interpretation of the photographic images. Radiographs and histological correlations are interspersed where appropriate.

The organization of the atlas is by organ system. The first chapter discusses the normal examination of the esophagus, stomach, small bowel, and colon. Subsequent chapters deal with each organ in detail, starting with a brief description of relevant technique and then a description of the diseases which affect that organ. The large number of photographs cover most disorders of the gastrointestinal tract. This atlas and slide set will serve as an excellent introduction to the endoscopic appearances of normal and abnormal intestinal organs for those learning endoscopic techniques. The superb photographs will also be useful for all physicians specializing in the diagnosis and management of gastrointestinal diseases. These photographs, obtained with unusual and meticulous endoscopic and photographic techniques, provide the best in vivo images yet available of these organs in health and disease. This should also be an excellent resource for surgeons, radiologists, and pathologists who may utilize these endoscopic photographs in the teaching of gastrointestinal disorders. This atlas is indeed a superb new resource.

Kurt J. Isselbacher, M.D.
Mallinckrodt Professor of Medicine
Harvard Medical School;
Chief, Gastrointestinal Unit
Massachusetts General Hospital
Boston, Massachusetts

F.E.S.: This book is dedicated to
Ellie, Curt, Mark, Laura, and Christopher

G.N.J.T.: This book is dedicated to
Christiane, Kristien, Lieve, Stefaan, and Johan

Preface

Endoscopy is one of the most exciting and expanding fields in clinical medicine. It provides accurate diagnostic information and is being used increasingly to provide therapy for intestinal disorders. Furthermore, it is least invasive, safer than many other therapeutic approaches, and often can be accomplished on an outpatient basis to achieve a favorable cost-benefit ratio.

The success of endoscopy creates several dilemmas. How is one to learn these techniques? How can one learn to interpret the images? Many of us who teach endoscopy know that the mechanical performance of the procedure is only the beginning. Accurate interpretation of images is at least as important, and learning this skill requires the highest quality endoscopic images.

This *Atlas of Gastrointestinal Endoscopy* represents a significant effort on the part of several people. The purpose of writing the Atlas and developing the companion Slide Atlas is to provide an organized series of photographs documenting the appearance of gastrointestinal organs in health and disease.

Endoscopic photography is not simple. Many of us have taken thousands of photographs for teaching and for documenting a patient's abnormality. Unfortunately, most of these photographs turn out to be poor. The unique aspect of this Atlas is the high quality of the photographs and the vast clinical experience from which they are drawn. Dr. Tytgat has mastered the art of endoscopic photography. When his interest and skill are combined with his large clinical facility, the large number of patients, and a wide variety of gastrointestinal problems encountered, the result is an exceptional set of photographs. The majority of images in this Atlas are reproduced from Dr. Tytgat's collection. Carefully labeled line drawings and schematic diagrams were added to clarify the critical diagnostic information.

Fred E. Silverstein, M.D.
Guido N.J. Tytgat, M.D., Ph.D.

Acknowledgments

We have many people to thank for helping us prepare this Atlas. Dr. Tytgat would like to thank his colleagues at the Academic Medical Center and his ex-fellows in training who referred patients with uncommon abnormalities. In particular Drs. Kees Huibregtse, Joep Bartelsman, Frieda Den Hartog Jager, Lisbeth Mathus-Vliegen, Lok Tio, Willem Dekker, and Max Scheijver; Mrs. Hanna Tikkemeyer who assisted with the clinical procedures and photography; and the staff of the Department of Medical Photography. He would also like to thank the Board of Directors of the Academic Medical Center for their support and appreciation.

Dr. Silverstein would like to thank Mary Hill and Mary Wieckowicz who helped edit the text and organize the slide set; Abe Krieger of Gower Medical Publishing who provided guidance; and his colleagues who provided thoughtful comments and some excellent examples of unusual diseases. He would like to thank in particular Drs. David Saunders, Michael Kimmey, Charles Pope, Charles Rohrmann, Rodger Haggitt, and George McDonald. We selected Dr. Kurt Isselbacher, an outstanding internist and gastroenterologist, to write the Foreword because this Atlas is intended for gastroenterologists, internists, and other specialists as well as gastrointestinal endoscopists.

Finally, we would like to thank Ellie Silverstein and Christiane Tytgat who assisted us with this project. Our families encouraged us, provided critical comments, and allowed us to devote the time necessary to complete this Atlas.

Contents

11 Colon II: Inflammatory and Infectious Disorders   11.1

12 Colon III: Diverticular Disease, Vascular Malformations, and Other Colonic Abnormalities   12.1

1

The Normal Gastrointestinal Tract

In this first chapter we will review the endoscopic examination of the normal gastrointestinal (GI) tract. Recognition of the normal endoscopic appearance is essential if one is to learn to identify abnormal appearances. Pertinent anatomy will be presented, especially as relates to the endoscopic examination. Some aspects of technique will be included although a detailed discussion of endoscopic techniques is not intended. Other sources are available which review technical aspects in detail.

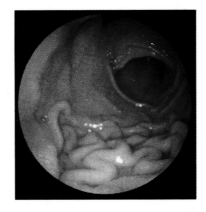

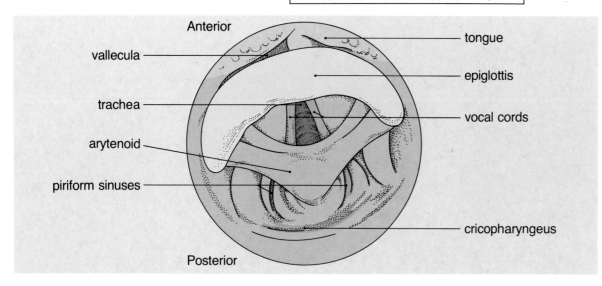

Figure 1.1 The anatomy of the hypopharynx.

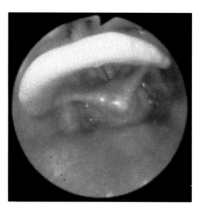

Figure 1.2 Endoscopic view of a hypopharynx, with the epiglottis, piriform sinuses, and closed vocal cords clearly evident. The cricopharyngeus muscle is closed and cannot be seen here, but is located posteriorly at the bottom of the field.

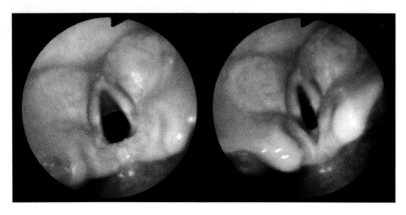

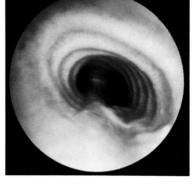

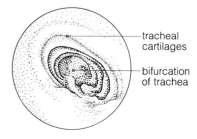

Figure 1.3 *Left,* In this closeup view of the larynx, the vocal cords are open. The arytenoid cartilages may also be observed. *Right,* The same vocal cords, this time partially closed.

Figure 1.4 This endoscopic view, seen at bronchoscopy, reveals the tracheal rings with a bifurcation in the distance. The endoscope should be immediately withdrawn so as not to block the airway. (Courtesy of Dr. Mark Richardson)

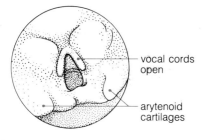

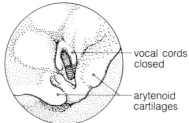

In addition, both the mouth and the pharynx should be checked for obvious oropharyngeal abnormalities such as tumors, scars, surgical deformity, mucosal inflammation, or infection. This inspection can be performed immediately prior to endoscopy.

THE NORMAL OROPHARYNX AND HYPOPHARYNX

We will begin our survey of the normal gastrointestinal tract with the oropharynx. In most patients, the fiberoptic endoscope can be easily passed through the mouth into the hypopharynx. Observations of structures in the mouth and posterior pharynx are rarely made by endoscopy, rather by simple direct inspection. It is important to be sure that the teeth are in reasonable repair, and that bridges are removed and loose teeth protected against breakage during endoscopy to prevent aspiration into the tracheobronchial tree.

ANATOMY

The anatomy of the hypopharynx may be observed upon advancing the endoscope or at the conclusion of the endoscopy as the instrument is removed from the esophagus (Fig. 1.1). These structures include:

The base of the tongue which ends at the epiglottis

The valleculae, the spaces lateral to the epiglottis

The larynx with vocal cords and arytenoid cartilages, just below the epiglottis

The piriform sinuses, on both sides of the larynx

The cricopharyngeus muscle, located posterior to the larynx, approximately 20 cm from the teeth

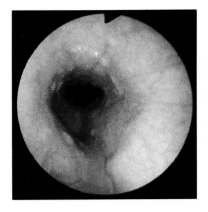

Figure 1.5 Normal pink-gray esophageal mucosa. A small amount of mucus is seen, as are the normal, fine, submucosal blood vessels.

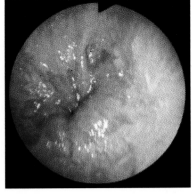

Figure 1.6 Note the ora serrata or Z line, the junction of the esophageal squamous mucosa and the gastric

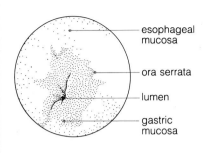

esophageal mucosa

ora serrata

lumen

gastric mucosa

columnar mucosa. The border is usually serrated, as seen here.

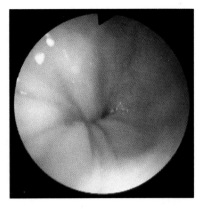

Figure 1.7 Four or five normal esophageal folds can be seen at the esophagogastric junction. These folds are pliable and can usually be distinguished from esophageal varices.

POSITIONING THE ENDOSCOPE

The tip of the endoscope is gently advanced through the mouth into the hypopharynx to approximately 18 cm from the incisors, the level of the upper esophageal sphincter or cricopharyngeus muscle. (For future reference, all distances mentioned during upper GI tract endoscopy will be in centimeters from the incisors.) The cricopharyngeus muscle is closed at rest but opens during swallowing (Figs. 1.2 and 1.3). We therefore ask the patient to swallow when the endoscope tip is at 18 to 20 cm. The endoscope can then be gently advanced into the esophagus.

There are several techniques for passage. One may guide the tip under direct endoscopic view down to and through the cricopharyngeus, or one may pass the instrument blindly using gentle manipulation. Some examiners place their fingers into the patient's mouth to keep the instrument midline in the oropharynx. Others place the correct bend on the endoscopic tip and are able to pass it into the patient's mouth and oropharynx without insertion of fingers. Regardless of which technique is employed, the endoscopist may encounter difficulty in passing the tip through the cricopharyngeus into the esophagus. Obstructing elements include cervical spine spurs, tumors, surgically modified anatomy, and abnormal neurologic function. If unusual difficulty is encountered, if pain or bleeding occurs, or if an abnormal hypopharyngeal area is seen or palpated, it is usually wise to stop the procedure and evaluate the area with the help of an otolaryngologist and/or radiologist.

Rarely, as the endoscope is being passed into the hypopharynx, the tip may inadvertently enter the trachea. You will know that this has occurred when tracheal cartilage or the tracheal bifurcation is visualized (Fig. 1.4). Should the endoscope lodge between the vocal cords, it can seriously compromise the patient's airway. Therefore, remove the endoscope immediately, either into the pharynx or completely out of the patient's mouth. If, during a difficult intubation, there is a question as to whether the endoscope has entered the trachea, the endoscopist can ask the patient to cough or phonate. If the endoscope is inserted between the vocal cords, the patient will be unable to cough or speak, and the endoscope should be withdrawn immediately.

THE NORMAL ESOPHAGUS

ANATOMY

The esophagus is a tubular organ which begins at the slitlike opening of the cricopharyngeus muscle (20 cm) and extends to the esophagogastric junction in the area of the diaphragmatic hiatus (approximately 40 cm). This hiatus can be identified endoscopically by having the patient sniff, which accentuates the location of the diaphragm, or by simply watching the esophageal wall during quiet respiration to observe the impression of the diaphragm. The level of the diaphragm is important when one tries to identify the presence of a hiatal hernia.

The esophageal diameter is 1.5 to 2.0 cm. Its wall has a muscle layer composed of striated muscle in the upper one-third and smooth muscle in the lower two-thirds. The entire esophagus is lined by stratified squamous epithelium which appears nearly white or pinkish-gray (Fig. 1.5). This lining extends to or below the level of the diaphragmatic hiatus where it meets the salmon-pink mucosa of the stomach. The distinct wavy or undulated line at this junction is called the ora serrata or "Z" line (Fig. 1.6). Note that the line may appear to straighten if the area is distended with air during endoscopy.

The esophageal lumen is usually free of debris, and normally has longitudinal mucosal folds which are pliable and flattened with distension. These folds can be easily distinguished from esophageal varices which appear beaded and may have a bluish color. Four or five longitudinal folds usually form a symmetrical, rosette-like structure at the esophagogastric junction (Fig. 1.7). This junction is normally

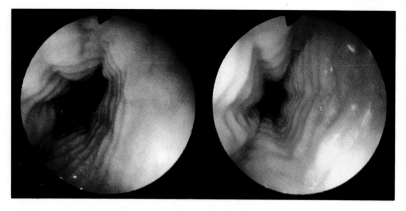

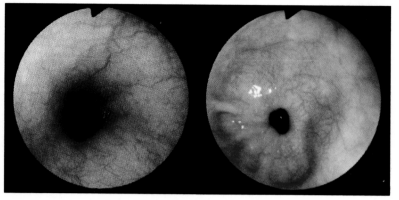

Figure 1.8 *Left,* Transverse ridging of a normal esophagus immediately prior to vomiting. *Right,* Transverse ridging of the esophagus with retching.

Figure 1.9 Views of normal distal esophageal mucosa with a delicate vascular pattern.

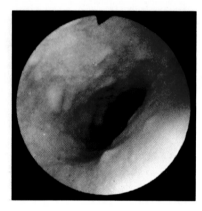

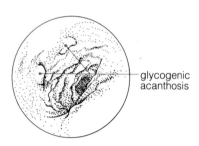

glycogenic acanthosis

Figure 1.10 Glycogenic acanthosis of the esophagus.

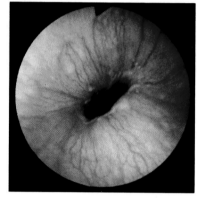

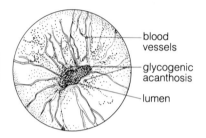

blood vessels

glycogenic acanthosis

lumen

Figure 1.11 This endoscopic view of the distal esophagus demonstrates normal blood vessels and glycogenic acanthosis of the mucosa.

closed but can be easily opened with gentle air insufflation. No resistance is usually encountered at this junction as the endoscope passes into the stomach. In addition to longitudinal folds, transverse ridges may occasionally be seen, especially prior to vomiting (Fig. 1.8).

The longitudinal folds gradually taper over a 2 to 3 cm section of distal esophagus and extend to the Z line. The squamocolumnar junction is usually located at the distal end of the lower esophageal sphincter (LES), 0.5 cm below the diaphragmatic hiatus, though it may be observed 1 cm above the hiatus due to variations which occur with respiration. Gastric folds extend up from below and end just below the squamocolumnar junction.

The submucosal vasculature of the esophagus can be seen at endoscopy as fine, small, delicate blood vessels. These vessels are only visible on the esophageal side of the ora serrata (Figs. 1.5 and 1.9).

In older individuals, one may commonly see glycogen granules in the esophageal squamous mucosa, a condition referred to as glycogenic acanthosis. The presence of these granules is of uncertain significance (Fig. 1.10). Such areas may also be seen in the distal esophagus (Fig. 1.11).

Motility in the esophagus is difficult to appreciate at endoscopy. Occasionally, contractions will be seen, especially tertiary contractions. Likewise, in certain diseases which involve the esophageal muscle, the lack of motility can be observed by endoscopy (e.g., a nonperistaltic esophagus in a patient with scleroderma). In general, esophageal motility should be evaluated with manometry or with fluoroscopic motion recordings with videotape.

A variety of normal and abnormal conditions will cause narrowing of the esophageal lumen. These include intrinsic structures such as rings, webs, tumors, or strictures, and extrinsic structures such as normal and abnormal blood vessels adjacent to the esophagus, mediastinal tumors, etc. The intrinsic lesions will be dealt with in the following chapters on esophageal pathology.

The importance of extrinsic compression on the esophagus is best understood when one remembers that the esophagus is positioned in a central location within the thorax: immediately posterior to the heart; between the lungs; and adjacent to the vertebral column, the inferior vena cava, and the aorta. It is attached at its upper end to the cricopharyngeus and at its lower end to the diaphragm. Normal (Fig. 1.12) and abnormal (Fig. 1.13) structures may impinge on the esophagus and can be seen during esophagoscopy. The normal structures include the aorta, approximately 25 to 30 cm from the teeth (Fig. 1.14), and the left mainstem bronchus, slightly below the aorta. Both of these structures cause a smooth indentation of the

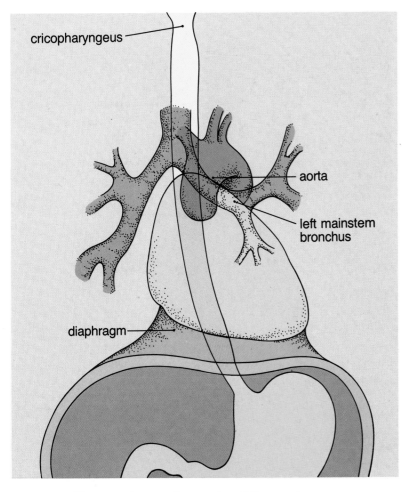

Figure 1.12 The normal areas of narrowing of the esophagus.

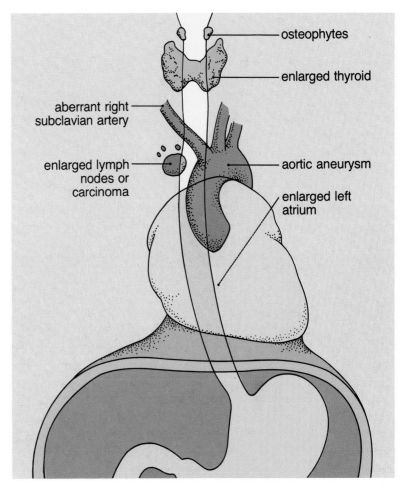

Figure 1.13 The abnormal areas of narrowing of the esophagus.

esophageal wall. The abnormal structures include osteophytes from the cervical spine, an enlarged thyroid gland, an enlarged aorta, an enlarged left atrium, bronchogenic tumors, lymph nodes, and abnormal vascular structures. In addition, an anomalous takeoff of the right subclavian artery from the descending aorta may cross behind the esophagus and compress it anteriorly against the trachea, causing difficulty in swallowing. This condition is referred to as dysphagia lusoria. In each case, the esophageal mucosa is indented but otherwise appears normal.

The esophagus terminates at the ora serrata and at the lower esophageal sphincter (LES). Anatomically, the LES appears as a slight thickening of the smooth muscle of the esophageal wall. It is normally closed at rest, and functions to keep gastric contents out of the esophagus.

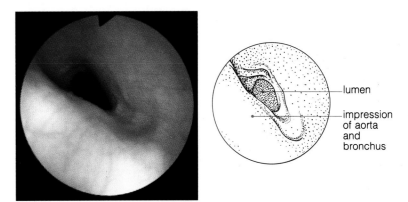

Figure 1.14 Normal esophagus with an impression caused by the adjacent aorta and left mainstem bronchus. The covering mucosa is normal.

POSITIONING AND ENDOSCOPIC EXAMINATION

The endoscope is passed under direct vision from the esophagus into the stomach. When using a forward-viewing endoscope, advancement should be accomplished with the lumen constantly in view; blind passage is not desirable. This passage often requires a turn to the left and anteriorly to track the esophagus as it enters the stomach. The lumen can usually be easily and gently followed into the stomach.

The area of the stomach just below the esophagogastric junction is the cardia. Endoscopic examination of the esophagus should include careful inspection of the cardia, which can only be partially accomplished during insertion of the instrument into the stomach. For complete and accurate examination, the instrument must be placed into the stomach and the tip bent back on itself, or retroflexed, to

1.5

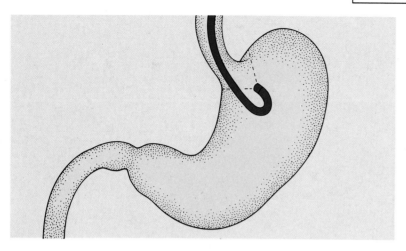

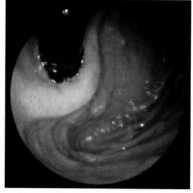

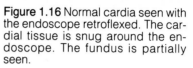

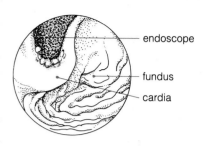

Figure 1.15 Diagram demonstrates retroflexion to inspect the gastric cardia, fundus, and lesser curvature.

Figure 1.16 Normal cardia seen with the endoscope retroflexed. The cardial tissue is snug around the endoscope. The fundus is partially seen.

see the gastric tissue of the cardia as it surrounds the endoscope (Figs. 1.15 and 1.16). This is the only reliable method of viewing ulcers, mucosal tears, or tumors in the cardia. When a hiatal hernia is present, a large, incompetent cardia will be observed in the retroflexed view, with a space surrounding the endoscope as it enters the stomach. A longitudinal ridge, mucosal fold, or sling can often be seen on retroflexed view and is thought to identify the end of the esophagus just below the level of the diaphragmatic hiatus as seen from below.

The retroflexion maneuver is also essential to permit adequate inspection of the gastric fundus and the lesser curve of the stomach. These areas are inspected by retroflexing the endoscope and then moving the endoscope in and out with rotation clockwise and counterclockwise. If one limits an endoscopic examination to direct endoscopy without performing careful retroflexion, significant lesions in the stomach can be missed.

THE NORMAL STOMACH

ANATOMY

The stomach is divided into several anatomic areas (Fig. 1.17): the fundus (Fig. 1.18), the cardia (seen in Fig. 1.16), the body (Figs. 1.19 and 1.20), and the antrum (Figs. 1.21 and 1.22). There is a lesser curve and greater curve. Endoscopically, the angularis, or incisura, usually marks the entrance into the antrum on the lesser curvature. This anatomic division is different than the histologic or physiologic boundary because of the distribution of the antral and fundal mucosa. The antral mucosa may extend high up on the lesser curvature to within a few centimeters of the cardia. This is higher than the incisura, the anatomic boundary for the beginning of the antrum. The significance of antral mucosa high in the lesser curvature is mainly for the surgeon who wishes to remove all or most antral mucosal tissue during

peptic ulcer surgery. To do this, he or she must extend the resection up the lesser curvature of the stomach, proximal to the anatomic incisura. For the endoscopist, this mucosal boundary is important because benign gastric ulcers often occur at the margin of the antral and fundal mucosa. Since this boundary can occur high on the lesser curvature, this is an area where gastric ulcers may be encountered.

POSITIONING AND ENDOSCOPIC EXAMINATION

Stomachs have a variety of normal shapes. Some are long and vertical while others are transverse. Most of these distinctions are not important to the endoscopist. The general principles for inspection are the same for all configurations.

The tip of the endoscope is passed through the distal esophagus and cardia into the upper body of the stomach. At this point, gentle inflation with air is necessary to inspect the stomach wall. The gastric pool is inspected and observations made as to the amount of fluid and the presence of blood, bile, and food (Fig. 1.23). Recently ingested antacid may compromise the endoscopic examination (Fig. 1.24), while other debris may suggest abnormal gastric emptying. A bezoar may be seen consisting of retained food residue or other material. After inspecting the gastric pool, it is usually wise to aspirate as much fluid as possible in order to prevent reflux and aspiration during the procedure and to facilitate the further inspection of the stomach.

The gastric mucosal surface is briefly inspected for color, surface appearance, blood vessels, and fold thickness. The complete gastric examination is usually performed after the duodenum has been intubated and inspected. An exception is if an abnormality is encountered during the initial exam, in which case the area is carefully inspected immediately. In this way the endoscopist knows that erythema or bleeding was present before endoscopy and was not caused by the shaft of the endoscope during inspection of the duodenum.

Although it seems that the area just below the cardia should be easy to inspect endoscopically, this is often not the case. In the high lesser curvature position, even large

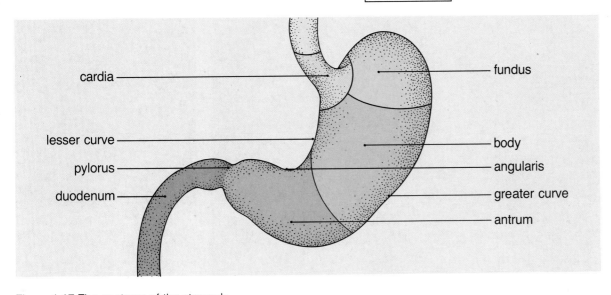

Figure 1.17 The anatomy of the stomach.

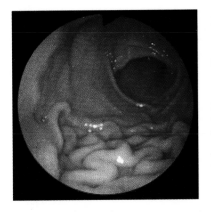

Figure 1.19 In this view of the stomach with the endoscope straight, one can appreciate the normal rugal folds in the body of the stomach and observe that these folds do not extend into the antrum in the distance.

Figure 1.18 In this retroflexed view, the normal fundus of the stomach is seen in addition to the cardia.

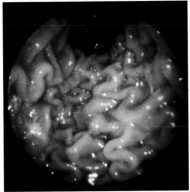

Figure 1.20 The normal mucosa of the stomach is glistening and moist, and normal rugae are also seen. The white spots are highlights of the endoscope lights reflecting off the mucosa.

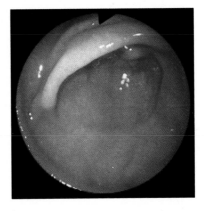

Figure 1.21 Normal antrum and angularis. The pylorus is located under the angularis (or incisura) and is therefore not seen in this view. There are no rugal folds.

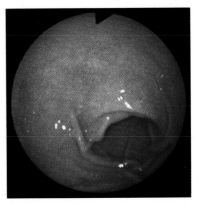

Figure 1.22 Normal antrum, with smooth mucosa and no rugae.

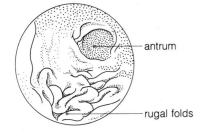

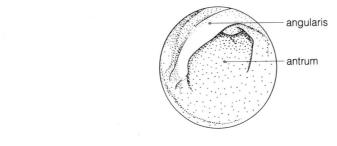

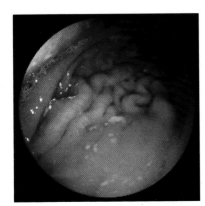

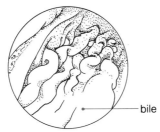

Figure 1.23 Normal stomach, with bile present in the gastric pool.

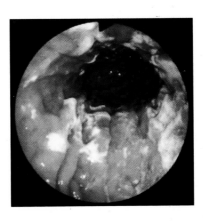

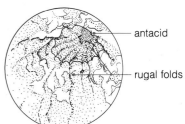

Figure 1.24 Normal stomach. The normal mucosa of the midbody is covered with antacid taken by mistake just before endoscopy. The rugal folds are normal.

1.7

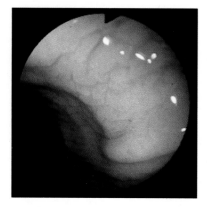

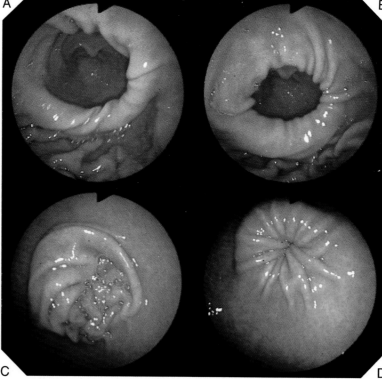

A

B

C

D

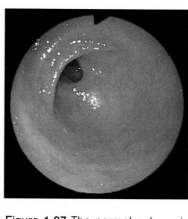

Figure 1.25 In this view one can observe normal areae gastricae. The gastric pits empty into these glandular structures.

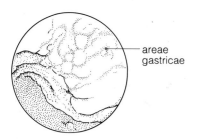

areae gastricae

Figure 1.26 This sequence demonstrates a normal antrum with a contraction wave moving toward the pylorus. If one watches this wave as it progresses, areas of decreased contractility can be identified and studied. The final view shows the wave ending at the pylorus.

Figure 1.27 The normal pylorus is seen just distal to the angularis.

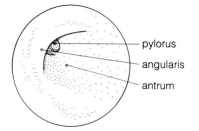

pylorus
angularis
antrum

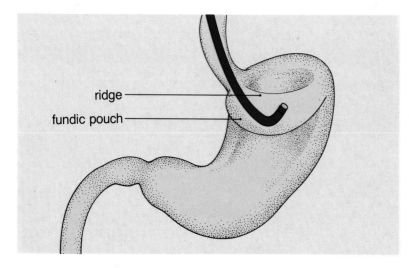

ridge
fundic pouch

Figure 1.28 Diagram of a "cup-and-pour" stomach demonstrates the problem this can create for the endoscopist.

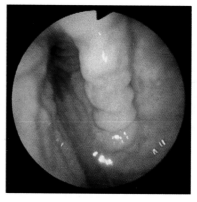

Figure 1.29 "Cup-and-pour" stomach. The fundic pouch, which may confuse the endoscopist, is seen to the right. In the center is the ridge separating the pouch from the main body of the stomach to the left.

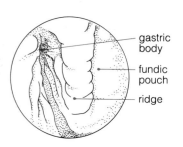

gastric body
fundic pouch
ridge

gastric ulcers can be missed with a forward-viewing endoscope. A similar problem occurs with other lesions of the cardia such as tears and tumors. Therefore, it is essential that these areas be observed on retroflexed view (see Figs. 1.16 and 1.18).

When fiberoptic endoscopes were first developed, complicated maneuvers were necessary to perform the retroflexion maneuver to inspect the cardia and fundus. This is no longer the case. The new fiberendoscopes can mechanically turn 180° with motion on the control handles. In fact, most can turn 210°, allowing simple retroflexion for inspection of the cardia and fundus. With experience, the retroflexion maneuver can be easily performed, allowing complete inspection of the lesser curvature, cardia, and fundus.

Normally, the gastric mucosa is a uniform salmon color (see Fig. 1.20). With careful inspection one can observe the areae gastricae, the macroscopic patterns of gastric glandular structures (Fig. 1.25). This pattern is absent in patients with atrophic gastritis, and accentuated in patients with hypersecretion and duodenal ulcers. Blood vessels are not usually

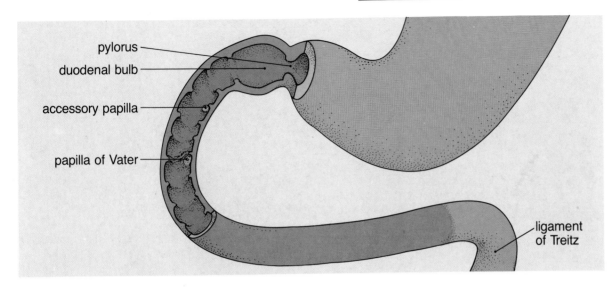

pylorus
duodenal bulb
accessory papilla
papilla of Vater
ligament of Treitz

Figure 1.30 Anatomy of the duodenum.

seen through the mucosa. The folds, or rugae, begin in the upper body of the stomach near the entrance to the esophagus and course distally to the antrum. They may be seen in the fundus but are often not longitudinally oriented. These folds are normally soft and pliable, and in most cases will flatten almost completely with distension of the stomach.

The antrum is usually smooth and free of folds (see Figs. 1.21 and 1.22). Gastric peristalsis begins in the midbody and progresses down into the antrum. Contractions, at a frequency of three per minute, continue to the gastric outlet or pylorus where they stop (Fig. 1.26). The pylorus is usually open (Fig. 1.27) but closes when the contraction wave reaches it. This probably allows for mixing of food, and for liquid contents to pass into the duodenum while the stomach retains and continues to liquefy solids. It is often useful to endoscopically watch a contraction wave move from the body to the antrum to determine if there is an area which is asymmetrical, stiff, and doesn't move well. If such an area is observed, it should be carefully inspected for signs of an abnormality. An ulcer or tumor may first be noted as an area which does not move well during an antral contraction wave.

There are several organs adjacent to the stomach which can cause extrinsic impressions of the gastric lumen. The most commonly seen is the spleen, whose impression may be noted in the posterior greater curvature area. Abnormalities of other structures such as aneurysms of the splenic artery, pancreatic pseudocysts, etc. may also appear as extrinsic pressure.

For the person using a forward-viewing endoscope, the various gastric configurations are not especially important. This is not true, however, when side-viewing endoscopes are used. With the latter instrument, one may get somewhat lost in the proximal stomach and have difficulty finding the antrum and pylorus. This is occasionally a problem during endoscopic retrograde cholangiopancreatography (ERCP) when a side-viewing endoscope is passed via the esophagus and stomach into the duodenum to locate and cannulate the papilla of Vater. This problem is especially noted in the "cup-and-pour" stomach, where a pouch of fundus lies

directly below the cardia. The tip of the endoscope enters this pouch, and the endoscopist is then unable to locate the route to the gastric body, antrum, and pylorus. The endoscope may turn around in the pouch presenting a retroflexed view, but the anatomy is confusing (Fig. 1.28).

Although the "cup-and-pour" or cascade stomach is mainly a problem for side-viewing endoscopes, it is also occasionally a problem with forward-viewing endoscopes. The instrument may be damaged because of extreme angulations and, more importantly, a complication such as a perforation can result because of the confusing anatomy. This problem may be solved by pulling the endoscope back to just below the esophagogastric junction and then looking to the left. One often sees a ridge which separates the fundic pouch from the rest of the stomach (Fig. 1.29). A turn to the left will then allow the endoscope to pass easily into the gastric body and down into the antrum.

The angularis is a useful marker to locate the lesser curvature, as well as the pylorus. The pylorus is found several centimeters distal to the angularis. Although it is usually not difficult to find the pylorus, it may be a problem with a side-viewing endoscope, or with any endoscope if the area is distorted by current or past peptic ulcer disease or surgery.

THE NORMAL DUODENUM

ANATOMY

The duodenum, measuring 25 to 30 cm in length, marks the beginning of the small bowel. It is composed of four portions (Fig. 1.30). The first is the duodenal bulb, which is 4 to 5 cm long and begins at the pylorus and runs to the right and posteriorly. The bulb is in the peritoneal cavity; the other portions are retroperitoneal. The second portion is approximately 7 to 8 cm in length and runs caudally. The third portion is approximately 10 cm long and runs to the left across the spine and great vessels. The fourth portion

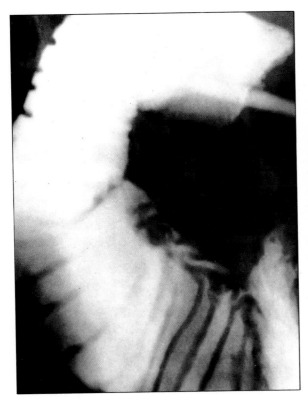

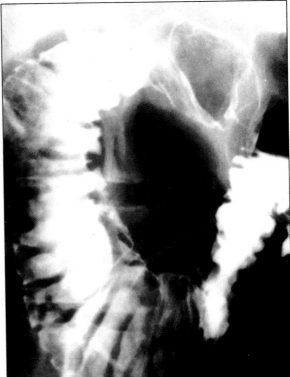

Figure 1.31 In this hypotonic duodenogram, barium outlines the papilla on the medial portion of the descending duodenal wall. The intramural common bile duct (CBD) and the plica duodeni longitudinalis can be seen along with a gathering of folds just distal to the papilla. (Courtesy of Dr. C. Rohrmann)

Figure 1.32 In this duodenal X-ray study, the papilla and the longitudinal fold distal to it are easily seen. This anatomy can orient the endoscopist and help locate the papilla. (Courtesy of Dr. C. Rohrmann)

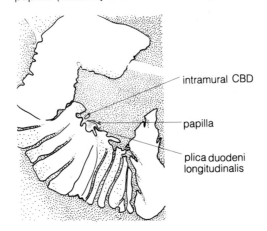

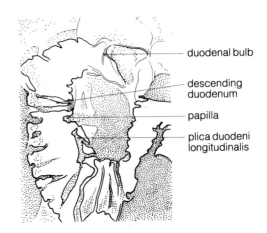

is 4 to 5 cm long and runs cephalad and to the left where it turns and joins the jejunum at the ligament of Treitz.

The mucosa of the duodenal bulb is free of folds, but the other portions demonstrate characteristic folds of Kerckring. The mucosal villi are similar to those found in the jejunum and ileum. Special to the duodenum are Brunner's glands which occur in the submucosa of the first half to two-thirds.

The papilla of Vater, located on the medial wall of the descending duodenum 3 to 6 cm distal to the apex of the bulb, is the main papilla which drains both the bile duct and the pancreatic duct in most patients. An accessory papilla (papilla of Santorini) may be located 2 to 4 cm proximal to the papilla of Vater on the medial duodenal wall. It is important to understand the anatomy of the duodenum around the papilla of Vater if one is to be able to find the papilla and cannulate it with a side-viewing endoscope. The papilla is often located at the distal end of a bulge in the medial duodenal wall. This bulge is the intramural portion of the distal common bile duct. Just distal to the papilla there is a characteristic longitudinal fold, the plica duodeni longitudinalis. Likewise, there may be several folds which converge proximally at the papilla. The experienced endoscopist will focus on the area at the distal end of the bulging intramural common bile duct and the proximal end of the longitudinal fold to locate the papilla. This anatomy may be appreciated on barium contrast X-ray studies of the duodenum, especially during hypotonic duodenography with air contrast (Figs. 1.31 and 1.32).

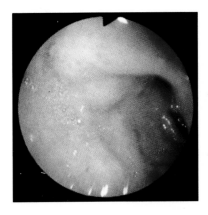 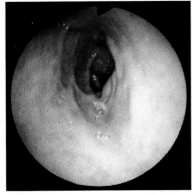 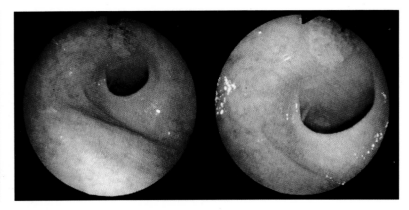

Figure 1.33 Normal duodenal bulb. The mucosa is slightly reticulated, and no blood vessels are seen. The apex of the bulb and the entrance into the descending duodenum are seen to the right.

Figure 1.34 Normal duodenal bulb. Folds of Kerckring can be seen in the distance just beyond the apex of the bulb.

Figure 1.35 *Left,* The apex of a normal duodenal bulb is seen; bile is present. *Right,* A closeup view.

POSITIONING THE ENDOSCOPE

Once the pylorus is located, the tip of the endoscope is advanced into the duodenal bulb. In most instances the tip passes easily, but occasionally persistence is required. Touching the pylorus, backing away, and then touching it again will sometimes assist passage. Force should never be used, as there may be an organic cause for an obstruction to passage and excessive force could result in a tear or perforation. In a vertically oriented or J-shaped stomach, the endoscopist may have to create a long, greater curvature gastric loop before the tip of the instrument can be advanced up to and through the pylorus into the duodenal bulb.

In some cases, the duodenal bulb is first inspected with the endoscope tip at the pylorus. This is referred to as the transpyloric view. This view may be useful if there is difficulty passing the pylorus or if, as the tip of the endoscope is passed into the bulb, it slips immediately down into the second or descending portion of the duodenum. This latter problem may occur in a patient with a J-shaped stomach, because once the tip of the endoscope passes the pylorus, pressure from the gastric loop pushes the tip beyond the duodenal bulb, not allowing adequate inspection of the bulb. As the endoscope is withdrawn in an attempt to see the bulb, the reverse problem occurs. First the gastric loop is removed. Then, when the instrument is straight, the tip begins to move back up the duodenum and comes out through the bulb very rapidly into the stomach, again not allowing adequate inspection of the bulb. One can repeat this in-out sequence several times and never adequately inspect the bulb. The solution is to stop the forward advance at the pylorus, inspect the bulb transpylorically, and then very slowly advance into the bulb. Similarly, when the tip is in the descending duodenum, pulling out very slowly will often allow the tip to come back into the bulb for adequate inspection of the area.

ENDOSCOPIC EXAMINATION

Nearly the entire surface of the duodenal bulb can usually be well-visualized with a small-caliber fiberendoscope. The most difficult areas to inspect are the fornices, just distal to the pylorus. The mucosa of the bulb often has a slightly reticulated appearance when contrasted with the stomach, though the color is often similar (Fig. 1.33). There are usually few if any folds (Fig. 1.34). Bile is often present (Fig. 1.35) and may cause a bubbly foam that can interfere with duodenal inspection. Using a wash fluid with simethicone or other surfactant will immediately break up these bubbles and permit excellent inspection of the mucosa. Active peristalsis may also make endoscopy of the duodenum difficult. Here, a hypotonic agent such as glucagon will rapidly cause duodenal hypotonia and allow endoscopic inspection of the duodenal bulb and descending duodenum.

If a red, reticulated area of mucosa is noted, careful inspection is essential because it may be adjacent to a duodenal ulcer which might otherwise be missed. This is especially problematic if heavy folds from previous peptic disease are present. Blood vessels are not visible in the duodenal bulb, nor are they visible further down in the descending duodenum. In addition to inspection for ulcers and erosive disease, surgical anastomoses such as a choledochoduodenostomy may be located. Using an end-viewing instrument, this orifice can be inspected and, if appropriate, cannulated for contrast X-ray studies of the common bile duct.

The endoscope is then routinely passed by the apex of the bulb and the superior duodenal angle into the descending duodenum. Since this portion of the duodenum is posterior and retroperitoneal, a turn to the right and down is usually required. In most cases this can be accomplished under direct vision, with the lumen maintained in view at all times. Occasionally, it may be necessary to turn the tip to the right and down without advancing the instrument

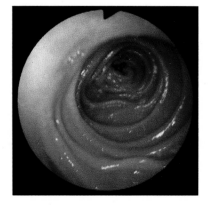 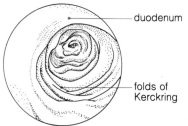

Figure 1.36 Normal descending duodenum, with the transverse folds of Kerckring clearly evident.

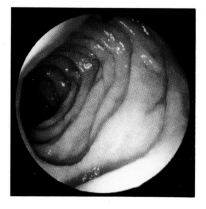

Figure 1.37 Normal descending duodenum. Circular folds are seen.

Figure 1.38 Normal descending duodenum, with a reticulated or velvet mucosal surface. In this case, some of the folds are longitudinally oriented.

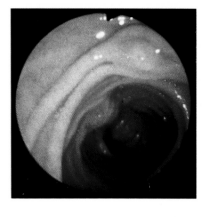 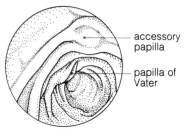

Figure 1.39 Descending duodenum, with the main papilla of Vater seen in the distance. The smaller accessory papilla is seen proximal to the main papilla.

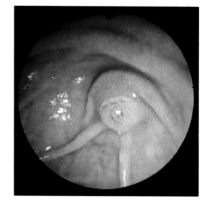 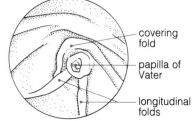

Figure 1.40 Normal papilla of Vater, with its characteristic red, reticulated surface. Two longitudinal folds distal to the papilla can be appreciated.

to see if one can enter the descending duodenum blindly. This maneuver may pass the tip gently into the descending duodenum. As soon as the descending duodenum is intubated, the lumen can again be imaged and the rest of the examination performed with the lumen clearly in view. (It is always preferable to perform all endoscopy with the lumen in view.)

The descending duodenum can be recognized by the folds of Kerckring which run transversely around the lumen (Figs. 1.36 and 1.37). There is considerable variability in the fold pattern, and in some patients longitudinally oriented folds connect the transverse folds (Fig. 1.38). The mucosal surface is smooth, and blood vessels are not seen. With magnification fiberoptics, it may be possible to see duodenal villi. Bile is often present and may help locate the papilla of Vater.

Inspection of the descending duodenum is usually performed to determine the presence of a postbulbar ulcer, as may be seen in gastric hypersecretory states, or to examine the papilla of Vater. Other indications include possible inflammatory disease in the postapical portion of the duodenum (Crohn's disease) or to evaluate masses noted on barium upper-GI X-ray studies. Examination of the postbulbar duodenum is usually brief, part of routine upper endoscopy.

Location and inspection of the papilla of Vater is not as easily accomplished with a forward-viewing endoscope as with a side-viewing endoscope. With a forward-viewing endoscope, the intramural portion of the common bile duct may be seen bulging into the duodenal lumen. One may also see the papilla of Vater protruding into the lumen (Fig. 1.39), as well as the vertical fold below the papilla, the plica duodeni longitudinalis. It is not usually possible to cannulate the papilla with an forward-viewing endoscope. On occasion, one will see the accessory papilla in the duodenum (see Fig. 1.39). This structure is usually on the same side of the duodenum as the main papilla but is located several centimeters closer to the pylorus. The accessory papilla is smaller, less red, and is usually not reticulated as is the main papilla.

The papilla of Vater is more easily located and inspected using a side-viewing endoscope. The papilla may have several shapes, varying from a prominent papillary projection to a flat appearance. The surface of the papilla has a characteristic red, reticulated appearance which clearly distinguishes it from surrounding duodenal mucosa (Fig. 1.40). In some cases, yellow or golden bile is seen flowing from the papilla or is noted on the mucosa adjacent to the papilla.

The endoscope is slowly withdrawn from the descending duodenum, inspecting the descending duodenal surface, the apex of the bulb, the duodenal bulb, the pylorus, and the stomach along the way. The detailed gastric exam is usually performed at this point. Once the stomach exam is completed, gentle suction is used to remove air, reducing the patient's discomfort after the procedure.

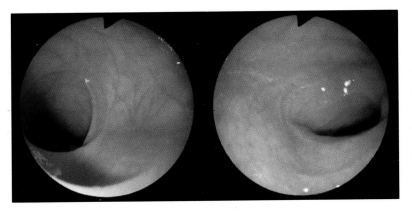
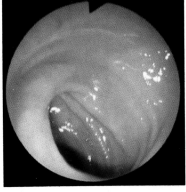
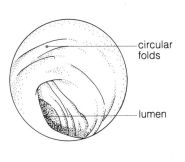

circular folds

lumen

Figure 1.41 Views of a normal terminal ileum. A fine vascular pattern can be seen with inflation of the lumen. Folds are subtle and the mucosa less glistening than in the colon.

Figure 1.42 Normal terminal ileum with less inflation. Folds are seen although they are less prominent than in the duodenum. The lumen tends to collapse readily with suction.

The endoscope is then pulled back into the esophagus, and the observations which were made as the endoscope was first passed are confirmed. If one moves slowly and gently as the tip of the endoscope passes up through the crico-pharyngeus, the anatomy of the hypopharynx and vocal cords can be observed. The instrument is then removed from the mouth and the endoscopy is complete.

THE TERMINAL ILEUM

ANATOMY

The terminal ileum, the end of the small bowel, attaches to the colon at the ileocecal valve. The colonoscopist may place the tip of the colonoscope in the cecum and then enter the terminal ileum for a short distance. This distal segment of ileum is not as mobile as is the rest of the ileum because it is attached to the cecum which is usually not mobile. The circular folds characteristic of the duodenum and jejunum are often absent in the terminal ileum whereas lymphoid aggregates may be seen.

POSITIONING THE COLONOSCOPE

The tip of the colonoscope is routinely passed retrograde into the cecum, the most proximal portion of the colon. In many cases the ileocecal valve can be identified.

Endoscopy of the terminal ileum is not easy and is often not indicated in routine colonoscopy. In some diseases, such as inflammatory bowel disease, it may be useful to inspect the terminal ileum, though it may not be possible to pass the valve because of narrowing. The technique is to pass the tip of the colonoscope just beyond the proximal lip of the ileocecal valve and then turn into the valve, often medially and posteriorly, to lift the lip of the valve and permit entry of the tip of the colonoscope. In some cases one can then gently withdraw the colonoscope in this hooked

position to advance the tip into the ileum. It may then be possible to gently insert more colonoscope length and further intubate the terminal ileum.

Fluoroscopy can confirm this position by demonstrating that the endoscope tip is oriented in a left and often cephalad direction (in contrast to a downward and to the left orientation noted when the tip of the endoscope is in the cecum). Location in the terminal ileum can also be suspected when a villus pattern is observed endoscopically. On occasion, a biopsy may be used to identify villi on the mucosa of the terminal ileum to be certain that the tip of the instrument is in place in the distal small intestine. Minimal amounts of air insufflation should be used to reduce patient discomfort. The technique should be gentle, with minimal force and intermittent removal of air to help the tip advance into the ileum.

ENDOSCOPIC EXAMINATION

Colonoscopy of the terminal ileum is useful in the differential diagnosis of radiographic abnormalities of the terminal ileum and in patients presenting with suspected Crohn's disease. Normally, the terminal ileum mucosa is smooth, and blood vessels may be seen, especially with air insufflation (Fig. 1.41). Kerckring folds or ringlike contractions are less marked in the terminal ileum than in the duodenum and jejunum (Fig. 1.42; compare with Figs. 1.36 to 1.38). The appearance of the mucosa is not glistening as in the colon but more villous and dull as in the duodenum. The lumen tends to collapse more readily than in the colon and is usually of smaller caliber than is the ascending colon or cecum. All of these factors can be clues to the fact that the tip of the instrument is, in fact, in the terminal ileum.

Occasionally, lymphoid nodules covered with normal mucosa are seen. These nodules can vary in size from 1 to several mm and may cause a nodular surface. The appearance of active peristalsis also helps distinguish the terminal ileum from the colon. Mucosal changes may indicate the presence of Crohn's disease or other inflammations of the terminal ileum, including tuberculosis and infection with Yersinia.

1.13

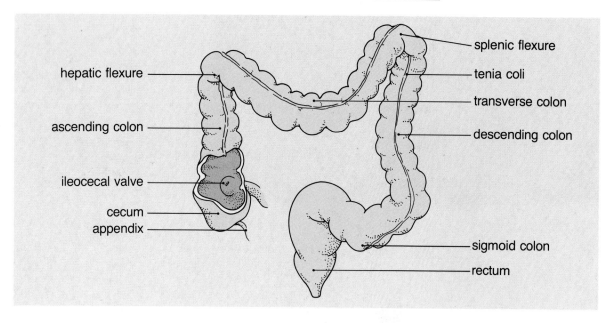

Figure 1.43 Anatomy of the colon.

THE NORMAL COLON

ANATOMY

The colon is a tubular organ which runs from the cecum in the right lower quadrant to the rectum (Fig. 1.43). It is widest in the cecum and ascending colon and gradually narrows as one approaches the rectum. The colon is divided into the following sections: the cecum; the ascending colon, which runs from the cecum cephalad to the hepatic flexure; the transverse colon, which runs from the hepatic flexure in the right upper quadrant to the splenic flexure in the left upper quadrant; the descending colon, which runs from the splenic flexure caudad to the left lower quadrant; the sigmoid colon, which runs from the left lower quadrant to the rectosigmoid junction; and the rectum, which extends down to the anal canal.

The longitudinal muscle in the wall of the colon is fused into three bands, the teniae coli. These bands start at the base of the appendix and run in the wall of the colon down to the rectum where they diffuse into the muscular coat. The three teniae cause the colon to have a triangular appearance endoscopically, which is especially prominent in the ascending and transverse colon. The haustra are outpouchings of the colon, separated by folds. In the descending colon the endoscopic appearance is often tubular.

POSITIONING THE COLONOSCOPE

The patient's perianal area is inspected and a digital exam performed. The colonoscope is then placed into the patient's rectum. A colonic cleansing preparation is required. For upper endoscopy, simply having the patient fast for 8 to 12 hours is sufficient to provide an adequate examination. However, for colonoscopy, a preparative program is essential. There are two approaches: The first is to give the patient clear liquids for 1 to 2 days and a purge with oral magnesium and enemas the day of the examination. The second, increasingly used technique is to purge the gut with a nonabsorbable electrolyte solution. This can be accomplished the night before or the morning of the examination. Either prep removes both fecal material and potentially explosive hydrogen and methane gases.

Most experienced colonoscopists use similar endoscopic techniques. As little air as possible is introduced to prevent overdistension. The pressure on the device is gentle to avoid stretching the colonic wall or mesentery which can cause pain, a vasovagal episode, or a perforation. The lumen is kept in view at all times; little or none of the examination is performed blindly. A variety of in and out maneuvers are used to "accordion" the colon on the colonoscope, keeping the colonoscope as free of loops as possible. In the difficult colon, special maneuvers such as creating an alpha loop in the sigmoid colon is used to pass the sharply angulated sigmoid/descending colon junction. This maneuver requires fluoroscopic guidance and training in the technique.

The colonoscope is advanced to the cecum under direct vision. The detailed examination of the mucosa is usually performed as the colonoscope is slowly removed from the cecum. If the colonoscope has been kept free of loops, the tip responds well and the examination is facilitated. This is especially true if a therapeutic procedure such as polypectomy is to be undertaken, because large, redundant loops of colonoscope can make control of the tip difficult.

Understanding the colonic anatomy is important for several reasons: first, to determine where the tip of the colonoscope is located to help decide on further techniques for passage and to determine the location of an abnormality if one is encountered; second, to determine whether a structure encountered is normal or not; and third, to determine whether the tip is in the cecum and that the entire surface has therefore been inspected. The latter point is critical, for in most indications for colonoscopy the endoscopist should examine the entire length of the colon. For example, if a patient presents with blood in the stool, the entire length of the colon

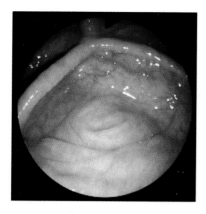

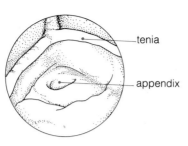

Figure 1.44 Crescent-shaped opening of a normal appendix, seen in the base of the cecum.

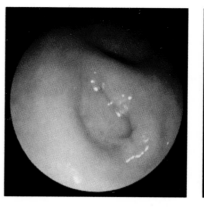

Figure 1.45 Slitlike opening of the appendix in base of cecum.

Figure 1.46 Crescent-shaped opening of the appendix on the wall of the cecum. The normal colonic vasculature can be appreciated.

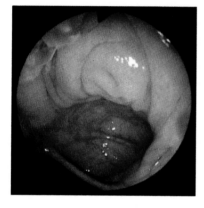

Figure 1.47 Opening of the appendix in the protruded type of configuration. The orifice appears closed.

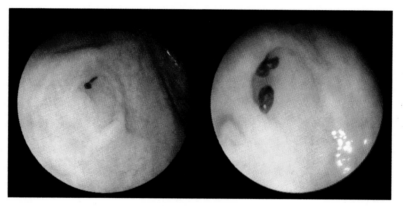

Figure 1.48 *Left,* Normal crescent-shaped appendiceal orifice with seeds noted. *Right,* A closeup view.

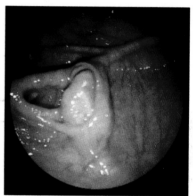

Figure 1.49 Normal appendix with a fecalith in the orifice. Convergence of the teniae can be seen at the orifice.

must be examined for a bleeding source. If one encounters a polyp in the descending colon, it is necessary to look higher for the possible presence of a synchronous polyp or cancer. There are circumstances where total colonoscopy is not possible; e.g., when it is impossible to safely advance the colonoscope tip proximal to the area because of diverticular disease or previous operations, and further proximal intubation of the colon is not possible mechanically.

It is imperative then to determine whether the tip of the colonoscope is in the cecum or whether it is unable to advance at a difficult flexure. Several clues can be used. Light from the tip of the colonoscope may transilluminate the patient's right lower quadrant when the tip is in the cecum. This may be more easily observed if the lights in the room are turned down and if the patient is not greatly obese. Note, however, that this may also occasionally occur when the tip is in the sigmoid colon or transverse colon, especially if a redundant transverse colonic loop is present. When in doubt, observe with X-ray fluoroscopy.

ENDOSCOPIC EXAMINATION

The first characteristic aspect of the cecum is the presence of the appendiceal orifice, a slitlike or crescent-shaped opening located near the coalescence of the three teniae coli (Figs. 1.44 to 1.46). The appendiceal orifice may present two general forms: flat where the orifice is open, and protruded where the base protrudes into the cecum and the orifice is usually closed (Fig. 1.47). Occasionally, small bits of food residue such as seeds or pits may be seen at the orifice (Fig. 1.48), as may a fecalith (Fig. 1.49).

The cecum, located just beyond the ileocecal valve, may be difficult to evaluate radiographically during barium enema examination. Likewise, polyps and cancers can be missed colonoscopically. Therefore, careful inspection of this area is essential. In some patients one may observe an area appearing to be a prominent haustral valve at the level of the ileocecal valve. One must pass this haustrum to enter the cecum.

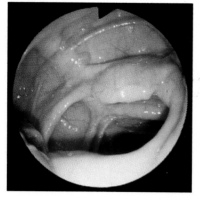
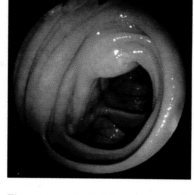
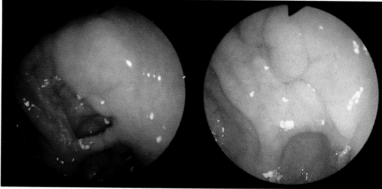
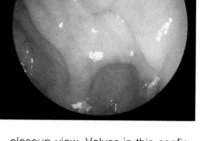

Figure 1.50 Normal ileocecal valve in the labial configuration. The cecum can be seen distal to the valve. This area should be carefully inspected endoscopically, since the fold marking the valve is subtle.

Figure 1.51 A slightly more prominent ileocecal valve of the semilabial type.

Figure 1.52 *Left,* A very prominent ileocecal valve with a papillary or multilobed appearance. *Right,* A closeup view. Valves in this configuration may be difficult to enter with the colonoscope.

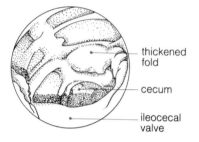
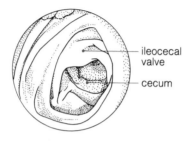
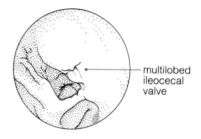
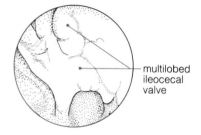

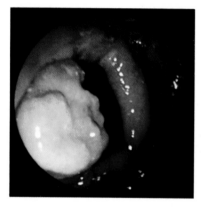
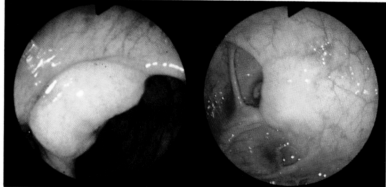
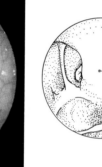

Figure 1.53 Prominent ileocecal valve in the papillary configuration.

Figure 1.54 Views of two normal ileocecal valves covered with slightly yellow adipose tissue (often referred to as lipomatous transformation of the ileocecal valve).

The ileocecal valve may provide another clue to the location of the colonoscope tip. The valve presents several appearances, varying from a subtle flattening of a colonic fold, referred to as the labial appearance (Fig. 1.50), to a prominent liplike structure bulging into the lumen, often referred to as the intermediate semilabial or "flower petal" appearance (Fig. 1.51), to the most prominent papillary or multilobed appearance (Figs. 1.52 and 1.53). The ileocecal valve may also have a fatty, or lipomatous, appearance (Fig. 1.54). In some cases, green ileal fluid (succus entericus) may be seen entering the colon through the ileocecal valve. Occasionally, air in the small intestine from colonoscopy insufflation can distend an adjacent loop of small bowel and cause an impression on the cecal wall which may be confused with the ileocecal valve (Fig. 1.55).

As the colonoscope is pulled out, it is advanced up the ascending colon. In this area, the typical colonic appearance is noted. The mucosa is smooth; normal, fine, delicate blood vessels are apparent (Fig. 1.56). Occasionally, bluish submucosal veins are seen (Fig. 1.57). The teniae coli cause the colon to occur in sacculations or haustra. It may be necessary to look carefully beyond each haustral fold to detect the presence of a small lesion such as a polyp or cancer. The lumen in the cecum and ascending colon is often wide and clearly more capacious than the terminal ileum or the transverse, descending, or sigmoid colon. In the ascending

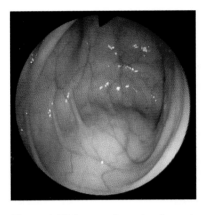

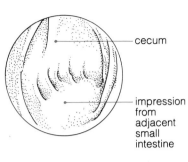

Figure 1.55 Impression of adjacent air-filled loops of small bowel on the wall of the cecum. This could be confused with the ileocecal valve but no orifice is seen.

cecum

impression from adjacent small intestine

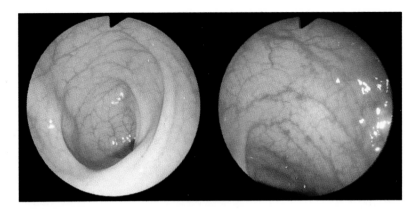

Figure 1.56 Views of the normal, delicate vascular pattern of the colonic mucosa.

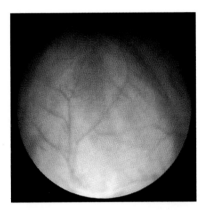

submucosal veins

Figure 1.57 Normal submucosal veins of the colon can be seen adjacent to small arterial structures.

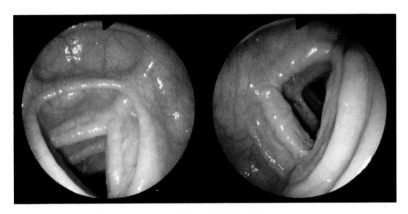

Figure 1.58 Views of the folds in the normal ascending colon. The folds are slightly thicker than in the transverse colon. The triangular configuration is evident, as is the normal colonic vascular pattern.

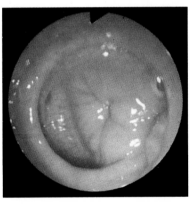

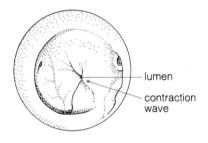

lumen

contraction wave

Figure 1.59 Normal colon with a contraction wave. With patience the orifice will open up and allow intubation. The colon just beyond the orifice may represent a relative blind spot and must be carefully inspected.

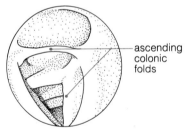

ascending colonic folds

and transverse colon the appearance is characteristically triangular because of the three teniae coli. The folds in the cecum and ascending colon (Fig. 1.58) are thicker than the folds in the transverse colon. The contents of the right colon are often slightly different in color than the rest of the colon because of the succus entericus, which imparts a dark green color. This change is only seen in the cecum and ascending colon.

Contractions of the colon may be noted, and in some patients with muscular colonic walls one may encounter a series of contracted haustrations with luminal orifices which must be intubated as the instrument is advanced proximally to the cecum. As the colonoscope is advanced up the colon, these haustral folds can usually be gently passed if attention is directed to keep the lumen in the center of the endoscopic visual field. Each area must then be carefully inspected as the instrument is withdrawn (Fig. 1.59). Rarely, antispasmodics such as glucagon are required. The tip may have to be passed through the area several times, and the colonoscopist must carefully inspect behind each fold to examine these blind spots and avoid missing a lesion.

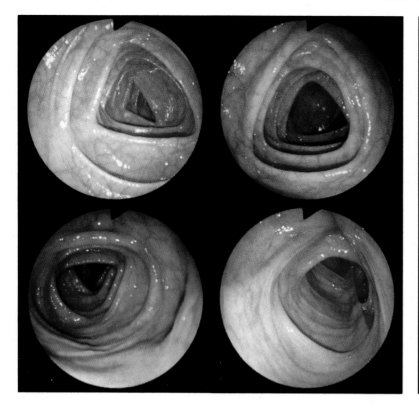

Figure 1.60 Views of a normal transverse colon demonstrate its typical configuration, caused by the three teniae.

Figure 1.61 Views of a normal transverse colon demonstrate its normal fine vascular pattern. The longitudinal teniae are seen.

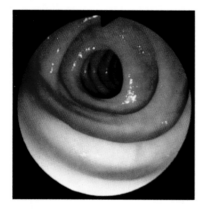

Figure 1.62 Normal descending colon. The haustra are less marked and the lumen is more tubular and less typically triangular.

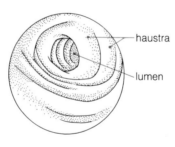

haustra

lumen

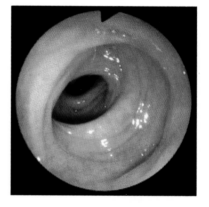

Figure 1.63 Normal sigmoid colon. The lumen has several bends and is tubular or circular.

The hepatic flexure is occasionally identifiable by a slightly bluish discoloration from the adjacent liver and/or gallbladder. The transverse colon has a typical triangular appearance with finer or thinner folds (Fig. 1.60), and may be seen to move readily with respiration. Here, as in the rest of the colon, the vessels are fine and delicate, and the mucosa is smooth (Fig. 1.61). The splenic flexure is difficult to identify endoscopically, except as a bend located between the obviously triangular transverse colon and the more circular, tubular descending colon.

The descending colon usually has less marked haustra and is usually not as triangular (Fig. 1.62). The colonoscope is pulled down the descending colon, past the sigmoid/descending junction, into the sigmoid colon. The sigmoid/descending junction is often a sharp angle with a potential blind spot, as are the hepatic and splenic flexures. These areas must be carefully examined to avoid missing a lesion. The sigmoid colon is also circular and may be of highly variable length from patient to patient (Fig. 1.63). The technique of withdrawal should allow inspection of the entire mucosal surface. If a sharp bend or fold is encountered, the colonoscope may have to be passed up again to carefully inspect the area.

At 16 to 18 cm from the anus one encounters the rectosigmoid junction. This is an acute bend which must also be carefully inspected to avoid missing a lesion.

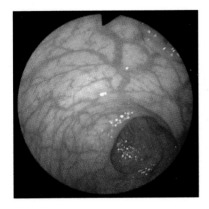 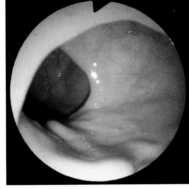 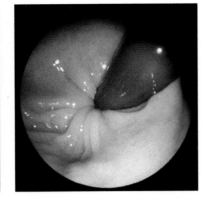 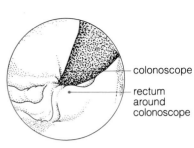

Figure 1.64 Normal prominent veins in the rectum.

Figure 1.65 Rectum distended with air. Two of the three normal rectal valves are seen.

Figure 1.66 The rectum just above the anal canal, as seen from the inside with the colonoscope retroflexed. This enables the endoscopist to see lesions just inside of the anal canal which can be easily missed otherwise.

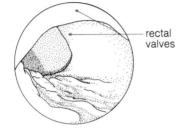

THE RECTUM

The colonoscope is now back in the rectum. The lumen here is wider than in the sigmoid, descending, and transverse colon. Blood vessels are easily observed and are more prominent than in other areas of the colon (Fig. 1.64). The mucosa is usually smooth and glistening.

Three rectal valves are seen (Fig. 1.65). A complete examination often requires that the endoscopist look behind each valve to be certain that a lesion is not missed. With new colonoscopes it is possible in many patients to retroflex the instrument in the rectum and, by rotating the shaft, look back at the rectal mucosa surrounding the endoscope as it passes through the anal canal (Fig. 1.66). This technique allows one to detect lesions which might go unnoticed by direct inspection with a straight tip. Lesions such as internal hemorrhoids, condylomata, and tumors can be seen with this maneuver. After retroflexion, the tip of the device is straightened and gas is gently suctioned from the colon. This makes the patient more comfortable at the conclusion of the procedure. The colonoscope is then slowly removed from the patient; the anal canal can be inspected directly during removal.

THE PERIANAL EXAMINATION

Examination of the rectum and colon is not complete without a careful inspection of the perianal area, a digital examination of the anal canal, and a stress test. Inspection of the perianal area may detect the presence of a bluish discoloration or lateral fissures, typical findings in Crohn's disease. The opening of fistulas or fissures may also be noted. The digital exam is essential prior to the introduction of the colonoscope to detect the presence of any low-lying rectal masses as well as areas of tenderness which might represent a fissure or abscess. Finally, diagnosis of rectal prolapse or internal hemorrhoids is best made using the stress test. The patient is asked to sit on a toilet and bear down. After 20 or 30 seconds, the patient leans forward and a mirror is placed under the patient's bottom to inspect the anal orifice. A flashlight is shined on the mirror to illuminate the area of the perineum. Using this technique, large, occasionally bleeding hemorrhoids can be appreciated, as can a rectal prolapse. This is a better technique than asking the patient to bear down while in the knee-chest or left-lateral decubitus position, for the patient will usually not bear down significantly because of fear of embarrassing himself.

TECHNICAL CONSIDERATIONS

Some general comments are now appropriate which relate to the endoscopic imaging of the GI tract. It is essential to ascertain that the endoscope is functioning properly before the procedure is started. If the endoscope is not working properly, the examination can be severely compromised, yield little or no information, and actually pose a higher risk of complication to the patient. Air insufflation is essential to gently inflate the luminal organ being exposed, thus allowing the endoscopist to see. If the water wash is not working and the endoscopist is unable to clean the lens, the field may be

1.19

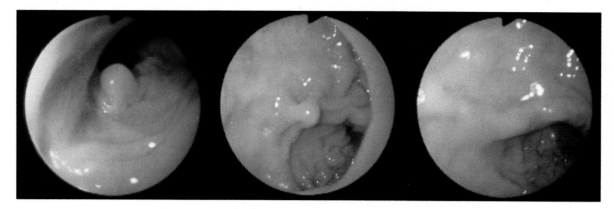

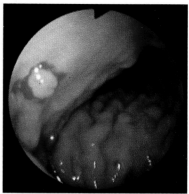

Figure 1.67 *Left,* Iatrogenic "polyp" caused by pulling the mucosa of the colon into the biopsy channel in the tip of the endoscope. *Center,* After several seconds the polyp begins to fade. *Right,* After 1 or 2 minutes the suction artifact is gone.

Figure 1.68 Bleeding suction artifact in the stomach. This can be very confusing for the endoscopist, especially in the patient being examined because of gastrointestinal bleeding.

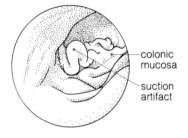

colonic mucosa

suction artifact

partially obscured with blood or mucus, markedly interfering with the endoscopy. If the suction channel is plugged, secretions or excessive insufflated air cannot be removed, which may interfere with the examination and increase the patient's discomfort. The mechanisms of the bending sections must be working so that retroflexion is possible to inspect the cardia, lesser curve, and fundus during upper endoscopy. Obviously, the optics must function correctly. If any of these problems exist, the endoscope should not be used until the problem is corrected.

Some additional comments are required regarding the use of the suction channel. As mentioned earlier, when used properly this channel is very helpful in reducing patient discomfort by preventing distension, and in the removal of secretions and blood which can cover lesions. In addition, the channel is essential for passing accessories during diagnostic procedures such as biopsy and cytology, or therapeutic procedures such as polypectomy, laser therapy, electrocoagulation, foreign body removal, etc. However, if used improperly the channel can confuse the endoscopist and interfere with the procedure. An example of this is the use of the channel for removing large objects such as a large blood clot or a large piece of stool. The suction channel is simply too small to accommodate these objects. Once such an object is pulled against the tip of the endoscope, it may be difficult to dislodge, and on occasion may necessitate removal of the endoscope for cleaning. Since the device must then be passed again, it causes significant inconvenience for both the patient and the examiner.

Another problem occurs if mucosa is sucked into the tip of the endoscope's biopsy channel. The experienced endoscopist often knows this has happened when he or she observes a crescent of red in the visual field and the suction stops working. The tip also moves less well. If this is recognized immediately, the tip can be maneuvered to release the mucosa, or the suction channel can be temporarily disconnected and the channel opened to room air, which will also immediately release the mucosa. If this problem is not recognized and the mucosa remains in the channel, a pseudopolyp or iatrogenic polyp may develop. If recognized early, one can see this polyp gradually fade (Fig. 1.67). However, if not recognized early, the polyp may appear red and "adenomatous" or may cause a small amount of bleeding (Fig. 1.68). This iatrogenic problem creates confusion and slows the endoscopic procedure. It is best prevented by learning about the problems and avoiding it by not pulling mucosa into the tip of the instrument or by releasing the mucosa immediately if the problem occurs. These considerations are essential to make endoscopy as complete, gentle, rapid, and informative as possible.

2

Esophagus I: Diverticula, Hiatal Hernias, Webs, Rings, Reflux, and Barrett's Metaplasia

This chapter is the first of three which will present diseases of the esophagus. In this chapter we will consider structural abnormalities such as diverticula, hiatal hernias, and esophageal webs and rings, as well as reflux, reflux-associated complications, and Barrett's metaplasia.

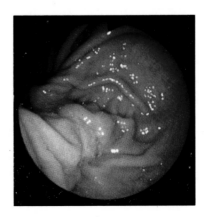

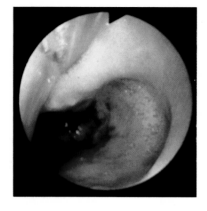

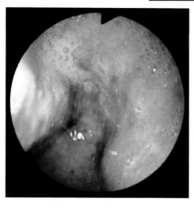

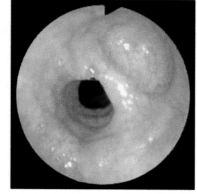

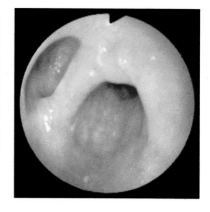

Figure 2.1 Zenker's diverticulum. A tube has been passed into the esophagus. The orifice into the esophagus is difficult to see.

Figure 2.2 Zenker's diverticulum. The small perforation resulted from blind intubation.

Figure 2.3 Midesophageal diverticulum. Small blood vessels are seen in the base of the diverticulum.

Figure 2.4 Midesophageal diverticulum. Here, the lumen fills in the direction of food moving down the esophagus.

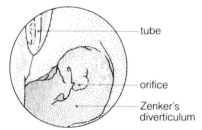

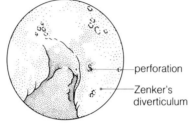

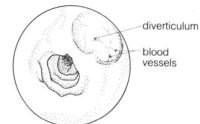

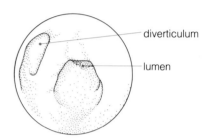

DIVERTICULA

Esophageal diverticula may be symptomatic or asymptomatic. Endoscopy does not play a primary role in their diagnosis or management; however, these entities are important to the endoscopist because a diverticulum can complicate endoscopy. For example, an unsuspected diverticulum can be perforated during intubation of the esophagus. Such a perforation can occur with both end-viewing or side-viewing endoscopes. A diverticulum of the upper esophagus can be perforated with the routine passage of an end-viewing endoscope because passage of the endoscope through the upper sphincter and upper part of the esophagus is often performed blindly. The routine passage of a side-viewing endoscope could perforate a diverticulum anywhere along the esophagus because it is difficult, if not impossible, to inspect the esophageal lumen as the instrument is being passed. It is important to remember that if the endoscope is not passing easily or is causing discomfort, one should stop the procedure and establish whether an organic obstruction or a proximal diverticulum is present (Figs. 2.1 and 2.2). This may be accomplished by obtaining and carefully examining a barium esophagram of the area. An alternative is to pass a small-caliber, end-viewing endoscope through the hypopharynx and on through the cricopharyngeus using a constant inspection technique where the lumen is always in view. Both radiologic and otolaryngologic evaluation may be necessary to study the hypopharyngeal area and the very proximal portion of the upper esophagus.

Diverticula may be observed in three possible configurations: (1) where the diverticulum empties into the esophagus in a downstream direction parallel to the esophagus; (2) where the diverticulum is located at a 90° angle to the esophagus (Fig. 2.3); and (3) where the diverticulum is dependent, meaning that the entrance to the lumen of the diverticulum points toward the stomach (Fig. 2.4). Of these three configurations, the dependent causes the most problems, as food and/or GI instruments tend to enter the diverticulum rather than stay in the lumen (Fig. 2.5). These configurations can be applied to the three types of esophageal diverticula: upper esophageal (Zenker's), midesophageal, and epiphrenic (just above the diaphragm). Each will now be discussed in detail.

ZENKER'S DIVERTICULUM

Zenker's diverticulum is an outpouching of the esophagus typically occurring just above or at the level of the cricopharyngeus sphincter (see Figs. 2.1 and 2.2). It usually presents in adults. The etiology of the diverticulum is not known, although motor dysfunction with incoordination

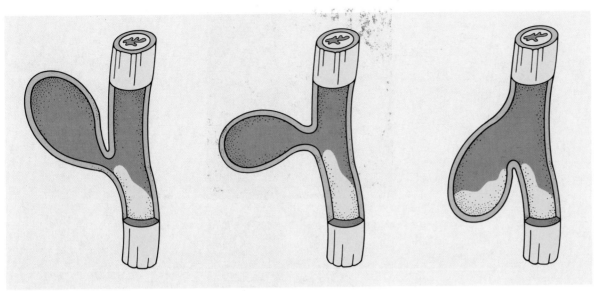

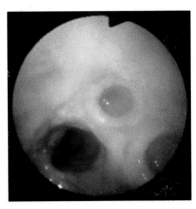

Figure 2.6 Multiple epiphrenic diverticula. The esophageal lumen adjacent to the diverticula has a benign stricture.

Figure 2.5 Configurations of esophageal diverticula. (1) The diverticulum empties caudad in a direction parallel to the esophagus; (2) the diverticulum fills at 90° to the esophageal long axis; (3) the diverticulum fills in the same direction as food passing down the esophagus. One can clearly see how food or instruments can be diverted into the lumen of the dependent diverticulum.

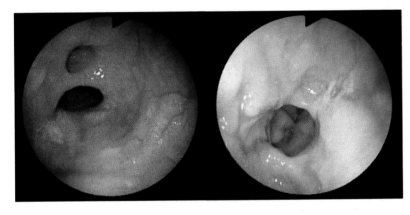

Figure 2.7 *Left,* Epiphrenic diverticulum in a patient with a motor disorder. After pneumatic dilation of the esophagus, the LES became incompetent, and reflux and a reflux-associated ulcer occurred. *Right,* A closeup view demonstrates the ulcer, but the diverticulum is less well seen.

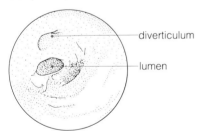

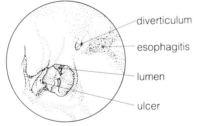

ticulum is suspected, endoscopy should be performed with utmost care and gentleness. The orifice of a diverticulum is usually difficult to visualize, and as one advances an end-viewing instrument, one may inadvertently enter the Zenker's diverticulum. Because further advancement could result in a perforation, the instrument should be withdrawn until the esophageal lumen is visualized. Then, the endoscope can be advanced with the lumen constantly in view. Alternatively, the endoscope can be passed over a guidewire which is introduced through the lumen of a sump tube placed in the stomach. The sump tube is removed, leaving the guidewire in place.

MIDESOPHAGEAL DIVERTICULA

Midesophageal diverticula are usually asymptomatic, and their cause is unclear. These diverticula are usually single but may be multiple. They are often associated with motor abnormalities of the esophagus.

EPIPHRENIC DIVERTICULA

Epiphrenic diverticula are frequently associated with motor abnormalities such as diffuse esophageal spasms and achalasia. Symptoms are more common with this type of diverticulum than with the midesophageal type. Diagnosis is usually made radiographically or by endoscopy. These diverticula may be multiple (Fig. 2.6) or single (Fig. 2.7), often occurring in association with esophagitis with stricture or ulceration. An epiphrenic diverticulum may create difficulty

of the cricopharyngeus may be the cause. The initial presenting symptom is usually dysphagia, which may gradually increase with time. If the diverticulum is large, symptoms associated with fluid retention such as sudden regurgitation of liquid with choking or aspiration may be noted. Gurgling sounds may be heard in the neck.

Although diagnosis is usually made by barium esophagram, a Zenker's diverticulum can be missed unless careful attention is paid to the cricopharyngeal area. If this diver-

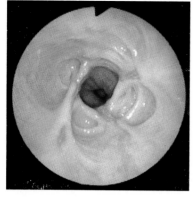
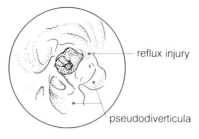

Figure 2.8 Bands in the distal esophagus creating pseudodiverticula. There is minimal associated reflux injury, with red streaks on the tops of the folds.

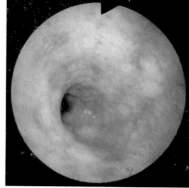
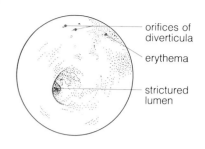

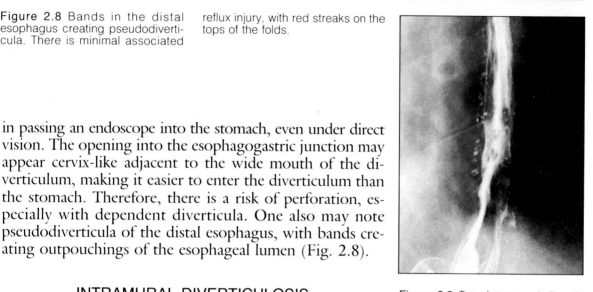

Figure 2.9 *Top,* Intramural diverticulosis. The mucosa appears pale, friable, and granular. Tiny orifices of the diverticula or outpouchings are seen. *Bottom,* A barium esophagram confirms the diagnosis.

in passing an endoscope into the stomach, even under direct vision. The opening into the esophagogastric junction may appear cervix-like adjacent to the wide mouth of the diverticulum, making it easier to enter the diverticulum than the stomach. Therefore, there is a risk of perforation, especially with dependent diverticula. One also may note pseudodiverticula of the distal esophagus, with bands creating outpouchings of the esophageal lumen (Fig. 2.8).

INTRAMURAL DIVERTICULOSIS

This is an unusual condition in which many small diverticula of the esophagus are seen. Patients often present with dysphagia. Diagnosis is usually made by barium esophagram, demonstrating numerous small outpouchings or irregularities of the esophageal wall, each approximately 1 to 2 mm in diameter. They are thought to represent dilated submucosal esophageal glands. Endoscopically, the mucosa may appear granular and friable, with tiny orifices of the diverticula visible (Fig. 2.9). In many cases these diverticula are associated with esophageal candidiasis, including the mucocutaneous type, and may be associated with motor disorders.

HIATAL HERNIA

There are two types of hiatal hernias: axial and paraesophageal. Each will be identified and discussed below.

AXIAL HIATAL HERNIA

An axial (sliding) hiatal hernia is the more common type of hernia encountered in clinical medicine. There are two issues regarding diagnosis: first, how to define what appears to be a small hiatal hernia; second, how to relate the presence of an axial hiatal hernia to symptomatic gastroesophageal reflux.

Radiologically, diagnosis of an axial hiatal hernia is usually made when a barium esophagram demonstrates a portion of the stomach above the diaphragm (Fig. 2.10). Endoscopically, diagnosis requires recognition of the squamocolumnar junction and the level of the diaphragmatic hiatus. If, during quiet respiration and without excessive air insufflation, the squamocolumnar junction is located more than 2 or 3 cm above the diaphragmatic impression, some will diagnose an axial hiatal hernia. Often, the hernia appears as a pouchlike area just below the mucosal junction and above the diaphragm. The squamocolumnar junction may be patulous, allowing the endoscopist to look through into the hiatal hernia pouch (Fig. 2.11).

To inspect the cardia, the endoscope is passed into the stomach and retroflexed. Normally, the tissue of the cardia appears snug around the endoscope. With an axial hiatal hernia, a space is evident around the instrument as it passes

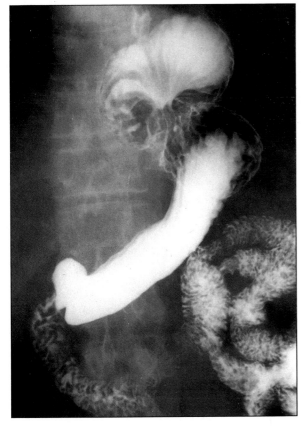

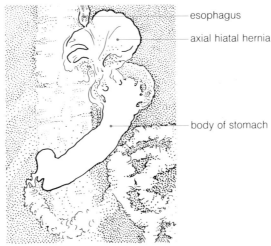

esophagus

axial hiatal hernia

body of stomach

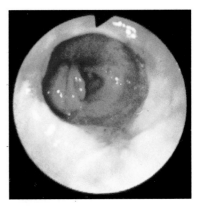

Figure 2.11 An axial hiatal hernia is seen just beyond the squamocolumnar junction, with minimal erythema on one rim of the junction. Gastric mucosa is seen in the pouch. (Courtesy of Dr. Eric Harder)

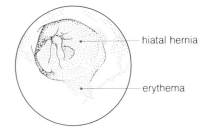

hiatal hernia

erythema

Figure 2.10 Barium esophagram demonstrates a large axial hiatal hernia. The proximal stomach has herniated through the diaphragm into the thorax. (Courtesy of Dr. Charles Rohrmann)

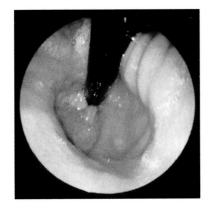

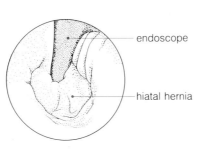

endoscope

hiatal hernia

Figure 2.12 An axial hiatal hernia, seen with the endoscope retroflexed. The tissue of the gastric cardia is not snug around the endoscope, and one can see into the hernia.

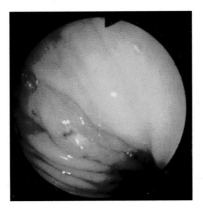

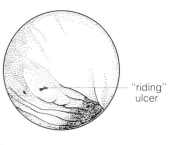

"riding" ulcer

Figure 2.13 A small "riding" ulcer is seen on the lower aspect of a hiatal hernia. A small blood clot can be seen in the base.

through the cardia (Fig. 2.12). Small ulcers may be seen in the hernia. These are referred to as "riding" ulcers if they occur on the gastric tissue separating the hiatal hernia from the remainder of the stomach (Fig. 2.13).

The symptoms of gastroesophageal reflux have little to do with the diagnosis of hiatal hernia. Reflux can occur without a hernia, and patients with a hernia may be free of reflux. These two diagnoses should not be automatically linked.

PARAESOPHAGEAL HIATAL HERNIA

A paraesophageal hiatal hernia is much less common than an axial hiatal hernia and may present a significant clinical problem. This hernia is defined as a pouch of stomach that has herniated up into the chest and is in a position adjacent to the esophagus. The esophagus does not necessarily empty into the most cephalad margin of the hernia. Patients present with a fullness in the chest after eating; they may also

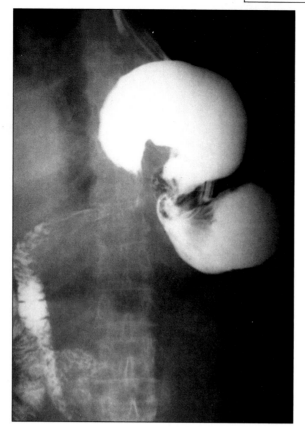

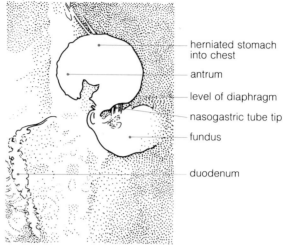

Figure 2.14 Barium esophagram reveals a large paraesophageal hernia. A nasogastric tube is seen with its tip below the diaphragm in the cardia of the stomach. The fundus is below the diaphragm, and the body and antrum are herniated into the chest. (Courtesy of Dr. Charles Rohrmann)

present with dysphagia, bleeding, and chest discomfort. Patients usually do not have gastroesophageal reflux. Paraesophageal hernias have been reported to cause obstruction, ulceration, and strangulation with infarction. Diagnosis is usually made radiographically (Fig. 2.14). Endoscopy may be problematic, as one may get lost inside the hernia pouch and have considerable trouble locating the main gastric lumen. However, the endoscope may be valuable in discovering the presence of an ulcer in the hernia, which may be the cause of bleeding.

WEBS AND RINGS

These structures are infrequently encountered in the esophagus but are of significance because they may cause symptoms which require therapy and because they can cause difficulty during endoscopy.

WEBS

A web is usually defined as a thin, membranelike structure containing mucosa and submucosa but without inclusion of muscle layers (Figs. 2.15 and 2.16). Webs can occur anywhere in the esophagus and may be single or multiple. Patients may present with dysphagia if the diameter of the lumen through the web is less than 12 mm. Etiology is unknown, though they may occur in chronic graft-versushost disease.

Webs may be noted incidentally on barium esophagrams (Fig. 2.17) or during endoscopy. Distension of the esophagus is necessary to see a thin web radiographically. A watersoluble bolus, such as a marshmallow, is usually swallowed with barium to determine if there is obstruction to passage. Endoscopically, the web can usually be seen if the esophagus is gently distended with air (see Fig. 2.15). Occasionally, the web may be difficult to see. This will occur if the endoscope gets caught in a web but the web is out of the field of view (Fig. 2.18). As the endoscope is advanced, the web may be inadvertently ruptured (Fig. 2.19). This may cure the problem because treatment for these webs is disruption using dilation with an esophageal dilator or with an endoscope.

Plummer-Vinson syndrome is an unusual condition in which a web occurs in the proximal 4 or 5 cm of the esophagus (Fig. 2.20). The syndrome may be associated with dysphagia, aspiration, and iron deficiency anemia, and has an increased incidence of hypopharyngeal carcinoma. The web is often eccentric. Such webs may be difficult to see on standard radiographs and may require a barium esophagram with video recordings. They can be difficult to see endoscopically if they are located in the upper esophagus

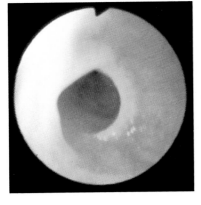 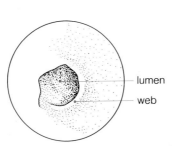

Figure 2.15 This thin esophageal web does not extend around the circumference of the esophagus. (Courtesy of Group Health Hospital)

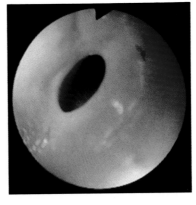 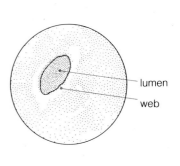

Figure 2.16 Web in the proximal esophagus.

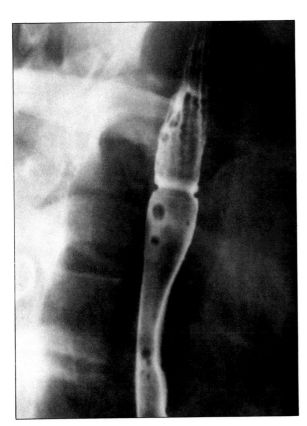 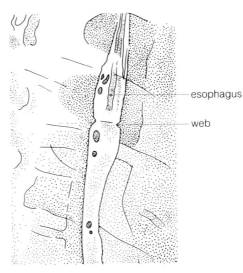

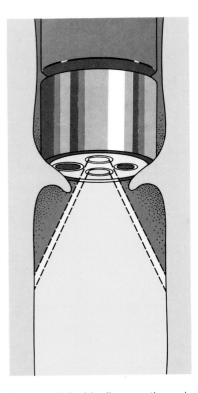

Figure 2.18 In this diagram, the web is preventing the passage of the endoscope while remaining out of view. If the endoscope is advanced, the web may be ruptured.

Figure 2.17 In this air-contrast view of the esophagus, a relatively thin web is seen in the proximal third. This patient presented with dysphagia. (Courtesy of Dr. Charles Rohrmann)

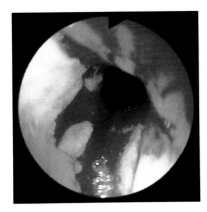 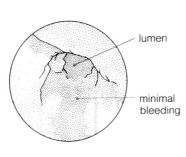

Figure 2.19 Web after rupture with Savary dilator. Mild bleeding is noted.

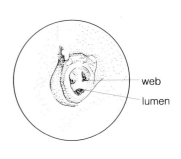

Figure 2.20 Web in the proximal esophagus of a patient with Plummer-Vinson syndrome. This is a complicated web with small lumen on either side. (Courtesy of Dr. George McDonald)

2.7

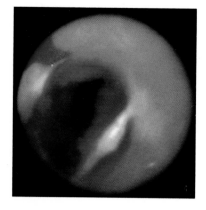
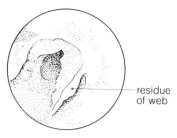

residue
of web

Figure 2.21 The web seen in Fig. 2.20, ruptured for therapy. Residual strands of the web can be seen.

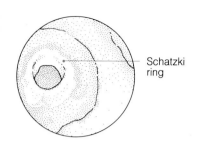

Schatzki
ring

Figure 2.22 Schatzki (B) ring in the distal esophagus. The proximal mucosa is stratified squamous, the mucosa below the ring is gastric columnar epithelium. This ring is sufficiently tight to cause dysphagia.

just beyond the cricopharyngeus muscle. In this position the web may be ruptured as the endoscope is passed through the cricopharyngeus muscle into the upper esophagus (Fig. 2.21). In addition to iron therapy, these patients with Plummer-Vinson syndrome must be screened periodically for hypopharyngeal cancer.

Webs in the midesophagus and distal esophagus may be asymptomatic or may be associated with dysphagia; they are usually not associated with reflux. Diagnosis is by careful radiology or endoscopy. Endoscopically, these webs appear the same as those in the upper esophagus. Some have suggested treatment using endoscopic biopsy forceps to incise the margin of the web or diathermy electrosurgical current to radially incise the structure, but most prefer routine dilation.

RINGS

Esophageal rings are often thicker than webs and are most often seen in the distal esophagus. There are two types of lower esophageal ring: the A ring and the B ring. The A ring occurs in the distal esophagus at the proximal margin of the lower esophageal sphincter (LES). It is covered with squamous mucosa and is usually located 2 or 3 cm proximal to the squamocolumnar junction. This ring does not cause symptoms except in rare instances.

The B, or Schatzki, ring is more common than the A ring. It is located at the squamocolumnar junction, with squamous mucosa on the upper side of the ring and columnar mucosa on the lower side (Fig. 2.22). The thickness of a B ring is usually 2 or 3 mm, rarely larger; it is usually symmetrical. The B ring is only seen endoscopically if the LES is located in the chest above the diaphragmatic hiatus. This may be accomplished by gently insufflating the distal esophagus, causing the LES to move upward into the chest. Having the patient sniff may also accentuate a B ring. In addition, the B ring is usually seen when a hiatal hernia is present because the hernia displaces the LES above the diaphragm. Therefore, the B ring is a dynamic structure which changes configuration with a variety of factors. If the diameter of the lumen through the ring is less than 12 or 13 mm, dysphagia may be present.

Only rarely is a ring seen with reflux esophagitis. The B ring is not seen after a Nissen fundoplication because the LES is intra-abdominal (below the diaphragm), nor with Barrett's metaplasia because the squamocolumnar junction is displaced proximally.

The most common symptom of a ring is dysphagia, but a somewhat unique form of dysphagia: The patient frequently complains of intermittent dysphagia which may occur with the first swallow of solid food in a meal, but then does not recur with the next swallow or for the rest of the meal. These symptoms may occur periodically over a period of several years. Obviously, these symptoms must be differentiated from those caused by a reflux-related peptic stricture or other obstructive lesions such as a carcinoma.

Diagnosis of a ring is radiographic or endoscopic. As with a web, it is important to have the patient swallow a water-soluble bolus during a barium esophagram to determine if there is obstruction to passage. Endoscopically, rings can be seen by gently distending the distal esophagus with air. They are usually more symmetrical around the esophageal lumen than are webs. It is important to differentiate a ring from a short, reflux-related peptic stricture. Rings usually do not have the associated mucosal changes of reflux injury such as erythema, erosion, ulceration, exudation, and bleeding. Also, with gentle pressure, the endoscope will usually pass a ring whereas a tight fibrous peptic stricture will usually not permit passage of the endoscope. With both rings and strictures, care should be taken not to accidentally injure the esophageal wall while passing the endoscope.

Food can impact above a ring and may require endoscopic removal. Inspection after removal of the impacted food may reveal a ring, though sometimes the endoscopic appearance is inconclusive. Only later, when a history consistent with a ring is noted, can careful radiology or repeat endoscopy diagnose the ring.

REFLUX

Reflux of gastric contents into the esophagus is a common but complex clinical disorder which is not completely understood. Most information relating to reflux has little to do with endoscopy. On the other hand, in cases of severe reflux, endoscopy is important to assess damage to the mucosa and to diagnose and manage the complications. We will now briefly discuss the clinical problem of reflux and reflux-related complications, comment on diagnosis, and then focus on the endoscopic features.

DEFINING THE CONDITION

A significant problem has been defining the disorder. Most gastroenterologists define reflux as the passing of gastric contents up into the esophagus with the subsequent development of symptoms. Reflux occurs to some degree in most people. However, if it is frequent, persistent, and injures the esophageal wall, symptoms may occur. Reflux is not related per se to a hiatal hernia; the definition of a hiatal hernia and the relationship of the hernia to reflux are not well understood. If a radiologist diagnoses a small hiatal hernia and the patient happens to experience chest discomfort from reflux, the patient may undergo surgery for a hernia which may not have been significant and had not caused the symptoms. Therefore, we shall concentrate here only on reflux, whether or not a hiatal hernia is present.

When symptomatic reflux occurs, the patient will usually complain of heartburn, a substernal burning discomfort. Other associated symptoms include dysphagia (which may be related to reflux esophagitis and/or a stricture caused by reflux); odynophagia (pain on swallowing); and regurgitation of fluid into the oropharynx, especially at night (which may be associated with laryngospasm, coughing, or a choking sensation).

Reflux is common in the adult population: It is estimated that between one-third and one-half experience intermittent heartburn, and in approximately 10% it is a daily occurrence. Even higher incidences are noted in pregnant women. Mechanical and postural factors (bending over, obesity) may exacerbate symptoms, as will certain foods (fats, citrus juices, alcohol) and smoking. The cause of reflux is not known, but sudden relaxing or total incompetence of the LES seems to be an important factor, especially in conjunction with poor acid clearing.

In the great majority of patients, diagnosis is made based on the history. No abnormalities are found on physical examination and no further tests are necessary. A therapeutic plan is devised, and the patient's symptoms are noted. This assumes the patient has heartburn without dysphagia. If dysphagia is present, a full workup, including endoscopy, is always indicated. Likewise, if the symptoms are severe, atypical, or suggest a complication, further workup is necessary.

There are several tests that can be used to evaluate the esophagus. These tests are generally oriented toward determining:

1. If reflux is present.
2. If the symptoms are caused by reflux.
3. Whether the esophageal mucosa is injured.

IS REFLUX PRESENT?
The tests to determine if reflux is present include a barium esophagram, radioisotope studies, pH studies, and manometry.

The barium esophagram is of limited usefulness in determining the presence of reflux, as many symptomatic patients will have pH-probe–proven reflux but not demonstrate this reflux on X-ray. If maneuvers are used to increase the sensitivity of the X-ray, reflux is then seen in 20 to 30% of otherwise normal patients. A barium esophagram is important in evaluating the complications of reflux: for example, strictures or ulcerations.

Radioisotope scans involve the ingestion of an isotope and the use of a gamma camera to detect reflux from the stomach into the esophagus.

Currently, the best method is considered to be esophageal pH-probe studies, where reflux of endogenous gastric acid or 0.1 N HCl instilled into the stomach can be detected in the esophagus, either at rest or after provocative maneuvers. Constant (24-hour) pH monitoring may be especially useful to determine how frequently reflux occurs, how long the acidic pH persists, and whether symptoms occur in association with reflux. These parameters can also be followed after therapy is instituted.

Manometry is less useful in the evaluation of reflux. Low pressure in the LES and inappropriate relaxation of the LES may be associated with reflux, but further tests are necessary to confirm the diagnosis.

IS REFLUX CAUSING SYMPTOMS?
When it is unclear whether the reflux is causing symptoms, an acid perfusion (Bernstein) test is often performed. This test can determine whether the infusion of 0.1 N HCl into the esophagus reproduces the patient's symptoms.

HAS REFLUX DAMAGED ESOPHAGEAL MUCOSA?
To assess whether reflux has damaged the mucosa, three approaches are available: a barium esophagram, biopsy, and endoscopy.

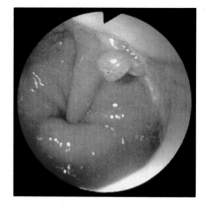

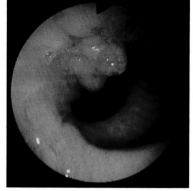

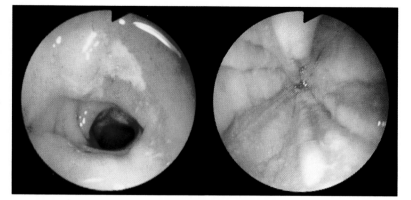

Figure 2.23 Sentinel fold in the proximal stomach of a patient with reflux symptoms. The fold is polypoid and is located just below the squamocolumnar junction.

Figure 2.24 Polypoid sentinel fold just below the squamocolumnar junction. The fold appears multilobulated.

Figure 2.25 This patient presented with a duodenal bulb ulcer (*left*) in conjunction with stage II reflux

esophagitis (*right*). This is a common manifestation associated with increased gastric acid production.

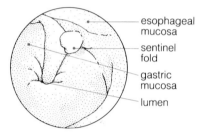

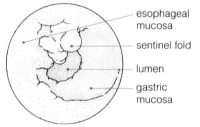

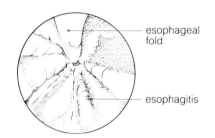

ENDOSCOPIC FEATURES

A barium esophagram is least likely to answer this question. As mentioned earlier, X-ray is useful in evaluating reflux complications such as stricture and ulcer but not in the diagnosis of simple reflux injury to the esophagus. Superficial ulcerations or erosions are usually not well seen radiographically, even with air contrast. Indeed, moderate to severe mucosal injury, noted endoscopically, may appear normal or only show nonspecific changes on X-ray.

The appearance of heavy folds has been associated with reflux, as has an increased incidence of sentinel fold and polyp. The sentinel fold is a gastric fold, usually located on the greater curvature side which ends just below the squamocolumnar junction. At the cephalad margin of the fold, a polypoid-appearing structure may be noted, often with a small central erosion on the tip (Figs. 2.23 and 2.24). This fold should not be removed endoscopically.

Esophageal mucosal biopsies using manometric placement may demonstrate abnormalities caused by the reflux of acid. These abnormalities include thickening of the basal cell layer and extension of the vascular pegs almost up to the luminal surface of the biopsy. These biopsies must be taken from an area 2 to 3 cm above the LES because the area of the sphincter itself may have changes suggesting reflux even when no reflux is present. Biopsy may occasionally be useful in some patients when the radiographic and/or endoscopic appearance is normal, yet the symptoms and pH-probe studies indicate reflux. Characteristic changes in the biopsy may clarify the clinical situation.

Endoscopically, the esophagus may appear entirely normal in a patient with symptoms of reflux and objective evidence of reflux by pH studies. This is the case in approximately 20% of patients with reflux. In other patients, endoscopic abnormalities are noted. Most investigators feel that some endoscopic abnormalities in the distal esophagus are not reliably correlated with reflux esophagitis and should not be used to make diagnosis. These include erythema of the mucosa and blurring of the usually distinct squamocolumnar junction at the ora serrata.

Reflux injury to the esophagus begins with mild changes and advances to severe damage with stricture formation, bleeding, ulceration, etc. In many cases a hiatal hernia is present. Reflux esophagitis may occur in association with an active duodenal ulcer, since both are manifestations of excess acid secretion (Fig. 2.25). Savary and Miller have proposed a four-stage scheme to quantify the mucosal changes seen in reflux esophagitis.

In stage I, nonconfluent red patches or streaks are noted at and just proximal to the squamocolumnar junction. The shape of these patches may be longitudinal, triangular, or oval. They often occur along a fold and may be covered with a fine white exudate. Patches may occur singly or may appear in multiple nonconfluent areas (Figs. 2.26 to 2.32).

As the damage progresses, the injury becomes confluent but still does not extend around the entire esophageal circumference. This marks stage II mucosal damage (Figs. 2.33 to 2.36). The typical appearance involves fingerlike lesions, with a white exudate in the center of the lesion and

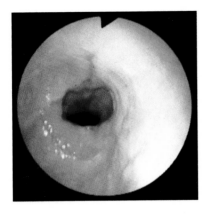

Figure 2.26 Stage I (mild) reflux esophagitis in a patient with an incompetent LES. The ora serrata is seen, and there is a single erosion extending up the esophagus.

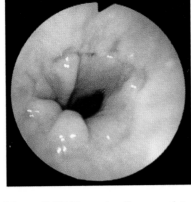

Figure 2.27 Stage I reflux esophagitis. Several small red streaks can be seen at the ora serrata.

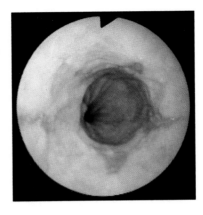

Figure 2.28 Stage I reflux esophagitis. Here, the reflux is slightly more extensive, with several linear, nonconfluent red streaks extending up the esophagus.

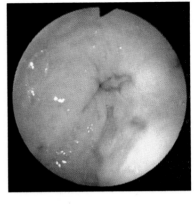

Figure 2.29 Stage I reflux esophagitis. A single erosion with a red perimeter and a white exudative base is seen, as are several small erythematous areas.

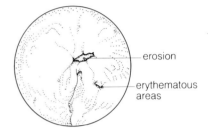

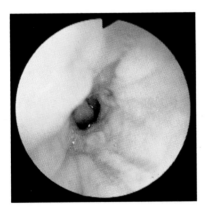

Figure 2.30 Stage I reflux esophagitis. Nonconfluent erythematous areas are seen extending up the esophagus.

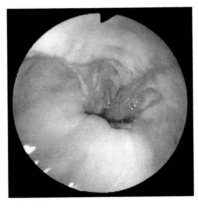

Figure 2.31 Stage I reflux esophagitis. This patient with a hiatal hernia and reflux demonstrates limited erosions.

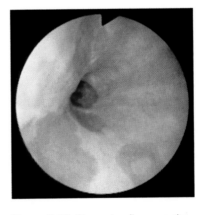

Figure 2.32 Stage I reflux esophagitis. Patches of erythematous mucosa are seen in the distal esophagus. There is minimal exudate, and the lesions are nonconfluent.

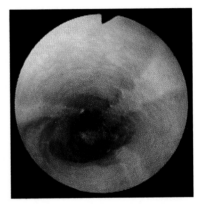

Figure 2.33 Stage II reflux esophagitis. Linear, confluent ulcerations can be seen involving part of the circumference of the esophagus. Note a white exudate on the lesion.

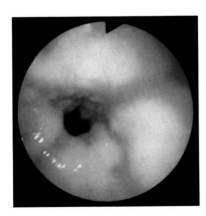

Figure 2.34 Stage II reflux esophagitis. Note the nonconfluent erythematous areas which do not in-

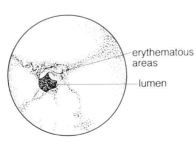

volve the entire circumference of the esophagus.

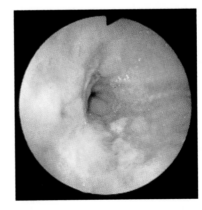

Figure 2.35 Stage II reflux esophagitis. These early confluent erosions have a white base and erythematous surrounding mucosa.

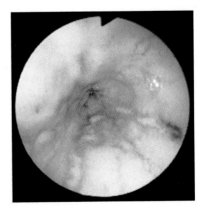

Figure 2.36 Stage II reflux esophagitis. White-based erosions extend up the esophagus. Confluence but noninvolvement of the entire circumference is noted.

2.11

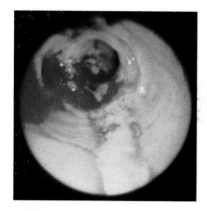

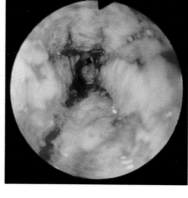

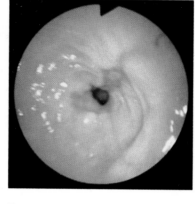

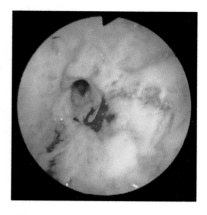

Figure 2.37 Stage III reflux esophagitis. In this severe case, a linear ulcer is seen involving the entire distal circumference of the esophagus. Some bleeding is evident, but there is no stricture.

Figure 2.38 Stage III reflux esophagitis. Denudation and friability are observed.

Figure 2.39 Stage IVa reflux esophagitis. An early stricture and associated small ulcerations or erosions on the esophageal side of the stricture can be noted.

Figure 2.40 Stage IVa reflux esophagitis. Here, a stricture and evidence of esophagitis are apparent. Bleeding is also present just proximal to the stricture over an area of ulceration.

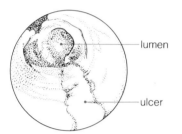

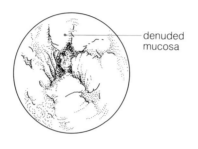

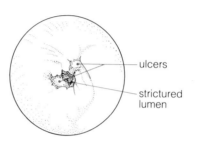

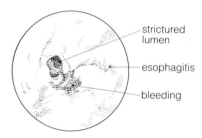

surrounded by erythematous mucosa, extending cephalad up the esophagus. They may be friable and bleed. If there is no exudate on the area of esophagitis, it may be difficult to distinguish this lesion from patches of columnar epithelium. Stage II reflux changes characteristically involve the distal esophagus at the squamocolumnar junction and extend proximally. If the esophageal mucosa just above the squamocolumnar junction is normal but inflammation is noted proximally in the esophagus, this favors a diagnosis of candidal infection, herpetic infection, drug injury, etc. rather than reflux.

In stage III, the inflammatory lesion extends to the entire circumference of the esophagus and is accompanied by edema, hyperemia, and friability. Bleeding and denudation of the mucosa may be noted; however, no stricture is present (Figs. 2.37 and 2.38).

Stage IV is divided into IVa and IVb. In IVa there are one or several esophageal ulcers which may be associated with circumferential stricturing, esophageal shortening, or Barrett's metaplasia (Figs. 2.39 to 2.43). In IVb a peptic stricture is noted, but there is no evidence of erosion or ulceration in the strictured area (Fig. 2.44). Food chronically impacted above a stricture may be associated with an irritated esophageal mucosa.

THERAPY

In most patients with reflux, medical therapy relieves symptoms. In a small number of patients, surgery is necessary due to severe reflux or complications of reflux that do not respond to medical therapy. The most popular procedure at this time is the Nissen fundoplication. In this operation, the fundus is wrapped around the distal esophagus to create a barrier to the reflux of acid from the stomach into the esophagus. The competence of the fundoplication can be assessed endoscopically by determining whether the esophagitis is healing and by passing the instrument through the esophagogastric junction and retroflexing the endoscope to examine the cardia. One can then determine if the tissue of the cardia is snug around the endoscope as a result of the surgery (Figs. 2.45 to 2.47).

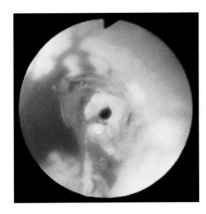

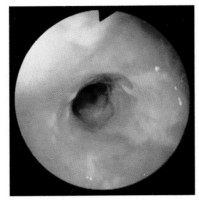

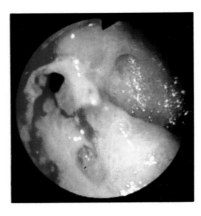

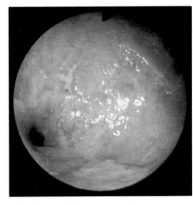

Figure 2.41 This patient with Zollinger-Ellison syndrome presents with severe stricture and stage IVa reflux esophagitis. The residual esophageal lumen is very stenotic. Blood covers the area of ulceration or erosion.

Figure 2.42 Stage IVa reflux esophagitis. An ulcer associated with this severe form appears in the distal esophagus. The ulcer has a white base and covers approximately one-third of the circumference. At the time of this endoscopy, this ulcer had been treated and was beginning to heal, thus accounting for the relative inactivity of the surrounding mucosa.

Figure 2.43 Stage IVa reflux esophagitis. The tight esophageal stricture has associated ulceration and pseudodiverticula formation.

Figure 2.44 Stage IVb reflux esophagitis. Note the reflux-associated benign esophageal stricture. The mucosa is slightly red and demonstrates inflammation due to stasis. No ulcers are present.

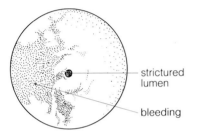

strictured lumen

bleeding

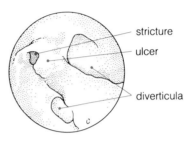

stricture

ulcer

diverticula

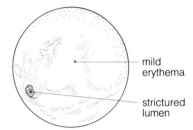

mild erythema

strictured lumen

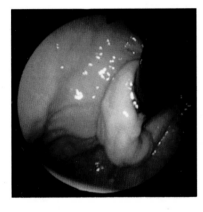

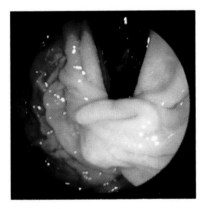

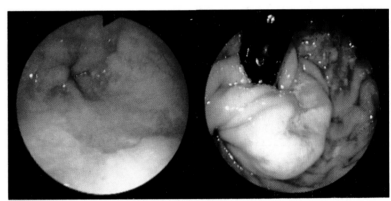

Figure 2.45 Nissen fundoplication for reflux. The endoscope is retroflexed in the stomach to examine the cardia. Abundant cardial tissue is snug around the endoscope, indicating that the Nissen wrap is competent.

Figure 2.46 Nissen fundoplication for reflux. Here, cardial tissue again appears snug around the endoscope. In fact, this Nissen wrap was supercompetent, causing the patient some difficulty with belching and some dysphagia. It is not possible to determine whether the Nissen wrap is too tight using this endoscopic inspection; symptoms are a better correlative factor.

Figure 2.47 *Left,* This patient with severe reflux esophagitis had a Nissen fundoplication performed. The ora serrata appears in the distal esophagus, and there is little evidence of esophagitis as healing

continues. *Right,* This same case viewed from below with the endoscope retroflexed reveals that the cardial tissue is snug around the endoscope.

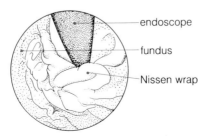

endoscope

fundus

Nissen wrap

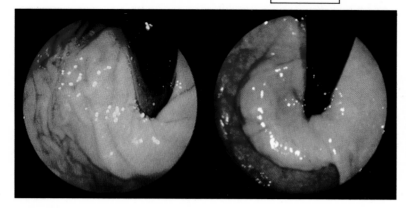

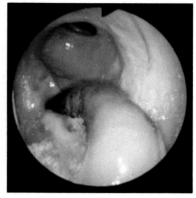

Figure 2.48 Two views of the Angelchik prosthesis around the distal esophagus, from below with the endoscope retroflexed.

Figure 2.49 This is a complication of the Angelchik prosthesis. The entire prosthesis has migrated into the stomach and is free in the gastric lumen.

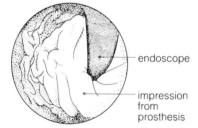

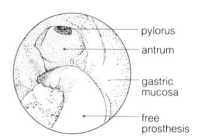

Another surgical approach to reduce reflux is to insert a silicone (Angelchik) prosthesis into the tissue surrounding the distal esophagus. The effect of this prosthesis is to make the gastroesophageal junction competent. This can be assessed endoscopically by retroflexing the tip of the endoscope to perform the U-turn maneuver to visualize the cardial tissue. The tissue with the prosthesis should be snug around the endoscope (Fig. 2.48). Complications have been reported with the use of this prosthesis, including migration of the prosthesis into the stomach (Fig. 2.49).

REFLUX-ASSOCIATED COMPLICATIONS

Several complications of reflux can occur, including strictures, ulcers, and Barrett's metaplasia.

STRICTURES

Strictures develop in approximately 15% of patients with reflux esophagitis. Characteristically, there is a long duration of reflux symptoms, an incompetent LES, and impaired esophageal clearing. The usual presenting symptom is dysphagia, initially to solid foods but gradually progressing to liquids as the lumen narrows. Where dysphagia is present and there are no other symptoms of reflux, one must consider a peptic stricture and esophageal cancer in the differential diagnosis because some patients may develop a reflux-related stricture with little or no reflux symptoms.

Strictures occur when circumferential inflammation of the esophageal wall extends to the submucosa and a fibrous reaction takes place, resulting in the formation of scar tissue which can narrow the esophageal lumen and shorten the esophagus. In the absence of Barrett's metaplasia, strictures usually occur in the distal esophagus, often proximal to a hiatal hernia. If Barrett's metaplasia is present, the squamocolumnar junction may migrate proximally in the esophagus, and a stricture may be noted proximal to the displaced junction. Proximal strictures may also be found in esophageal injury resulting from trauma to the esophagus, such as with caustic ingestion or medication-related esophageal injury associated with ulceration.

Strictures are usually short, although they may occasionally be 5 or 10 cm long, especially in nasogastric-tube–related strictures. A barium esophagram will usually detect the stricture, but careful observation is required to define its length. As with webs and rings, a bolus swallow may be required during the X-ray study to demonstrate the obstruction.

A small-caliber endoscope may be helpful in evaluating strictures because it can be passed through the stricture to permit biopsies and cytologies along the entire length of the stricture. Also, when retroflexed, the endoscope will allow visualization of the esophagogastric junction below the stricture. Endoscopy combined with biopsy and brush cytology allow one to differentiate a benign reflux stricture from a cancer. Occasionally it may be necessary to dilate a stricture so that biopsies and cytologies can be obtained along its length. By knowing the instrument's diameter, one can calibrate the diameter as well as the length of the stricture and determine the distance from the incisors. Observed endoscopically, strictures vary from predominant involvement of a portion of the wall, seen as a white crescent-like

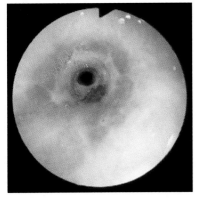
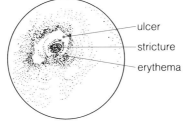

Figure 2.50 In this case of stage IVa reflux esophagitis, we see ulceration and very tight stricture of the lumen.

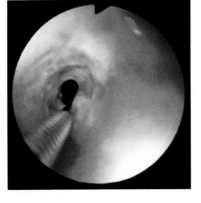
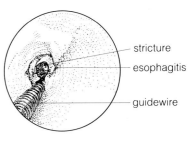

Figure 2.51 Tight esophageal stricture caused by reflux. A guidewire has been passed under endoscopic guidance to direct dilators and reduce the likelihood of a perforation during dilation.

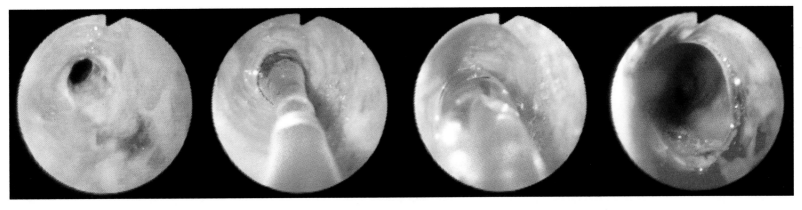

Figure 2.52 Tight esophageal stricture caused by reflux (*left*). Dilation by passage of mercury-filled bougies would be difficult, so a balloon-tipped catheter has been passed into the stricture under endoscopic guidance. Then, the balloon is inflated to stretch the stricture. Finally, inspection of the stricture after dilation shows that the lumen is open (*right*). The minimal bleeding was caused by the dilation. (Courtesy of Dr. Eric Harder)

area covered with an exudate, to circumferential involvement. There may also be varying amounts of reflux-associated change and superficial ulceration. The caliber of the lumen varies from fairly wide with minimal dysphagia (1.2 to 1.3 cm in diameter) to very tight with nearly complete esophageal obstruction (Fig. 2.50).

The initial treatment for reflux strictures is to treat the underlying reflux esophagitis. Some feel that all strictures should be dilated initially over a guidewire. Others try to dilate a stricture initially with rubber mercury-filled bougies. In the latter method, a series of graduated sizes are used to gently stretch the stricture. If the stricture is exceptionally tight or tortuous, one may pass a springtip guidewire through the stricture under endoscopic guidance (Fig. 2.51). Fluoroscopy confirms that the tip of the wire is in the stomach. Then, metal, olive-shaped dilators of gradually increasing size are passed over the wire. There are also dilators which can be passed over a guidewire in which several sizes are built onto the same dilator tube. The guidewire reduces the chances of an esophageal perforation. Endoscopy immediately after dilation will often reveal a small amount of bleeding when the stricture has been stretched. Endoscopy is rarely helpful immediately after dilation except to permit biopsy and cytology in the strictured area if these examinations could not be adequately obtained before dilation.

There are now new approaches to dilation of strictures in which the endoscope is used to guide a balloon-tipped, Gruntzig-type catheter. The catheter is passed into the stricture and then expanded under direct vision to dilate the stricture (Fig. 2.52).

ULCERS

Ulcers in the esophagus are rare. They commonly occur as the result of injection sclerotherapy for esophageal varices, but also appear in association with reflux esophagitis, Barrett's metaplasia, and esophageal infections such as Candida and herpes. Quite often ulcers are deep and extend into the muscle layers of the esophagus (see Fig. 2.53). Manifestations include severe pain or moderate-to-severe upper GI bleeding.

Ulcers may also develop in patients on medications (e.g., antibiotics, especially tetracycline) if the pills are ingested without liquid and remain in the esophagus for a prolonged period of time. This cause of ulceration will be dealt with in detail in Chapter 4.

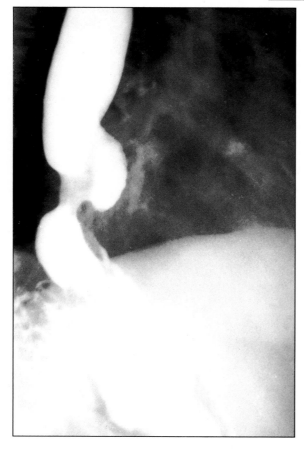

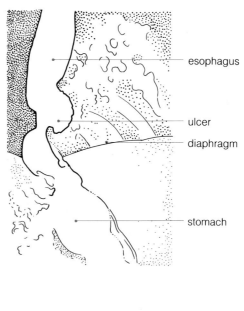

Figure 2.53 Barium esophagram shows a large esophageal ulcer in the distal third of the esophagus. The ulcer extends into the tissue adjacent to the esophagus. (Courtesy of Dr. Charles Rohrmann)

Esophageal ulcers can usually be detected by barium esophagraphy (Fig. 2.53). Endoscopic examination reveals deep, white-based ulcers, usually in the distal esophagus. There may be an associated stricture or reflux mucosal injury. Bleeding may be noted; occasionally, it may be massive.

BARRETT'S METAPLASIA

This is an abnormality of the esophagus which is not completely understood at the present time. In patients with chronic reflux esophagitis, the normal squamous esophageal mucosa is replaced with columnar epithelium. This occurrence has been associated with a number of conditions, including esophagitis, proximal esophageal strictures, esophageal ulcers, mucosal dysplasia, and adenocarcinoma.

The cause of this abnormality is unknown. Some feel that one type of Barrett's metaplasia is caused by a congenitally short esophagus in the presence of a hiatal hernia. Many now feel that nearly all cases of Barrett's are acquired. The current theory is that chronic reflux esophagitis produces a chronically inflamed esophageal mucosa which desquamates and is gradually replaced by columnar epithelium. As this replacement occurs, the squamocolumnar junction (ora serrata) migrates in a cephalad direction and may be found in the upper third of the esophagus in patients with this condition. The junction may appear normal or it may be indistinct. In other cases, the junction may be very irregular, with mixed islands of squamous and columnar mucosa (Figs. 2.54 to 2.57).

The columnar epithelium is of three types: (1) fundal mucosa, identical to that found in the gastric fundus, with parietal and chief cells and with a foveolar surface; (2) cardial mucosa, with pylorocardial glands and a foveolar epithelial surface; and (3) metaplastic mucosa of the specialized Barrett's type. It is this latter metaplastic mucosa which is felt to be the tissue in which dysplasia and adenocarcinoma may develop. The characteristic distribution of these types of mucosa seems to be metaplastic mucosa cephalad, just distal to the proximally migrated squamocolumnar junction; then, moving distally, a variable segment of cardial mucosa; finally, most distally, fundal-type mucosa. The cardial and fundal mucosa usually occur in the distal 2 to 3 cm of the esophagus. The pathophysiologic sequence is thought to be the following: reflux, which causes inflammation followed by desquamation, replacement with metaplastic mucosa, and finally dysplasia and carcinoma. Biopsies along the length of the esophagus are essential to identify the types of mucosa present and to establish the presence of Barrett's metaplasia.

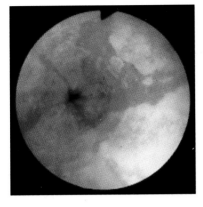
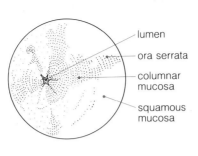

Figure 2.54 Barrett's metaplasia. The squamocolumnar junction has moved proximally in the esophagus.

It is distinct but irregular, with islands of columnar mucosa.

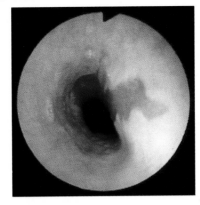

Figure 2.55 Barrett's metaplasia. Here, the proximally located junction is less irregular.

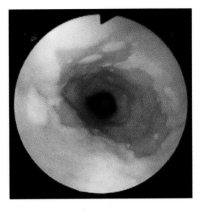

Figure 2.56 Barrett's metaplasia. The proximal junction is slightly irregular, with islands of squamous and columnar tissue.

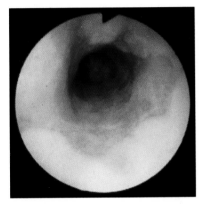

Figure 2.57 Barrett's metaplasia. The squamocolumnar junction is located at 20 cm from the teeth. The ora serrata is regular and would appear normal except for its proximal position.

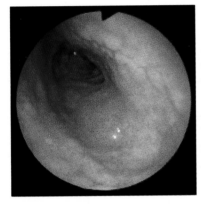

Figure 2.58 Segment of Barrett's mucosa in the midbody of the esophagus. The mucosa is salmon-pink, as is the normal gastric mucosa. The mucosa appears slightly irregular, but there are no areas suggesting carcinoma or adenoma. Vessels are not well seen.

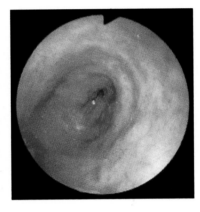
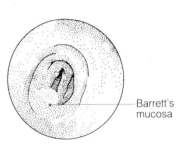

Figure 2.59 Barrett's metaplasia in the midesophagus, just below the ora serrata.

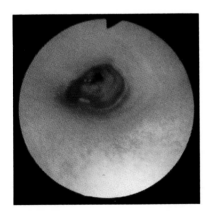
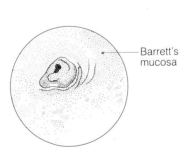

Figure 2.60 This Barrett's segment can be seen as a fine, erythematous mucosal pattern.

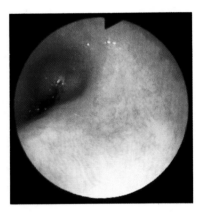

Figure 2.61 The color of this Barrett's mucosa is typical; atypically, blood vessels can be seen.

Figure 2.62 A fine reticulated pattern can be seen in the mucosa of this Barrett's segment.

The typical endoscopic appearance of Barrett's epithelium is normal, pink esophageal mucosa proximally, an ora serrata in the upper or middle third of the esophagus, and a salmon-pink segment of Barrett's metaplasia (with cardial and fundal segments) below the ora serrata. This latter mucosa runs down and joins the similar-appearing mucosa of the stomach (Figs. 2.58 to 2.62). The esophagus in the Barrett's segment is devoid of folds, and submucosal vessels cannot be seen.

In the distal esophagus one may see the zone where the ora serrata used to be located prior to its cephalad migration

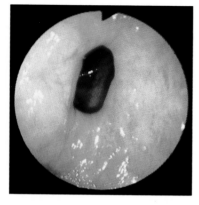
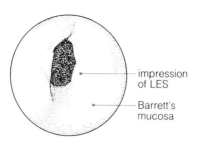

Figure 2.63 In this case of Barrett's metaplasia, the area of the former LES can be seen. This physiologic narrowing is not a stricture but represents the area where the ora serrata used to be located. The ora serrata is now located cephalad.

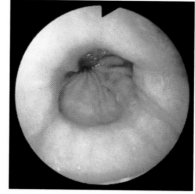
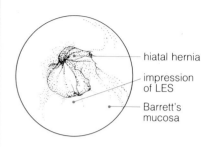

Figure 2.64 In this case, the LES can be seen. Although the typical squamocolumnar junction is not present, the narrow area can be appreciated. There is also a hiatal hernia just below the LES. The folds inside the hernia terminate just below the narrowed area.

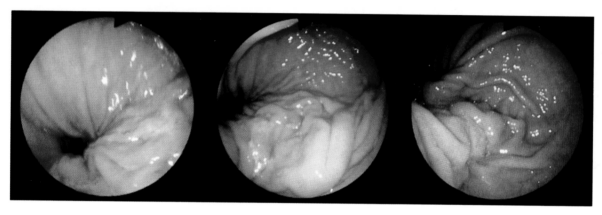
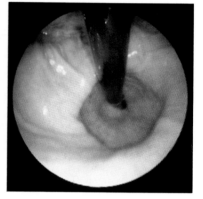

Figure 2.65 Examples of hiatal hernias in cases of Barrett's metaplasia, seen under direct endoscopic view as the tip is advanced past the area of the LES.

Figure 2.66 The hiatal hernia in this case of Barrett's metaplasia is seen from below with the endoscope retroflexed.

(Figs. 2.63 and 2.64). This is recognized by a semicircular ridge of tissue and by noting gastric folds which run vertically and end just below the ridge; no esophageal B ring is seen. A hiatal hernia may be seen—directly (Fig. 2.65) and with the endoscope retroflexed (Fig. 2.66)—just below the ridge. Therefore, if the ridge and folds are seen and identified but the squamocolumnar junction is more than 1 cm proximal to that area, the endoscopist should suspect Barrett's metaplasia.

Another technique by which one can identify the type of mucosa as columnar or squamous is by using Lugol's I₂ solution. (It is important to first be certain that the patient is not iodine-sensitive.) Lugol's solution will stain the squamous mucosa but not the columnar mucosa. Therefore, in cases of Barrett's metaplasia, the stain is seen on squamous mucosa extending to the new ora serrata which is located proximally in the esophagus and not at the level of the diaphragm. On occasion, one will see islands of whitish-pink squamous epithelium in the otherwise uniform salmon-pink–appearing Barrett's segment.

As mentioned earlier, a number of conditions have been associated with Barrett's epithelial change. Esophagitis may be noted in the squamous mucosa proximal to the squamo-columnar junction (Figs. 2.67 and 2.68). This esophagitis is similar in appearance to typical, distal reflux esophagitis. The mucosa may be red and friable, with erosions, exudation, and bleeding. There may be some degree of friability and erythema in the Barrett's segment as well.

Strictures typically occur in the esophagus at or just proximal to the ora serrata. Therefore, the mucosa distal to a stricture is always columnar. As the ora migrates cephalad, so does the location of strictures (Figs. 2.69 and 2.70). An exception is when a stricture occurs in the distal esophagus in association with a deep esophageal ulcer, with resulting fibrous tissue formation. In this case, the strictured area may remain in the distal esophagus, even as the squamo-columnar junction migrates cephalad (Fig. 2.71). If a stricture is found distally, the differential diagnosis should include a fibrous stricture which remained in the distal esophagus because of associated ulceration with fibrosis or an infiltrating adenocarcinoma presenting with a stricture.

Of patients with reflux, approximately 15% develop stricture. If the stricture is located in the distal esophagus, it is usually associated with a hiatal hernia or Barrett's metaplasia. If the stricture is in the middle or the upper third of the esophagus, it is almost always associated with Barrett's.

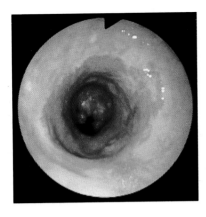
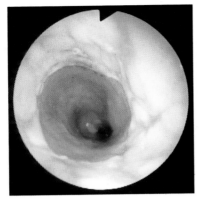
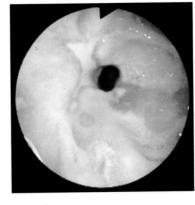
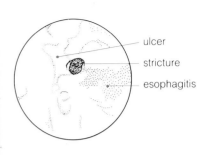

Figure 2.67 Barrett's metaplasia, with a proximal squamocolumnar junction and evidence of mild esophagitis proximal to the junction.

Figure 2.68 Barrett's metaplasia, with a mucosal junction proximal in the esophagus. There is evidence of inflammation and ulceration at the mucosal junction.

Figure 2.69 Barrett's metaplasia. A stricture is present at the proximal squamocolumnar junction, with associated evidence of esophagitis and ulceration. The stricture moved proximally with the mucosal junction.

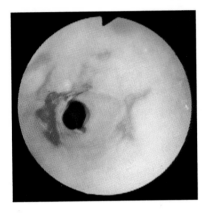
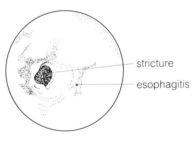
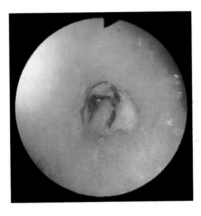
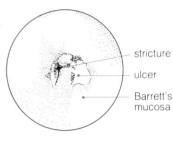

Figure 2.70 Barrett's metaplasia. This stricture is located at 20 cm, having migrated proximally with the mucosal junction. There is associated esophagitis, ulceration, and bleeding.

Figure 2.71 Barrett's metaplasia. The ora serrata has moved proximally, but this ulceration and associated stricture remain in the distal esophagus at the location of the LES.

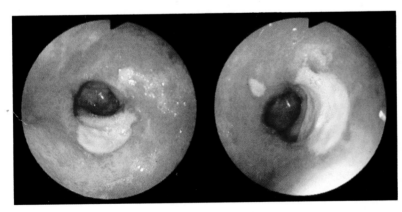
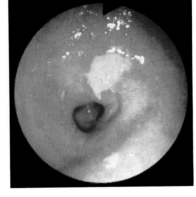

Figure 2.72 *Left,* Barrett's metaplasia, with kissing ulcers in the Barrett's segment. The ulcers appear benign, with white bases and smooth margins. Biopsy and cytology were performed to rule out a malignancy. *Right,* A closeup view.

Figure 2.73 White-based, benign-appearing ulcer in Barrett's segment, below the ora serrata. The mucosa surrounding the ulcer is columnar.

Ulcers occur in Barrett's metaplasia and may be found anywhere along the Barrett's segment (Figs. 2.72 and 2.73). These ulcers typically appear in the lower esophagus; they may be deep and may bleed. The ulcers are never totally surrounded by squamous mucosa; there is always at least a portion of the ulcer margin which is lined by columnar epithelium.

The ulcer may occur at the squamocolumnar junction. Then, as the junction migrates in a cephalad direction, the ulcer remains in its original position and is gradually and increasingly surrounded by columnar epithelium. In an area of Barrett's metaplasia, it may be difficult to differentiate an island of squamous mucosa from an ulcer, although one

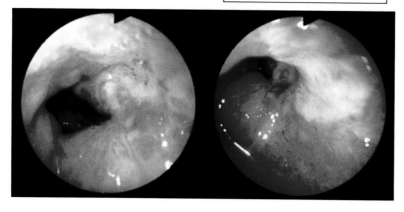

Figure 2.74 This patient had Barrett's metaplasia, with carcinoma and severe dysplasia proximal to the cancer. Here we see two views of the dysplastic area, demonstrating an irregular, discolored surface. A small amount of exudate appears to be present.

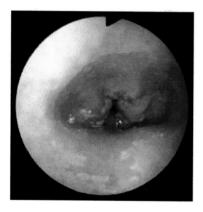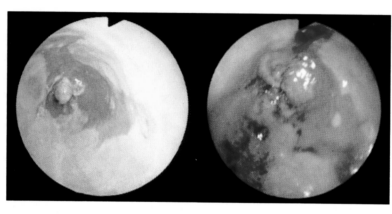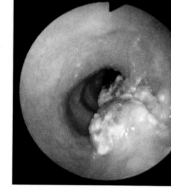

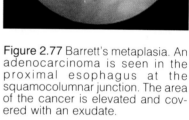

Figure 2.75 Barrett's metaplasia, with an irregular ora serrata and an adenocarcinoma just below the mucosal junction. The cancer is infiltrating and has caused a stricture.

Figure 2.76 *Left,* Esophageal adenoma in a patient with Barrett's metaplasia. Because of underlying medical problems, this was removed endoscopically using a polypectomy technique. *Right,* 2 years later, an adenocarcinoma is found in the same area. The tumor was superficial but had metastasized.

Figure 2.77 Barrett's metaplasia. An adenocarcinoma is seen in the proximal esophagus at the squamocolumnar junction. The area of the cancer is elevated and covered with an exudate.

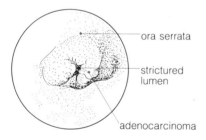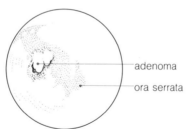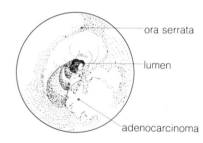

can usually make this distinction because the ulcer has depth while the squamous mucosa is flat.

Barrett's metaplasia seems to be a premalignant condition. In approximately 8 to 10% of patients who first present with Barrett's metaplasia, an adenocarcinoma is found to be present. In addition, dysplasia of the mucosa is also an associated condition. This raises the question as to whether all patients with Barrett's metaplasia need to be periodically screened for the development of dysplasia or adenocarcinoma.

Dysplasia seems to occur predominantly in the Barrett's segment, rather than in the fundal or cardial segments. The dysplastic area may appear irregular, with a villous surface (Fig. 2.74), or the mucosal surface may appear similar to the adjacent metaplastic mucosa. A mosaic of abnormalities may occur. If the dysplastic type of mucosa occurs in elevated bumps, some considered these ares to be adenomas—a rarity in Barrett's metaplasia.

Dysplasia is diagnosed histologically. In surveying patients with Barrett's metaplasia, some recommend a series of biopsies, starting in the area of the gastric cardia and extending throughout the length of the esophagus, to detect dysplasia and foci of adenocarcinoma. Some feel that adenocarcinoma of the cardia is similar to adenocarcinoma of the esophagus and that both occur in Barrett's metaplasia. One interesting observation is that cardial cancer often occurs in conjunction with a normal gastric fundal mucosa below the carcinoma. This is noted despite the fact that many of these patients are elderly and would be expected to have somewhat atrophic mucosa, which is also the case in the usual gastric cancer patient. In addition, these cardial cancers have Barrett's metaplasia above them in

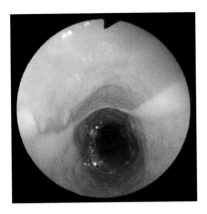

Figure 2.78 Ectopic gastric mucosa in the proximal esophagus. The color is similar to gastric mucosa.

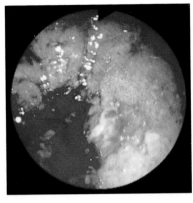

Figure 2.79 Adenocarcinoma in the Barrett's segment. The tumor is diffusely infiltrating and is bleeding.

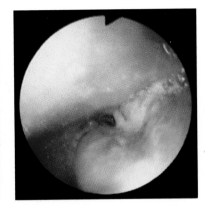

Figure 2.80 This Barrett's adenocarcinoma is in the distal third of the esophagus and caused an irregular narrowing and a tight stenosis.

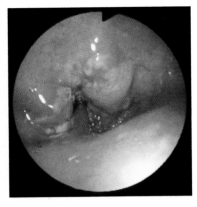

Figure 2.81 Obstruction of the distal esophagus by a Barrett's adenocarcinoma. Here, the tumor is friable and irregular.

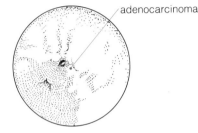

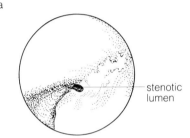

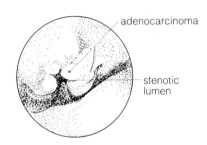

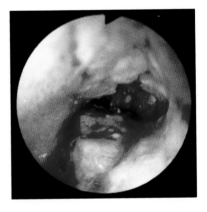

Figure 2.82 Barrett's adenocarcinoma in the distal esophagus, with tight stenosis and friability.

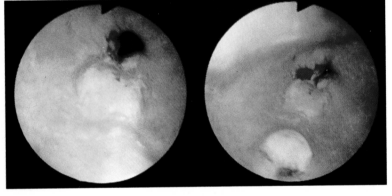

Figure 2.83 *Left,* Distal adenocarcinoma associated with Barrett's metaplasia. The tumor is diffusely infiltrating. *Right,* Intramural metastasis from the carcinoma at left.

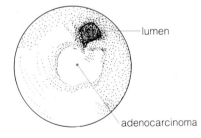

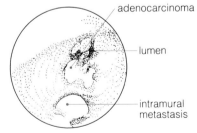

approximately 50% of cases. This evidence suggests a sequence of high acid production associated with a duodenal ulcer and chronic severe reflux esophagitis, which then progresses to Barrett's metaplasia, dysplasia, and eventually to adenocarcinoma.

Adenocarcinomas in Barrett's metaplasia are usually found in the middle or distal third of the esophagus (Figs. 2.75 and 2.76). Proximal esophageal cancer is less common but does occur (Fig. 2.77). Most esophageal adenocarcinomas are felt to be associated with Barrett's metaplasia. Other etiologies of adenocarcinoma are thought to be cancer in esophageal submucosal glands or congenital ectopic gastric mucosa in the esophagus (Fig. 2.78).

Adenocarcinomas vary in configuration from flat (infiltrating) to polypoid. They frequently ulcerate and may bleed (Fig. 2.79). Occasionally, the tumor may obstruct the lumen (Figs. 2.80 to 2.82). Metastases may occur in the esophageal wall adjacent to the carcinoma (Fig. 2.83). In some cases,

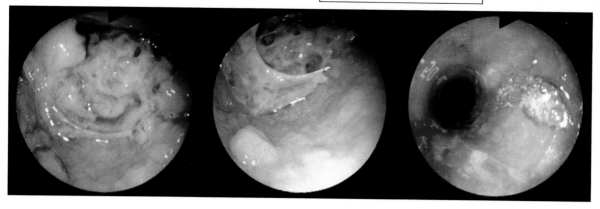

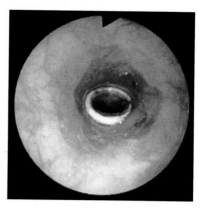

Figure 2.84 Barrett's metaplasia with multiple adenocarcinomas. *Left,* A large distal cancer is seen. This tumor is infiltrating and obstructing the lumen. *Center,* Proximal to the distal cancer, this smaller adenocarcinoma is seen. *Right,* The smaller, proximal adenocarcinoma is seen through the wall of a transparent Tygon prosthesis, placed for palliation.

Figure 2.85 In this case of Barrett's carcinoma with stenosis, an esophageal prosthesis has been passed. The proximal, wide flange of the tube can be seen just distal to the ora serrata. The tumor is located just beyond the flange.

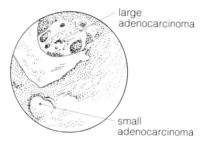

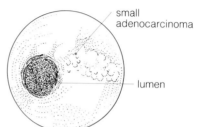

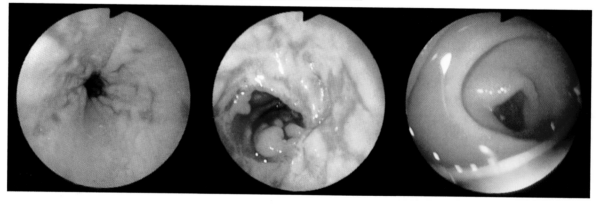

Figure 2.86 Alkaline reflux esophagitis. *Left,* Red streaks are seen, and there is an unusual amount of bile. *Center,* Another view of this esophagitis, caused by reflux from an esophagojejunal anastamosis formed after a total gastrectomy for gastric cancer. *Right,* A large amount of bile is seen in the jejunal segment.

multiple adenocarcinomas may be found (Fig. 2.84). In cases of stenosing carcinoma, an endoscopic prosthesis may be passed as palliative treatment (Figs. 2.84 and 2.85). The endoscopic appearance of esophageal and cardial adenocarcinomas will be considered in greater detail in Chapter 3.

Studies now underway will attempt to determine which patients with Barrett's metaplasia should undergo periodic surveillance for dysplasia and carcinoma.

ALKALINE REFLUX ESOPHAGITIS

The injurious fluid refluxing into the esophagus from the stomach is not limited to acid and pepsin. Alkaline bile salts may also reflux. In some cases, there is sufficient reflux of bilious secretions (often after gastric surgery such as a Billroth II gastrojejunostomy procedure) to diagnose bile reflux esophagitis (Fig. 2.86). The endoscopic appearance is similar to that of acid reflux, but a large amount of bile is usually noted in the distal esophagus.

3

Esophagus II: Neoplasms, Infections, and Involvement in Graft-Versus-Host Disease

In this chapter we will consider neoplasms of the esophagus, esophageal infections, and graft-versus-host disease involving the esophagus. The neoplasms may be benign or malignant, primary or metastatic. Infections include herpes, Candida, and cyto-megalovirus. Finally, we will consider esophageal problems which occur with chronic graft-versus-host disease.

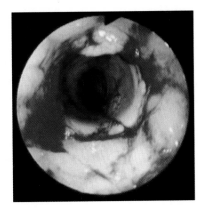

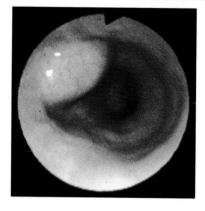

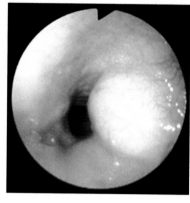

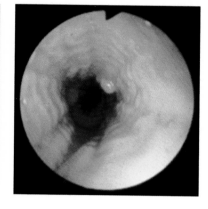

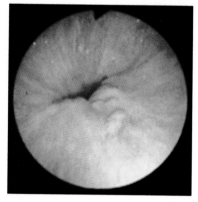

Figure 3.1 This esophageal leiomyoma is covered with normal mucosa. The lumen is seen in the distance.

Figure 3.2 This submucosal leiomyoma is covered with normal esophageal mucosa. Endoscopic ultrasound may be useful to study this lesion.

Figure 3.3 A small squamous papilloma of the esophagus. The covering mucosa appears normal, as does the transverse ridging.

Figure 3.4 Several small squamous papillomas in the distal esophagus.

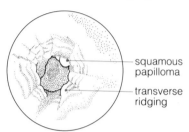

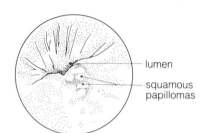

NEOPLASTIC DISEASES OF THE ESOPHAGUS

Tumors of the esophagus, a significant problem in both clinical medicine and gastroenterology, may be classified as benign or malignant. Clearly the most problematic neoplastic diseases of the esophagus are the malignancies. Despite recent advances in diagnosis, including endoscopy, CT scanning, double-contrast radiologic examinations, etc., esophageal carcinoma continues to have a dismal 5-year survival rate. Since endoscopy is currently the primary diagnostic method, we will explore its applications for each of the major esophageal tumors, beginning with the benign and continuing on to the malignant.

BENIGN ESOPHAGEAL NEOPLASMS

LEIOMYOMA

The most common benign tumor of the esophagus is a leiomyoma. These tumors are often found incidentally during postmortem examination, or during diagnostic endoscopy or radiologic examination for another problem. The typical endoscopic appearance of a leiomyoma is that of a submucosal bulge covered by normal-appearing mucosa (Figs. 3.1 and 3.2).

Leiomyomas rarely bleed and are usually asymptomatic unless very large. Biopsy of these lesions is often not productive since only normal surface mucosa is sampled.

If the lesion is large enough to cause symptoms or is worrisome in appearance, surgical removal is recommended. Some fear that biopsy performed at endoscopy prior to surgical enucleation of the lesion by an extraesophageal approach may result in a fistula through the biopsy site, and is another reason why some endoscopists do not biopsy the mucosa over leiomyomas. Exfoliative cytology and brush cytology are useful adjuncts in the diagnosis of a leiomyoma to be sure that a carcinoma is not present.

SQUAMOUS PAPILLOMA

This is an abnormality which may be seen in the esophagus as a small mucosal warty tumor covered with normal-appearing mucosa. They may occur singly (Fig. 3.3) or multiple (Figs. 3.4 and 3.5). Some may appear to have a stalk

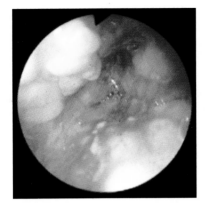

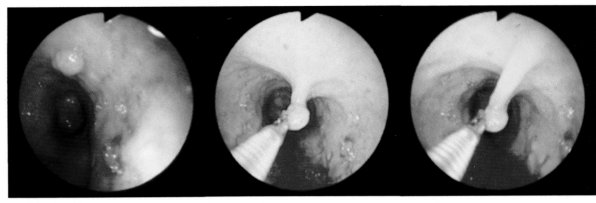

Figure 3.5 Multiple large squamous papillomas in the esophagus.

Figure 3.6 *Left,* This single squamous papilloma of the esophagus is covered with normal mucosa and no stalk is seen. However, when a biopsy forceps is placed over the papilloma and gentle traction is applied, a stalk appears to form *(center).* With continued traction, a longer stalk appears *(right).*

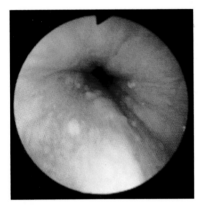

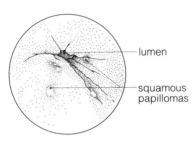

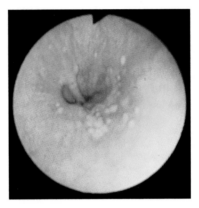

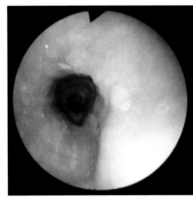

Figure 3.7 Small lesions in the distal esophagus which proved to be squamous papillomas but were differentially diagnosed as glycogenic acanthosis.

Figure 3.8 Multiple esophageal lesions of glycogenic acanthosis, similar in appearance to squamous papillomas.

Figure 3.9 White, plaque-like deposits, typical of glycogenic acanthosis.

or pseudostalk (Fig. 3.6). Squamous papillomas may be difficult to differentiate from glycogenic acanthosis or glycogen deposits (Figs. 3.7 to 3.9). These neoplasms tend to remain small and are rarely symptomatic.

ADENOMATOUS POLYP

Typical adenomatous polyps occur rarely in the esophagus, often in association with Barrett's metaplasia. When pedunculated, these polyps can be removed using a polypectomy snare with coagulating current. At endoscopy, the adenomas are usually covered with mucosa typically found on adenomas elsewhere in the GI tract, demonstrating an erythematous reticulated surface. When seen at the esophagogastric junction, these may be gastric adenomas prolapsing up into the distal esophagus (Fig. 3.10).

OTHER POLYPOID LESIONS

Other benign lesions of the esophagus include lipomas, inflammatory fibrous polyps, lymphangiomas, and epithelial esophageal cysts, all of which are difficult to differentiate by their endoscopic appearance. If the neoplasms are pedunculated and moderate in size, endoscopic removal may

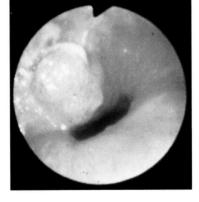

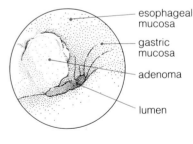

Figure 3.10 This adenomatous polyp is located in the distal esophagus at the esophagogastric junction, and is covered with erythematous, lacy mucosa. Biopsy revealed it to be an adenoma. (Courtesy of Dr. Eric Harder)

be possible. If the lesion is sessile or large, surgical removal may be required. Intramural hematomas may also occur in the esophagus in patients on anticoagulants or in patients with leukemia or lymphomas. These lesions should not be biopsied or removed.

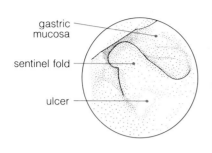

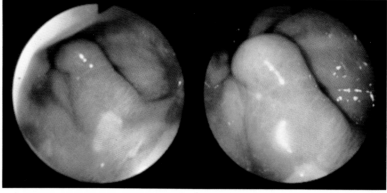

Figure 3.11 *Left,* This is the typical appearance of a sentinel fold, located in the proximal stomach just distal to the esophagogastric junction. A small ulceration can be seen on the cephalad margin. *Right,* A closeup view. The mucosa over the fold is gastric.

SENTINEL FOLD AND POLYP

This rarely noted longitudinal fold in a hiatal hernia pouch has been associated with reflux symptoms and may be confused with a polyp or mass. It is typically located on the greater curvature side of the stomach and ends proximally at the squamocolumnar junction. There may appear to be a small ulceration or erosion on the proximal tip of the fold (Fig. 3.11). The fold is actually a hyperemic gastric fold prolapsing above the diaphragmatic hiatus. Differential diagnosis includes a varix, adenoma, papilloma, and leiomyoma or carcinoma. These folds are not neoplastic and need not be removed endoscopically. Biopsy and brush cytology may be used to rule out a neoplasm.

MALIGNANT ESOPHAGEAL NEOPLASMS

There are two major types of malignant neoplasms of the esophagus: squamous-cell carcinoma and adenocarcinoma.

SQUAMOUS-CELL CARCINOMA

Most tumors of the esophagus are squamous-cell carcinomas, representing approximately 60% of esophageal and esophagogastric junction malignancies. The incidence of these tumors varies worldwide. In the United States, the rate is approximately 5 cancers per 100,000 population. In some areas of the world, rates as high as 100 cases per 100,000 have been reported. The reason for this variability in incidence is not clear, but a correlation has been suggested between the occurrence of esophageal carcinoma in some regions and the drinking of superheated beverages which cause chronic injury to the esophageal mucosa. In the United States, consumption of alcohol and cigarette smoking have both been correlated with carcinoma of the esophagus. Other known associations include tylosis which presents with thickening of the skin of the palms and soles, long-standing achalasia of the esophagus with stasis, lye injury to the esophageal mucosa, and esophageal webs of the proximal esophagus associated with Plummer-Vinson syndrome. In patients with Barrett's metaplasia of the esophagus resulting from chronic reflux esophagitis, there is an increased incidence of mucosal dysplasia and adenocarcinoma. Long-standing exposure to ionizing radiation has also been associated with esophageal carcinoma.

Patients with carcinoma of the esophagus usually present with dysphagia, which begins with solid food and progresses to liquids, including saliva. Unfortunately, dysphagia does not manifest itself until more than two-thirds of the esophageal circumference and a length of approximately 3 to 4 cm of the esophagus have been involved by the tumor. At this stage, the tumor has often grown into the mediastinum and is therefore unresectable.

Despite various combinations of radiation therapy, surgery, and chemotherapy, the 5-year survival rate for patients with squamous-cell carcinoma of the esophagus remains 5 to 15%. Part of the problem relates to the high operative mortality which results from the presentation of patients with advanced weight loss and debility. This is often a result of delay by both the patient and physician in evaluating the cause of dysphagia.

Swallowing is taken for granted by healthy people, but it is in reality a highly sophisticated physiological sequence. When this sequence is interrupted, significant problems occur. Difficulty swallowing may be divided into oropharyngeal (transfer) dysphagia, which occurs with oropharyngeal problems, and esophageal dysphagia, which originates in the esophagus. Transfer dysphagia occurs in patients after a stroke or in association with diseases such as pseudobulbar palsy. The patient with transfer dysphagia will complain of difficulty swallowing, but a careful history and observation of the patient swallowing some water will correctly identify the problem as oropharyngeal rather than esophageal. When the patient swallows water, he or she will gag and choke as some of the liquid enters the larynx or regurgitates through the nose. Oropharyngeal dysphagia is not an esophageal problem and does not usually merit esophageal endoscopy.

Esophageal dysphagia always merits a complete, thorough evaluation with a history, physical exam, barium esophagram, and nearly always endoscopic examination. Cytology and biopsy are called for if a lesion is found. It is not uncommon for a patient with dysphagia to present with a negative X-ray, yet at endoscopy a small esophageal cancer is found. Swallowing a bolus such as a 1-cm marshmallow will often help the ra-

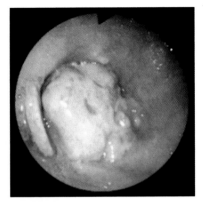
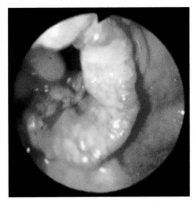
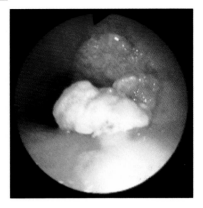

Figure 3.12 This polypoid squamous-cell carcinoma is deeply infiltrating.

Figure 3.13 This elevated squamous-cell carcinoma involves more than 75% of the esophageal circumference. The resulting narrowed lumen produced severe dysphagia. The transition between the uninvolved esophagus and the tumor is abrupt. (Courtesy of Dr. Eric Harder)

Figure 3.14 Typical squamous-cell carcinoma, with raised margins and a central ulcer presenting with a meniscoid sign.

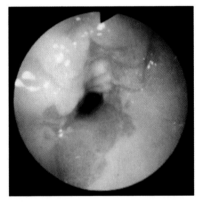
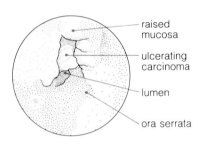

raised mucosa

ulcerating carcinoma

lumen

ora serrata

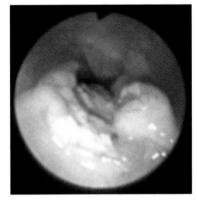
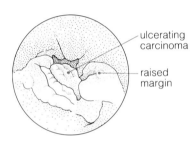

ulcerating carcinoma

raised margin

Figure 3.15 Squamous-cell carcinoma, just proximal to the ora serrata. Only a portion of the circumference is involved with this ulcerative lesion. The mucosa surrounding the ulcer is raised.

Figure 3.16 Squamous-cell cancer, with an ulcerated center and raised margin. Only a portion of the wall is involved.

diologist determine if an organic cause of dysphagia is present. True esophageal dysphagia usually has an identifiable, organic cause and must be thoroughly evaluated.

Any patient who presents with dysphagia should be considered to have esophageal carcinoma until proven otherwise. This is especially important for patients over 35 to 40 years of age, although cancer occasionally occurs in younger patients who have predisposing conditions.

Endoscopic Appearance and Diagnosis. The endoscopic appearance of squamous-cell carcinoma varies. Usually the tumor is advanced in its extent because the patient doesn't seek medical care until dysphagia develops and, at this point, the tumor is large and has extended into the periesophageal tissue.

Most squamous-cell carcinomas are located in the middle or distal third of the esophagus. However, they may also occur high in the esophagus, just below the cricopharyngeus sphincter. In a patient who presents with dysphagia, it may be helpful to obtain a barium esophagram prior to endoscopy to avoid passing the endoscope into an unsuspected proximal lesion as the instrument is being introduced into the esophagus.

There are three typical endoscopic appearances of squamous-cell carcinoma: (1) a polypoid, exophytic mass; (2) a mass with a central depressed ulceration; and (3) a diffuse infiltrating form often associated with a malignant stricture.

A polypoid mass is the configuration in approximately two-thirds of all squamous-cell cancers. The appearance is that of a bulky, wide-based mass which is firm and irregular on the surface and friable (Fig. 3.12). The covering surface is often gray-white in appearance, with some erythematous areas and occasionally superficial erosive or ulcerative features. As with each type of gross appearance, infiltration of the esophageal wall is noted by an abrupt margin to the tumor proximally (Fig. 3.13). This margin is seen radiographically as a shelf, one of the characteristic features of tumor involvement of the esophagus.

The second most common appearance of squamous-cell carcinoma is a mass with a central, meniscoid, depressed, and irregular ulcer. The margins surrounding the ulcer are raised, erythematous, and may appear nodular (Figs. 3.14 to 3.16).

With either of these first two types, the tumor initially involves just a portion of the esophageal wall. However, as

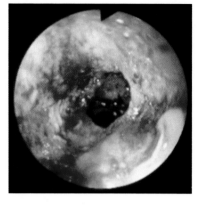
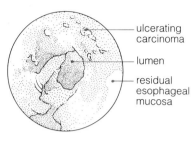
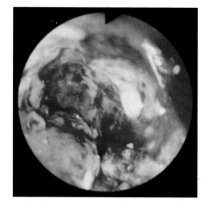

Figure 3.17 Circumferential involvement of the esophagus with friable squamous-cell carcinoma. Note the narrowed lumen.

Figure 3.18 This extensive squamous-cell cancer involves the entire lumen of the esophagus. Severe exudation and friability are also present.

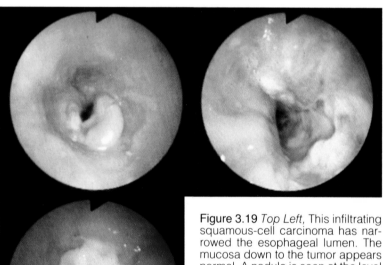
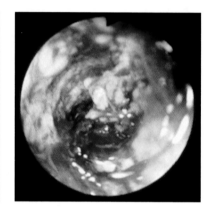
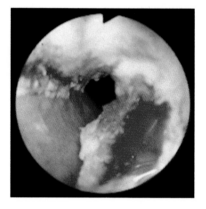

Figure 3.19 *Top Left,* This infiltrating squamous-cell carcinoma has narrowed the esophageal lumen. The mucosa down to the tumor appears normal. A nodule is seen at the level of stenosis. *Top Right,* When the endoscope is placed into the proximal stricture, an ulcer with a central meniscoid sign is observed. This proved to be a malignant stricture. *Bottom Left,* Another patient with malignant stenosis caused by squamous-cell carcinoma.

Figure 3.20 In this extensive carcinoma there is necrotic tissue over the surface of the cancer in addition to friability.

Figure 3.21 This extensive squamous-cell carcinoma demonstrates friability and bleeding.

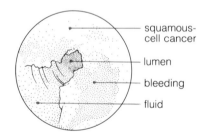

the tumor grows, it extends to involve the entire circumference (Figs. 3.17 and 3.18).

The third type of squamous-cell carcinoma is the diffuse infiltrating type. This scirrhous tumor causes thickening and rigidity of the esophageal wall and may spread submucosally. It is also the most common cause of malignant stricture; the lumen is often eccentric. The mucosa above the tumor usually appears normal, with an abrupt transition at the level of the stenosis (Fig. 3.19). The mucosa at the stenosis may be nodular, with evidence of tumor in areas around the

circumference of the stenosis, or the mucosa may appear normal. The fact that the tumor may not be obvious means that this type of malignant stricture can be confused with a benign, reflux-type stricture. Therefore, biopsy and cytology are essential in all strictures to differentiate a benign from a malignant etiology.

In all types of squamous-cell carcinomas, extensive necrosis and friability may be noted (Fig. 3.20), as may bleeding (Fig. 3.21). During endoscopy, one should use gentle technique to avoid injuring the esophageal wall.

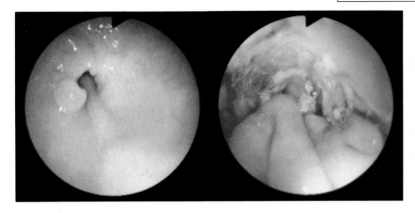

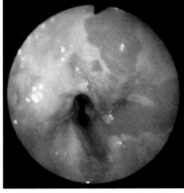

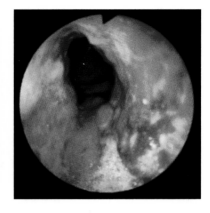

Figure 3.22 *Left,* A small, polypoid cardial adenocarcinoma is seen in the distal esophagus. *Right,* A closeup view. Friability and exudation are better appreciated in this view.

Figure 3.23 This subtle adenocarcinoma of the cardia is localized to a portion of the lumen and appears as an irregular area of elevated mucosa. The ora serrata is seen. The area should also be inspected with the instrument retroflexed.

Figure 3.24 This cardial adenocarcinoma narrowed the esophageal lumen, producing dysphagia. The tumor appears relatively flat, and appears to be friable and bleeding.

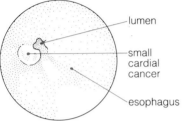

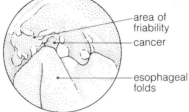

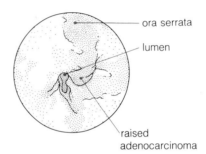

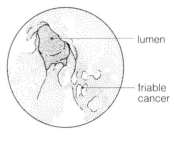

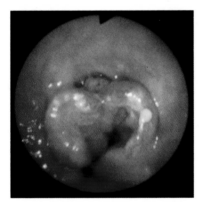

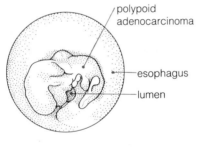

Figure 3.25 A large, polypoid adenocarcinoma of the cardia extending into the distal esophagus and involving most of the lumen.

ADENOCARCINOMA

Adenocarcinomas represent 1 to 5% of esophageal malignancies. These are usually cardial cancers which may have extended up into the distal esophagus. They seem to occur in association with Barrett's metaplasia, but may also represent a rare carcinoma arising from cells of esophageal mucous glands or a patch of congenital ectopic gastric mucosa. Symptoms are indistinguishable from those found in patients with squamous-cell carcinoma.

Adenocarcinoma involving the distal esophagus has a 5-year survival rate of 10 to 15%. For both adenocarcinoma and squamous-cell carcinoma, large controlled clinical trials are now underway to delineate the best approach to therapy, using combinations of chemotherapy, radiation therapy, and surgery.

Endoscopic Appearance and Diagnosis. There are two circumstances in which adenocarcinomas of the esophagus are encountered. The most common—and increasing in frequency—is a cancer of cardial origin at the esophagogastric junction extending up the esophagus. The second is adenocarcinoma in association with Barrett's metaplasia.

Cardial adenocarcinomas are usually infiltrative and appear with a narrowed lumen with or without an associated mass (Figs. 3.22 and 3.23). Often the adenocarcinoma may have a nodular shape, with friable, eroded mucosa having an erythematous or exudative surface. The mass may be flat and circumferential (Fig. 3.24) or large and polypoid (Fig. 3.25); narrowing of the lumen, friability, and bleeding are associated conditions.

It may be possible to directly visualize cardial adenocarcinomas as the endoscope enters the distal esophagus, but frequently the area is better evaluated with the instrument passed into the stomach and the tip retroflexed to examine the cardia from below. A nodular, irregular mass will be

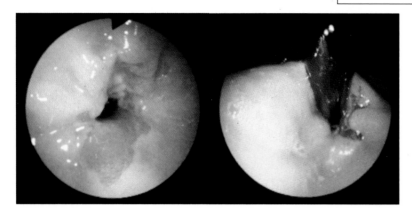

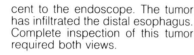

Figure 3.26 *Left,* A small cardial adenocarcinoma, seen from above. *Right,* With the instrument retroflexed in the stomach, the tumor can be better observed immediately adja- cent to the endoscope. The tumor has infiltrated the distal esophagus. Complete inspection of this tumor required both views.

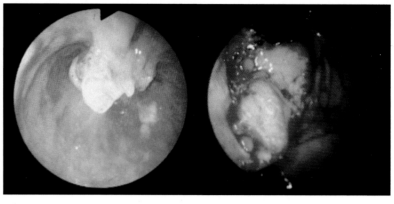

Figure 3.27 *Left,* This cardial adenocarcinoma is seen from above and appears as a small, polypoid mass. The mucosa over the mass is white from necrotic tissue. *Right,* With the endoscope retroflexed in the stomach, a more extensive, friable, and bleeding adenocarcinoma can be appreciated.

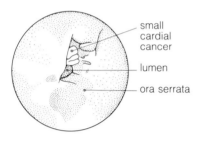

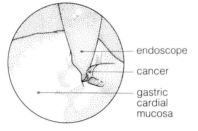

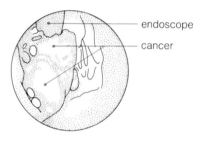

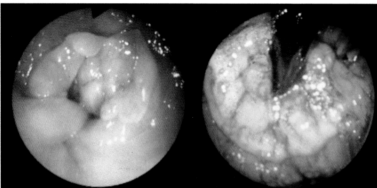

Figure 3.28 *Left,* On direct view, this adenocarcinoma in the distal esophagus demonstrates heavy folds, with a raised and somewhat irregular mucosa. *Right,* On retro- flexed view, the cancer is better seen. The tumor appears polypoid and friable. Now the cause of the obstruction and symptomatic dysphagia is evident.

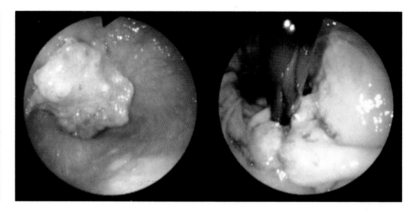

Figure 3.29 *Left,* Cardial adenocarcinoma from an elderly patient who presented with dysphagia, seen from above. *Right,* With the endo- scope retroflexed in the stomach, the infiltrating mass can be better observed adjacent to the instrument.

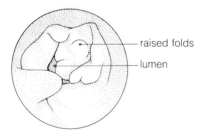

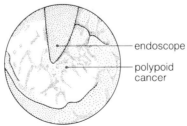

seen adjacent to the endoscope (Figs. 3.26 to 3.29). Some- times the endoscopic appearance is subtle. If any lesion or suspicious area is seen, biopsy and cytology are essential. In a patient presenting with dysphagia, it is essential to in- spect the cardia from above and below, and a cardial cancer should always be included in the differential diagnosis of a distal esophageal narrowing. Cardial cancers may simulate achalasia. Therefore, in patients with suspected achalasia, an endoscopic inspection of the cardia usually precedes bal- loon dilation, since this procedure is not performed for car- cinomatous obstruction of the esophagogastric junction. Also, with cardial adenocarcinoma one may find above-

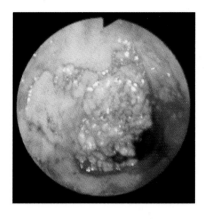
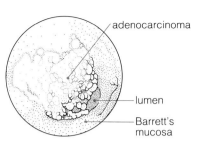

Figure 3.30 Adenocarcinoma of the esophagus, arising in an area of Barrett's metaplasia. The tumor is an exophytic, polypoid mass which was friable and bled.

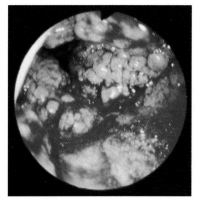
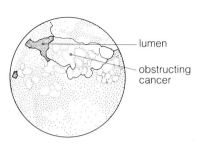

Figure 3.31 Extensive adenocarcinoma in Barrett's metaplasia, with obstruction of the lumen and bleeding.

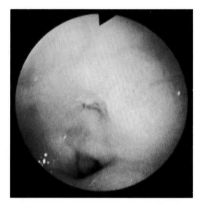
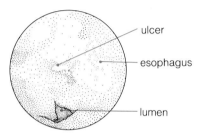

Figure 3.32 Early squamous-cell carcinoma. Note the tiny ulcer, which proved on biopsy to be malignant (1 of 20 positive).

normal gastric acid production (as noted with a history of duodenal ulcer and an endoscopic appearance of prominent areae gastricae in the fundus of the stomach) and Barrett's metaplasia.

Adenocarcinoma arising in Barrett's metaplasia may present as a polypoid, exophytic mass with exudation, friability, and bleeding (Figs. 3.30 and 3.31). A more common appearance is that of an infiltrated lesion causing a stricture. It is often located a few centimeters distal to the new proximal squamocolumnar junction; therefore, the cancer is often in the middle third of the esophagus. As with infiltrative squamous-cell carcinoma, the mucosa may appear intact down to the level of the stricture, making the endoscopic diagnosis of a malignant stricture difficult. Tumor nodules and abnormal mucosa with erythema and exudation may be visible at the cephalad margin of the stricture. The margin may be abrupt, suggesting tumor. In all cases of Barrett's-associated adenocarcinoma, biopsies of the mucosa adjacent to the tumor will determine whether Barrett's metaplasia is present. In some cases this diagnosis of Barrett's is obvious, but when the squamocolumnar junction is indistinct, biopsy is essential to diagnose Barrett's metaplasia. Biopsy and cytology of the mass is also essential to diagnose a carcinoma.

EARLY ESOPHAGEAL CANCER

At the present time the diagnosis of esophageal cancer is usually made when the cancer is at an advanced stage and surgical resection for cure is not possible. Clearly, the early diagnosis of esophageal cancer is essential. In certain geographic areas with a very high incidence of cancer, screening programs for symptomless patients have led to early detection and, consequently, to an excellent chance for surgical cure and a reasonable 5-year survival rate.

The appearance of early esophageal cancer is not as obvious as with larger, further-advanced squamous-cell and adenocarcinomas. In fact, there are early cancers which are invisible to the naked eye and cannot be detected endoscopically. These occult cancers may be encountered when a wash cytology is positive yet no lesion is seen endoscopically (squamous-cell), or in Barrett's metaplasia when dysplasia or a small focus of adenocarcinoma is detected on biopsy but the endoscopy does not reveal an area which suggests cancer.

According to Guo-Qing (1981), early squamous-cell carcinoma has four characteristic appearances. The first is that of localized mucosal erosions, seen in approximately 50% of cases (Fig. 3.32). The mucosa is red, eroded, and friable, often in a geographic pattern, surrounding areas of more normal mucosa. The second type consists of circumscribed mucosal protuberances, seen in 25% of cases. These lesions show an irregular, thickened mucosa with a polypoid, nodular, or papillary configuration. The mucosa over the surface is often eroded or ulcerated and friable. The third type is a focal area of erythema (occasionally with red spots), congestion, and coarseness of the mucosa which bleeds easily; this type is seen in approximately 13% of cases. Finally the fourth type, seen in approximately 9% of cases, presents with white mucosal plaques which are not friable, are single or multiple, and may be confluent. Where no lesion is visible, staining in vivo with toluidine blue may help locate areas of early squamous-cell cancer since these areas stain dark blue.

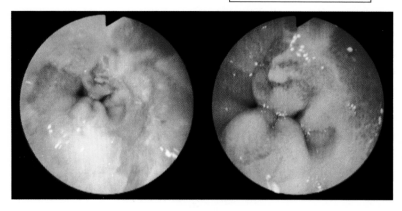

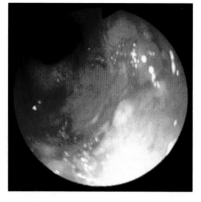

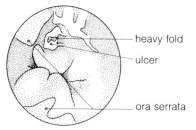

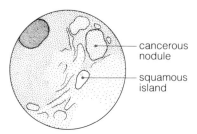

Figure 3.33 Early adenocarcinoma. *Left,* A slightly enlarged fold can be observed at the squamocolumnar junction of a patient with Barrett's metaplasia. Biopsy revealed malignancy. *Right,* A closeup view. The small ulcer resulted from a previous biopsy.

heavy fold
ulcer
ora serrata

Figure 3.34 Early adenocarcinoma. A slightly nodular, friable cancer can be observed in the Barrett's segment. The white plaque represents a squamous island.

cancerous nodule
squamous island

Early adenocarcinoma is occasionally noted in patients with Barrett's metaplasia of the esophagus (Fig. 3.33). Routine biopsies as part of a screening program may reveal dysplasia or a focus of invasive adenocarcinoma in an area which did not appear abnormal endoscopically. A small nodule, erosion, friable area, or ulcer may be noted, or the area may appear the same as the surrounding Barrett's metaplastic mucosa (Fig. 3.34). The only method to detect these early and potentially resectable cancers is to biopsy patients with Barrett's metaplasia as part of a screening program. The ideal frequency for this program is not known. Certainly, these patients should be examined periodically and endoscoped if symptoms change or if new symptoms develop. Some feel that dysplasia or carcinoma in situ in a patient with Barrett's metaplasia may be an indication for surgery.

Early cardial adenocarcinoma may present as a small polypoid mass at the squamocolumnar junction which may at first appear as a thickened fold (Fig. 3.35).

BIOPSY AND CYTOLOGY IN ESOPHAGEAL CANCER
The mucosa surrounding an esophageal cancer may have a marked inflammatory reaction. Therefore, biopsy of that mucosa may not reveal cancer cells but rather reactive tissue. If multiple biopsies are taken (up to 8 or 10) and if the biopsies are carefully planned to include areas which may contain tumor tissue, the true-positive biopsy rate may be as high as 80 to 90%. Rates of positive biopsies as low as

60% used to be reported, but this has improved considerably with current techniques.

Another essential aspect to diagnosis is the use of endoscopic sheathed brush cytology. The brush is passed down the channel, opened, and then passed over the surface of the lesion, sampling a wide area of tumor. When multiple biopsies are used in conjunction with this type of brush cytology, a true-positive diagnosis rate of 95% can be attained. Exfoliative wash cytology can also aid in precise diagnosis if an expert cytologist is available.

When a stricture is present, it may be difficult to biopsy and brush the area inside the narrowed segment. In such cases it may be possible to gently pass a cytology brush through the stricture to sample the mucosa. Occasionally, a biopsy forceps can be guided through the narrowed lumen to sample the narrowed segment. If these techniques are not possible or are negative while the endoscopic appearance is that of a cancer, another technique is to gently dilate the stricture and then repeat the biopsy and brushings along the length of the suspicious area (Fig. 3.36).

ENDOSCOPIC MANAGEMENT OF MALIGNANT STRICTURES
Patients with esophageal carcinomas may present with very tight, irregular strictures. Dilation of the stricture may be essential to allow adequate biopsy and cytology, but also to initiate treatment for relief of symptoms. The endoscope

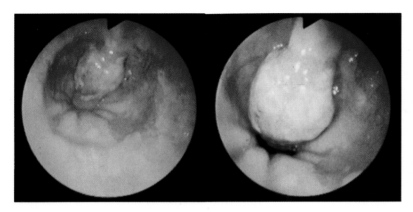

Figure 3.35 *Left,* Early adenocarcinoma of the cardia just distal to the ora serrata. What appeared to be a thickened fold is seen to be a mass as the endoscope is advanced into the distal esophagus. *Right,* A closeup view.

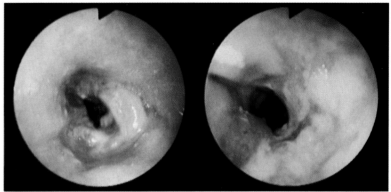

Figure 3.36 *Left,* This stricture was suspected of being caused by a squamous-cell carcinoma. The mucosa just proximal to the narrowed area is slightly nodular and red, but biopsies in this area failed to reveal tumor. *Right,* When the tip of the endoscope is advanced into the narrowing after gentle dilation, the obvious squamous-cell carcinoma with ulceration is seen.

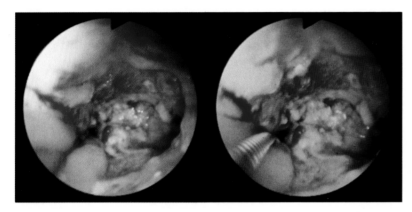

Figure 3.37 *Left,* A large necrotic tumor can be observed. The stenotic residual lumen is eccentric and not easily seen. *Right,* Under endoscopic guidance, a guidewire is introduced into the tumor. This wire can safely route dilators through the stenotic lumen and reduce the likelihood of a perforation.

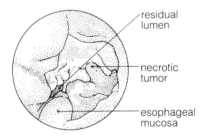

residual lumen

necrotic tumor

esophageal mucosa

necrotic tumor

lumen

guidewire

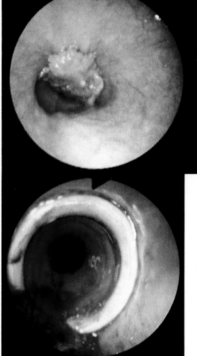

Figure 3.38 *Top Left,* Squamous-cell carcinoma of the esophagus, with an ulcerated area seen in the distance. *Top Right,* On closeup view, the ulcer is found to be deep and infiltrating. *Bottom Left,* Under endoscopic guidance, a prosthetic stent was placed through the narrowed area, with the top of the stent just above the tumor.

may be useful in dilating the stricture. Under endoscopic guidance, a guidewire with an atraumatic tip can be passed through the lumen of the stricture into the stomach (Fig. 3.37), the position of the wire confirmed radiographically. Metal, olive-shaped dilators or catheter dilators with single or multiple tapers can then be passed over the wire to dilate the stricture. The guidewire reduces the risk of perforation. By using dilators of gradually increasing size, it is possible to progressively dilate the stricture. The endoscope can also be used to guide balloon-tipped catheters into a tight stricture for balloon dilation under direct endoscopic guidance.

For patients with recurrent or unresectable carcinomas, palliative therapy is often appropriate. This is accomplished by dilating the esophagus and inserting a plastic, tubular esophageal prosthesis. The upper and lower margins of the tumor can be located and the distance from the teeth measured to determine the length and correct position of the prosthesis. The endoscope can then be used as a guide for insertion of the prosthesis (Fig. 3.38). After insertion, the endoscope can evaluate the position of the prosthesis relative

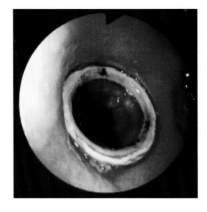

Figure 3.39 A prosthesis in position in the esophagus of a patient with adenocarcinoma associated with Barrett's metaplasia. The wide proximal flange of the prosthesis is located just cephalad to the stenosing carcinoma.

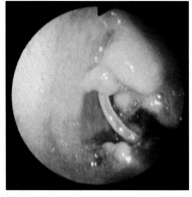

Figure 3.40 A carcinoma has grown extensively and is now obstructing

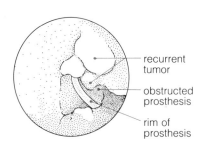

a prosthesis proximally. Only a small rim of the prosthesis is still visible.

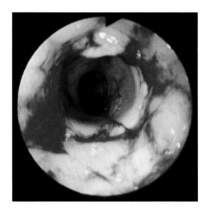

Figure 3.41 Reflux esophagitis above a prosthesis, with evidence of friability and bleeding.

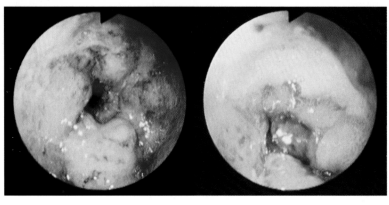

Figure 3.42 *Left,* This squamous-cell carcinoma had been treated with a prosthesis. However, the prosthesis has produced pressure necrosis of the esophageal wall. The mucosa is inflamed, and an ulcer can be faintly observed. *Right,* A closeup view of the area of pressure necrosis better demonstrates the mucosal ulceration.

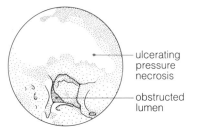

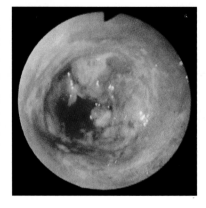

Figure 3.43 Squamous-cell carcinoma had produced total obstruction of the esophagus. However, after one Nd-YAG laser therapy session, the lumen is open. The white areas represent ulcers caused by the laser treatment.

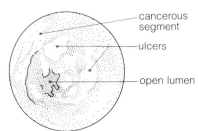

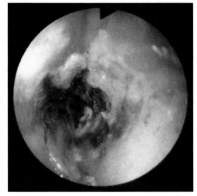

Figure 3.44 Recurrent esophageal carcinoma after radiation therapy. Nd-YAG laser treatment reestablished the lumen. The whitish areas are necrotic tumor, coagulated by the laser.

to the carcinoma (Fig. 3.39). This prosthesis may be useful in occluding a tracheoesophageal fistula, but should be avoided in very proximal esophageal lesions. Complications may include overgrowth of the tumor, obstructing the proximal lumen (Fig. 3.40), reflux with bleeding (Fig. 3.41); migration of the prosthesis; and pressure necrosis of the esophageal wall (Fig. 3.42).

Another approach to the palliation of recurrent or unresectable esophageal cancers is to use the endoscope to direct a Nd-YAG laser at the tumor. This laser can destroy tumor tissue and reestablish the lumen (Figs. 3.43 and 3.44).

OTHER ESOPHAGEAL MALIGNANCIES

These tumors include lesions which can be recognized because of characteristic endoscopic features, for example, pigment visible in a primary melanosarcoma (Fig. 3.45). In other instances tumors may be difficult or impossible to distinguish endoscopically, but the biopsy may permit diagnosis of tumors other than squamous-cell or adenocarcinomas, for example, esophageal myoblastoma granular (Fig. 3.46).

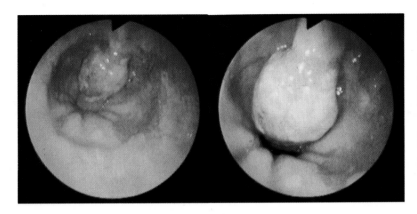

Figure 3.35 *Left,* Early adenocarcinoma of the cardia just distal to the ora serrata. What appeared to be a thickened fold is seen to be a mass as the endoscope is advanced into the distal esophagus. *Right,* A closeup view.

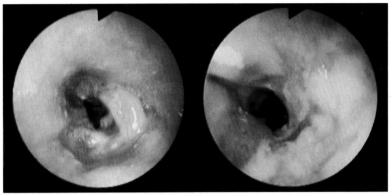

Figure 3.36 *Left,* This stricture was suspected of being caused by a squamous-cell carcinoma. The mucosa just proximal to the narrowed area is slightly nodular and red, but biopsies in this area failed to reveal tumor. *Right,* When the tip of the endoscope is advanced into the narrowing after gentle dilation, the obvious squamous-cell carcinoma with ulceration is seen.

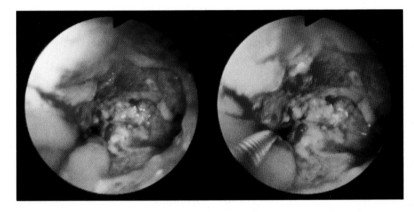

Figure 3.37 *Left,* A large necrotic tumor can be observed. The stenotic residual lumen is eccentric and not easily seen. *Right,* Under endoscopic guidance, a guidewire is introduced into the tumor. This wire can safely route dilators through the stenotic lumen and reduce the likelihood of a perforation.

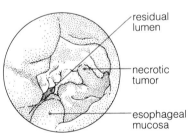

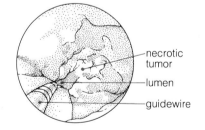

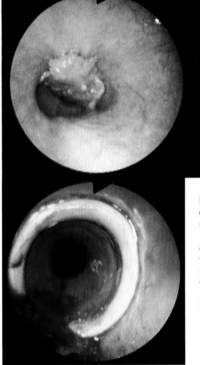

Figure 3.38 *Top Left,* Squamous-cell carcinoma of the esophagus, with an ulcerated area seen in the distance. *Top Right,* On closeup view, the ulcer is found to be deep and infiltrating. *Bottom Left,* Under endoscopic guidance, a prosthetic stent was placed through the narrowed area, with the top of the stent just above the tumor.

may be useful in dilating the stricture. Under endoscopic guidance, a guidewire with an atraumatic tip can be passed through the lumen of the stricture into the stomach (Fig. 3.37), the position of the wire confirmed radiographically. Metal, olive-shaped dilators or catheter dilators with single or multiple tapers can then be passed over the wire to dilate the stricture. The guidewire reduces the risk of perforation. By using dilators of gradually increasing size, it is possible to progressively dilate the stricture. The endoscope can also be used to guide balloon-tipped catheters into a tight stricture for balloon dilation under direct endoscopic guidance.

For patients with recurrent or unresectable carcinomas, palliative therapy is often appropriate. This is accomplished by dilating the esophagus and inserting a plastic, tubular esophageal prosthesis. The upper and lower margins of the tumor can be located and the distance from the teeth measured to determine the length and correct position of the prosthesis. The endoscope can then be used as a guide for insertion of the prosthesis (Fig. 3.38). After insertion, the endoscope can evaluate the position of the prosthesis relative

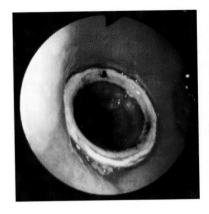

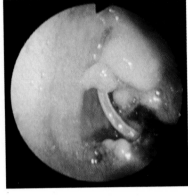

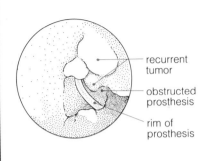

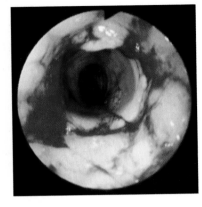

Figure 3.39 A prosthesis in position in the esophagus of a patient with adenocarcinoma associated with Barrett's metaplasia. The wide proximal flange of the prosthesis is located just cephalad to the stenosing carcinoma.

Figure 3.40 A carcinoma has grown extensively and is now obstructing a prosthesis proximally. Only a small rim of the prosthesis is still visible.

Figure 3.41 Reflux esophagitis above a prosthesis, with evidence of friability and bleeding.

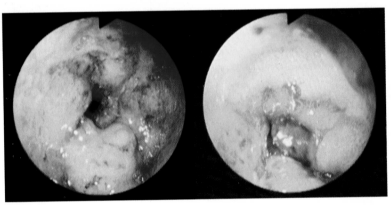

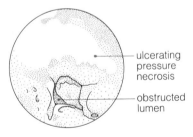

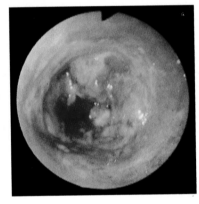

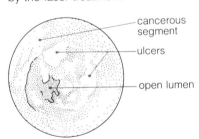

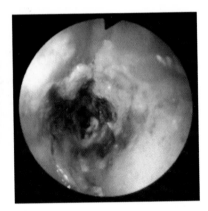

Figure 3.42 *Left,* This squamous-cell carcinoma had been treated with a prosthesis. However, the prosthesis has produced pressure necrosis of the esophageal wall. The mucosa is inflamed, and an ulcer can be faintly observed. *Right,* A closeup view of the area of pressure necrosis better demonstrates the mucosal ulceration.

Figure 3.43 Squamous-cell carcinoma had produced total obstruction of the esophagus. However, after one Nd-YAG laser therapy session, the lumen is open. The white areas represent ulcers caused by the laser treatment.

Figure 3.44 Recurrent esophageal carcinoma after radiation therapy. Nd-YAG laser treatment reestablished the lumen. The whitish areas are necrotic tumor, coagulated by the laser.

to the carcinoma (Fig. 3.39). This prosthesis may be useful in occluding a tracheoesophageal fistula, but should be avoided in very proximal esophageal lesions. Complications may include overgrowth of the tumor, obstructing the proximal lumen (Fig. 3.40), reflux with bleeding (Fig. 3.41); migration of the prosthesis; and pressure necrosis of the esophageal wall (Fig. 3.42).

Another approach to the palliation of recurrent or unresectable esophageal cancers is to use the endoscope to direct a Nd-YAG laser at the tumor. This laser can destroy tumor tissue and reestablish the lumen (Figs. 3.43 and 3.44).

OTHER ESOPHAGEAL MALIGNANCIES

These tumors include lesions which can be recognized because of characteristic endoscopic features, for example, pigment visible in a primary melanosarcoma (Fig. 3.45). In other instances tumors may be difficult or impossible to distinguish endoscopically, but the biopsy may permit diagnosis of tumors other than squamous-cell or adenocarcinomas, for example, esophageal myoblastoma granular (Fig. 3.46).

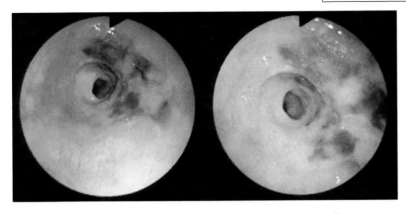

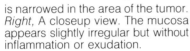

Figure 3.45 *Left,* This primary esophageal melanosarcoma has a characteristic appearance, with melanin pigment noted. The lumen is narrowed in the area of the tumor. *Right,* A closeup view. The mucosa appears slightly irregular but without inflammation or exudation.

melanosarcoma

lumen

esophageal mucosa

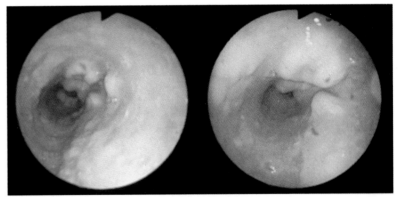

Figure 3.46 *Left,* This lesion in the distal esophagus presents with several masses, one of which has a depressed center suggesting that the tumor in the center might have outgrown its blood supply. The mucosa overlying the masses appears slightly pale. On biopsy, the tumor proved to be an esophageal myoblastoma granular. *Right,* A close-up view. The multiple masses can be seen, and the depressed center of the largest mass can be appreciated.

myoblastoma granular

esophageal mucosa

lumen

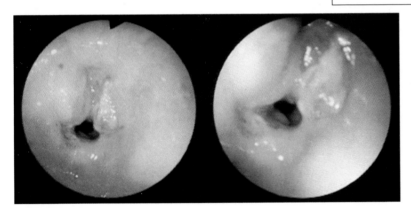

Figure 3.47 *Left,* Breast carcinoma which metastasized to the esophageal wall. The area of the metastasis is slightly erythematous, with a small nodule. The lumen is narrowed. A prosthesis which was inserted previously is invisible because of this overgrowing tumor. *Right,* A close-up view better demonstrates the narrowed lumen and the adjacent nodule.

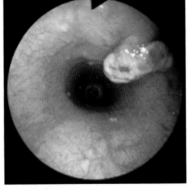

Figure 3.48 Esophageal metastasis of a melanosarcoma, as evidenced by a small amount of pigment.

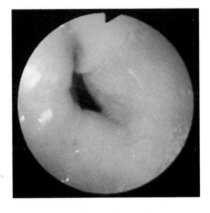

Figure 3.49 Narrowing of the esophageal lumen, caused by breast carcinoma metastasizing to the mediastinum adjacent to the esophagus. The overlying mucosa appears normal.

EXTRINSIC COMPRESSION ON THE ESOPHAGUS BY ADJACENT NEOPLASMS

Carcinomas of the thyroid or lung and metastases to the mediastinum may present with extrinsic compression of the esophagus, causing dysphagia. Endoscopically, the esophagus may appear to have a smooth indentation in one wall, while the overlying esophageal mucosa is usually normal.

Metastases may also involve the esophageal wall directly. These result from tumors of other organs such as breast cancer (Fig. 3.47) or other tumors (Fig. 3.48). Metastases to the tissue around the esophagus may cause extrinsic esophageal narrowing, though the mucosa through the area appears normal (Fig. 3.49). Lesions may occur at a distance

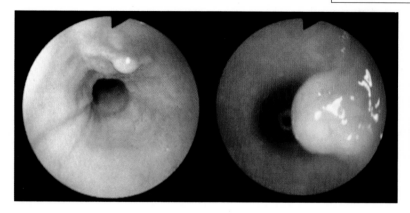

Figure 3.50 Intramural metastasis from esophageal squamous-cell carcinoma.

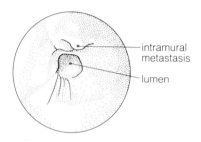

- intramural metastasis
- lumen

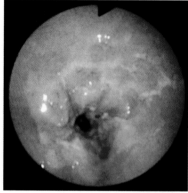

Figure 3.51 These tiny satellite lesions are intramural metastases from an adenocarcinoma in the distal esophagus. The primary tumor is located just distal to these lesions.

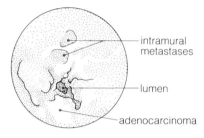

- intramural metastases
- lumen
- adenocarcinoma

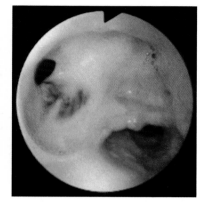

Figure 3.52 Tracheoesophageal fistula, caused by an ulcerating esophageal squamous-cell carcinoma. The fistulous tract orifice is clearly seen.

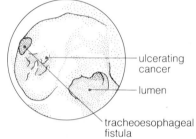

- ulcerating cancer
- lumen
- tracheoesophageal fistula

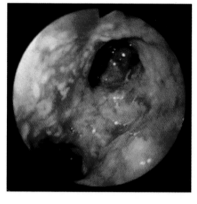

Figure 3.53 This squamous-cell carcinoma is seen as a large, necrotic tumor, with a narrowed lumen and a large fistula to the lung.

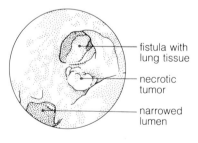

- fistula with lung tissue
- necrotic tumor
- narrowed lumen

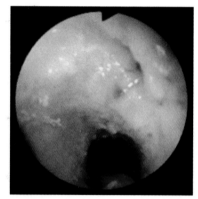

Figure 3.54 This flat squamous-cell carcinoma displays less exudation and friability than the cancer shown in Fig. 3.53. The mucosa appears diffusely abnormal, and the orifice of a small fistula to the lung is seen.

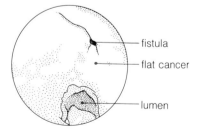

- fistula
- flat cancer
- lumen

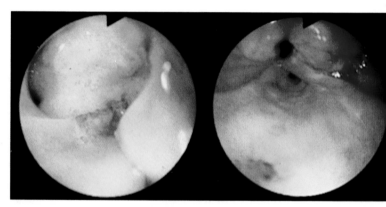

Figure 3.55 *Left,* This cancer presents with a large necrotic cavity in the lung and a tracheoesophageal fistula. *Right,* With the endoscope at a slightly different position, the fistula orifice is better seen.

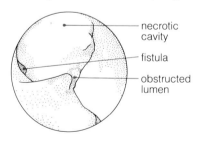

- necrotic cavity
- fistula
- obstructed lumen

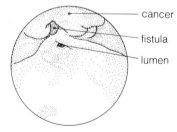

- cancer
- fistula
- lumen

from primary tumors (Fig. 3.50) or adjacent to the primary tumor, with satellite nodules and, in some cases, submucosal spread (Fig. 3.51).

One of the most feared complications of esophageal cancer is a tracheoesophageal fistula, which may cause very troublesome and disabling symptoms for the patient. These fistulas may occur after radiation-therapy–associated injury to the esophagus. Endoscopy may allow the physician to directly visualize the cancer and the fistula (Figs. 3.52 to 3.55). In some cases it may be possible to see the pleural

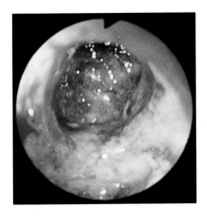

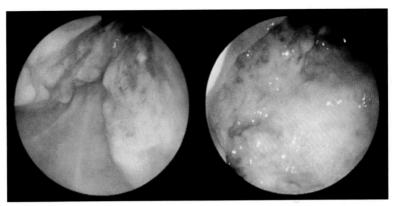

Figure 3.56 At the base of this large, ulcerating squamous-cell carcinoma is a tracheoesophageal fistula, with lung tissue also visible at the base.

Figure 3.57 *Left,* This large mesenchymal tumor with a necrotic cavity in the lung can be seen endoscopically from the esophageal lumen.

Right, Another view of the necrotic cavity. The base of the tumor cavity is irregular, with exudate and scattered erythema.

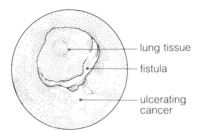

lung tissue

fistula

ulcerating cancer

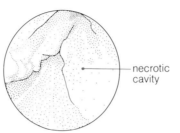

necrotic cavity

cavity and visualize lung tissue at the base of the fistula (Fig. 3.56) or look into the necrotic tumor cavity (Fig. 3.57). A tracheoesophageal fistula may be an indication for an esophageal prosthesis.

INFECTIOUS DISEASES OF THE ESOPHAGUS

Several types of infectious agents can involve the esophagus and produce symptoms which vary from mild discomfort to severe life-threatening clinical problems. These diseases often occur in patients who are immunosuppressed from underlying medical illnesses. For some of these infections, there are now specific therapeutic measures available, making precise diagnosis essential. For other infections, treatment of the underlying disorder may result in an improvement of the symptoms.

The three most commonly encountered infections of the esophagus are herpetic esophagitis, candidal esophagitis, and cytomegaloviral esophagitis. These diseases must be distinguished from esophagitis caused by gastroesophageal reflux and, in bone marrow transplant patients, from the

esophageal changes of chronic graft-versus-host disease. There are characteristic endoscopic features to each type of esophageal infection, but it is still often difficult to differentiate one from the other. Therefore, biopsies, brushings, and cultures may be necessary.

HERPETIC ESOPHAGITIS

One of the most commonly encountered infections involving the esophagus is caused by herpes simplex virus. This infection may be confused with or coexist with candidiasis of the esophagus or cytomegalovirus infection. The incidence of herpetic esophagitis is increasing, especially in the immunocompromised host with leukemia, lymphoma, a bone marrow transplant, etc. However, the infection may also occur in patients without severe underlying illness. The clinical presentation often includes odynophagia, dysphagia, and heartburn. There may be a history of a herpetic lesion on the lip preceding the onset of odynophagia by several days. Examination of the oral pharynx may be normal or may show vesicles in the mouth and pharynx. Radiologic examination of the esophagus may be normal depending on the severity of mucosal involvement.

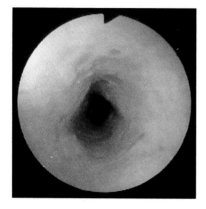

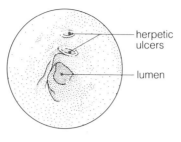

Figure 3.58 Early herpetic esophagitis. Ulcers are small and slightly depressed, with a minimally raised margin.

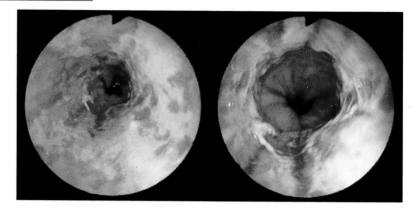

Figure 3.59 *Left,* Severe herpetic esophagitis. There is evidence of diffuse involvement of the mucosa with confluent ulcers, friability, and exudation. *Right,* A closeup view. One can see that the mucosa of the stomach, just distal to the ora serrata, is normal, but the esophageal mucosa is severely involved.

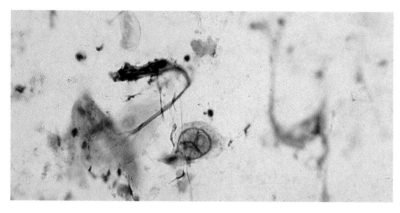

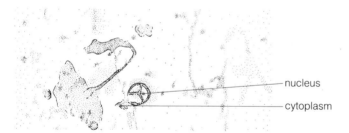

Figure 3.60 Photomicrograph shows cells with the typical cytopathic changes of herpes virus: intranuclear inclusions but no cytoplasmic inclusions. (Courtesy of Dr. George McDonald)

Herpetic esophagitis evolves in several phases. In the first phase, the lesion is vesicular (Fig. 3.58). The following phase is marked by sharply demarcated small ulcers with raised margins. These ulcers are typically in the middle or upper third of the esophagus, and may show a gray or yellowish necrotic material in the base. The mucosa surrounding the ulcer is often erythematous, with normal mucosa surrounding the erythema. These ulcers will enlarge and may begin to coalesce. Finally, there is a necrotic phase during which the infected epithelium is diffusely involved, resulting in a diffuse esophagitis with confluent ulcers (Fig. 3.59). Smear of the surface of the esophagus fails to reveal mycelia of Candida.

Diagnosis is made by examining tissue from the esophageal mucosa. Biopsy specimens reveal typical cytopathic changes of replicating viruses. Since these changes are most marked at the margin of the herpetic ulcer, biopsies should be taken there.

Biopsy specimens will reveal multinucleated giant cells and ballooning degeneration of cells; these cells are marked by basophilic nuclei with a "ground glass" inclusion and chromatin margination (Fig. 3.60). One may also observe cells with eosinophilic intranuclear inclusions surrounded by a halo. No cytoplasmic inclusions are seen.

These cytopathic changes may also be found on brushings obtained from the area at the margin of the ulcer, in cells obtained by exfoliative cytology, and in tissue culture after 1 week. Recently, the use of monoclonal antibodies in herpetic esophagitis has simplified the diagnosis, since these specific antibodies will identify the presence of herpes virus in the involved tissue. It is important to remember that cytopathic changes may not be obvious unless one is looking for them. Therefore, the pathologist should be alerted to the possibility of herpetic esophagitis so that these characteristic changes may be sought.

Clinically, the usual consideration is whether the patient has reflux esophagitis (which should be treated with appropriate antireflux measures), candidal esophagitis (which should be treated with antifungal drugs), or herpetic esophagitis (which can be treated with antiviral agents). In patients who have undergone a bone marrow transplant, chronic graft-versus-host disease (which can be treated with increased dosages of immunosuppressive agents) must also be included in the differential diagnosis.

CANDIDAL ESOPHAGITIS

Candida is a fungus which can proliferate anywhere along the GI tract, and candidal esophagitis is being increasingly diagnosed. This increase may be due to improved detection through fiberoptic endoscopy and the increasing number of immunosuppressed patients, including patients with organ transplants, those undergoing cancer chemotherapy,

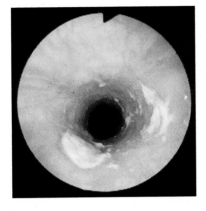

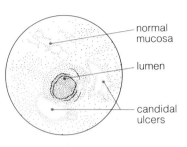

normal mucosa

lumen

candidal ulcers

Figure 3.61 *Candidal esophagitis. Ulcers are noted, with fairly normal* surrounding mucosa. A white exudate covers the ulcers.

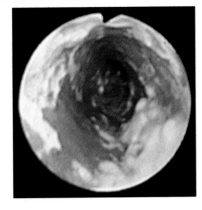

Figure 3.62 *Moderate to severe candidal esophagitis. Here the entire circumference of the esophagus is involved, with erythema of the mucosa and white exudate clearly evident.*

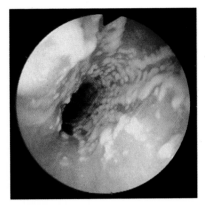

Figure 3.63 *Severe candidal esophagitis. Extensive exudation and erythema are noted.*

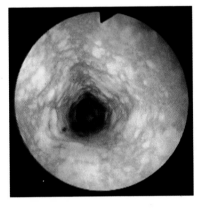

Figure 3.64 *In this severe case, diffuse Candida with exudation involving a considerable length of esophagus is seen.*

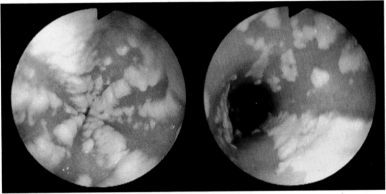

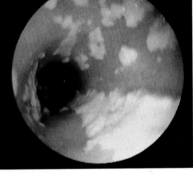

Figure 3.65 *Two cases of severe candidal esophagitis in patients with AIDS. The underlying mucosa is* erythematous, and the linear exudate is typical of this infection.

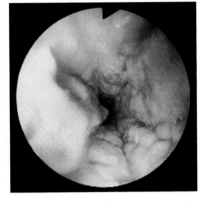

Figure 3.66 *Candidal esophagitis in a patient with AIDS. The combination of exudate and severe edema of the mucosa may compromise the esophageal lumen.*

and those with other causes for immunosuppression. Other predisposing illnesses to candidal infection include diabetes mellitus and malignancy. Significant symptomatic esophageal candidiasis has also been reported in patients with no underlying illness. In the years prior to the application of fiberoptic endoscopy, diagnosis was made by barium swallow radiograph which demonstrated irregular outlines of exudates, ulcers, strictures, aperistalsis, etc. However, for known cases of candidal esophagitis, such radiographs appeared normal 20 to 80% of the time.

The presenting symptoms of candidal esophagitis are usually dysphagia and odynophagia, but patients may also present with weight loss, back pain, and gastrointestinal bleeding. In addition, esophageal obstruction from debris may occur. Diagnosis is made from the endoscopic appearance of the esophageal mucosa and from examination of brushings taken with endoscopic guidance. The presence of oral Candida (thrush) is not required for the diagnosis

of candidal esophagitis, since it is present in only 20 to 80% of patients with the infection.

Endoscopic examination of early, mild candidal esophagitis demonstrates small amounts of a white, creamlike exudate; the underlying mucosa may be erythematous or fairly normal in appearance (Fig. 3.61). As the disease increases in severity, larger amounts of exudate become evident, with more obvious mucosal erythema and early ulceration. With further progression, the entire circumference of the esophagus becomes involved (Fig. 3.62). These changes are characteristic but not pathognomonic. The underlying esophageal mucosa becomes increasingly erythematous and friable, and exudation becomes severe (Figs. 3.63 to 3.65).

Ultimately, the increased inflammation and debris may narrow or obstruct the esophagus (Fig. 3.66). At this point marked friability, bleeding, and ulceration may be noted. The endoscopic differential diagnosis includes herpetic esophagitis and reflux esophagitis; each may present with sim-

3.17

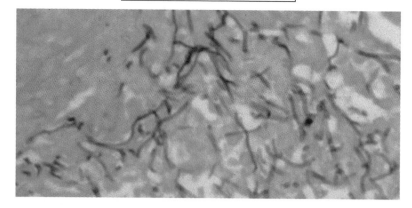

Figure 3.67 This stained brushing from the exudate of a patient with candidal esophagitis shows large numbers of candidal mycelia. (Courtesy of Dr. Eric Harder)

ilar endoscopic appearances. Other rare esophageal infections include *Torulopsis glabrata* and *Lactobacillus acidophilus*.

Diagnosis is usually made by examining the mucosal brushings obtained during endoscopy. A sheathed cytology brush is passed, and plaque or exudate is brushed. After staining the slides with Gram's stain, mycelia and/or yeast forms can be seen (Fig. 3.67). Biopsies can be obtained and examined for invasive Candida, especially in patients presenting with ulcerative mucosa, but this method is not as commonly used or as productive as the smear technique.

Cultures are not relied upon since Candida is normally found in 35 to 50% of oral pharyngeal washings and in 65 to 90% of stool samples. Thus, a positive culture is not indicative of disease. If a culture is desired, a sterile cytology brush can be passed and exudate sampled. The brush is then rubbed directly onto Sabouraud's agar or washed in normal saline followed by culture of the saline. Serology can also be used to determine invasive Candida, but the sensitivity and specificity of the serologic approach is still not satisfactory due to the occurrence of false-positives.

CYTOMEGALOVIRAL ESOPHAGITIS

Cytomegalovirus (CMV) is another viral agent which causes esophagitis. These infections may occur secondary to damaged epithelium, as is seen in chronic graft-versus-host disease. However, in primary CMV infections the esophageal mucosa has a relatively characteristic appearance: superficial erosions with a geographic, serpiginous, nonraised border (Fig. 3.68). This distinguishes CMV lesions from the raised lesions seen in herpes simplex virus. In CMV, the erosions may be large (1 to 3 cm in diameter) but very superficial. The centers of these erosions are diffusely involved and have a reticulated appearance (Figs. 3.69 and 3.70). When these changes are noted at the gastroesophageal junction, the appearance of the mucosa may be similar to that of reflux esophagitis. However, the mucosal changes are distinctive when surrounded by normal mucosa.

Diagnosis of cytomegalovirus is made by obtaining tissue from biopsies or cytologic brushings, and evaluating the tissue for typical cytopathic changes. The changes include a characteristic cellular appearance with a basophilic intranuclear inclusion, a clear halo surrounding the nucleus, and the presence of multiple, smaller intracytoplasmic inclusions (Fig. 3.71). Cultures for the virus can also be obtained; cytopathic effects are seen in tissue culture after 3 weeks. CMV may occur simultaneously with graft-versus-host disease and herpetic esophagitis.

GRAFT-VERSUS-HOST DISEASE

Bone marrow transplant is a therapeutic technique being used with increasing frequency for several hematologic disorders, including aplastic anemia and leukemia. After transplantation, patients often experience esophageal problems, including viral infections (herpes and cytomegalovirus) and fungal infections with Candida. Later in the course of recovery, these patients may develop severe retrosternal pain, dysphagia, and odynophagia caused by an epithelial reaction of the esophageal mucosa as part of chronic graft-versus-host disease.

Viral esophagitis occurs approximately 10 weeks after bone marrow transplantation. Chronic graft-versus-host disease involving the esophagus has a median onset of approximately 250 days following transplantation, with a range of approximately 70 days to more than 2 years. As a further complication, these patients may present with a combination of chronic graft-versus-host disease of the esophagus and viral or fungal infection.

In a recent study, 8 of 63 patients with chronic graft-versus-host disease developed severe esophageal symptoms. At endoscopy, 7 of the 8 patients showed mucosal changes characteristic of graft-versus-host disease. The first and most commonly seen change is desquamation marked by superficial peeling of the erythematous mucosa (Figs. 3.72 and 3.73). Severe involvement is marked by erythema and exudation, and may demonstrate mucosa hanging in shreds

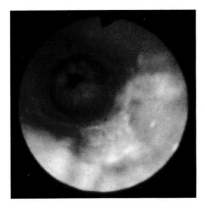
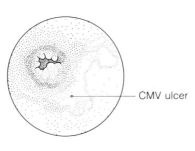

Figure 3.68 This is the characteristic appearance of esophageal mucosa infected with cytomegalovirus: large, superficial erosions with a geo- graphic pattern; the margins of the erosions are not raised. (Courtesy of Dr. George McDonald)

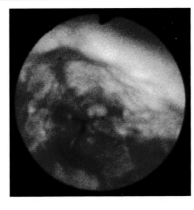
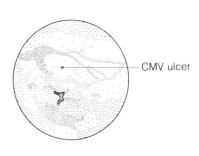

Figure 3.69 This is a typical large, superficial erosion caused by cy- tomegalovirus. The borders are nonraised, serpiginous, and geo- graphic; the mucosa is reticulated in appearance. (Courtesy of Dr. George McDonald)

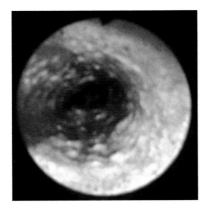
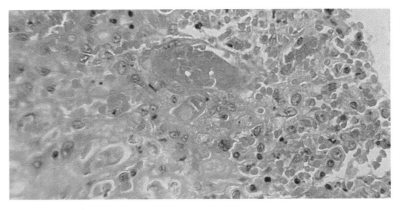

Figure 3.70 In this severe case of cytomegaloviral esophagitis, there is evidence of diffuse involvement of the esophageal mucosa, with a characteristic flat, reticulated sur- face. (Courtesy of Dr. George McDonald)

Figure 3.71 Photomicrograph shows the typical cellular changes asso- ciated with cytomegaloviral infec- tion. The cell has an intranuclear in- clusion, a halo surrounding the nucleus, and multiple intracyto- plasmic inclusions. (Courtesy of Dr. George McDonald)

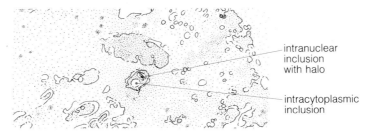

Graft-Versus-Host Disease

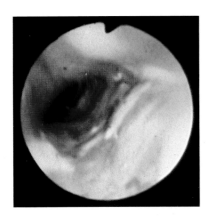
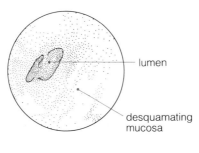

Figure 3.72 In the early stages of the disease, desquamation of the mu- cosa can be noted. (Courtesy of Dr. George McDonald)

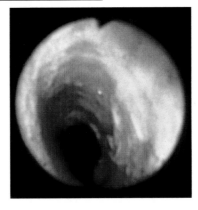
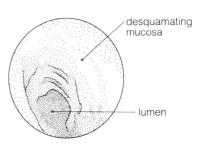

Figure 3.73 In this early stage, mu- cosal desquamation and erythema are evident. (Courtesy of Dr. George McDonald)

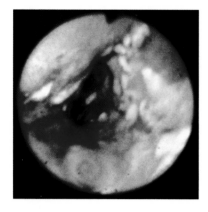
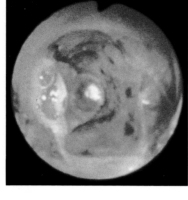
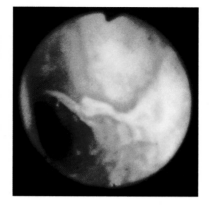
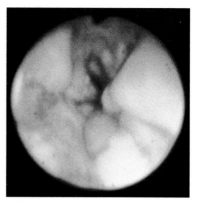

Figure 3.74 As the disease progresses, one may note severe desquamation, with erythema, shredding mucosa, bleeding, and marked exudation. (Courtesy of Dr. George McDonald)

Figure 3.75 In severe disease, one will note marked, diffuse mucosal erythema in association with severe desquamation. (Courtesy of Dr. George McDonald)

Figure 3.76 This patient presented with substernal esophageal pain and dysphagia approximately 250 days after bone marrow transplantation. Endoscopic examination reveals shredded desquamated mucosa, indicative of graft-versus-host disease. (Courtesy of Dr. George McDonald)

Figure 3.77 Note that despite desquamation in the upper and middle esophagus, the esophagogastric junction remains normal. This finding is characteristic of graft-versus-host disease. (Courtesy of Dr. George McDonald)

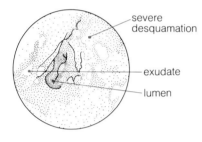
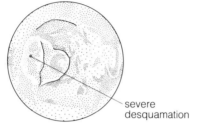
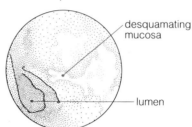

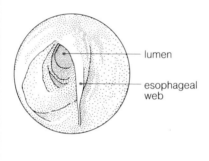
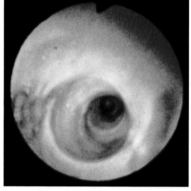
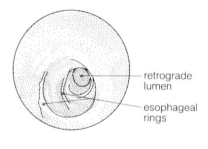

Figure 3.78 An esophageal web with mucosal erythema, a characteristic finding in graft-versus-host disease. (Courtesy of Dr. George McDonald)

Figure 3.79 Retrograde study via a gastrostomy reveals that multiple esophageal rings with evidence of mucosal erythema caused total obstruction of the upper third of the esophagus. (Courtesy of Dr. George McDonald)

(Figs. 3.74 to 3.76). This latter change is often found in the upper esophagus and is occasionally confluent with chronic graft-versus-host disease involving the oral mucosa. Even in the presence of these severe changes, the distal esophagus may appear normal (Fig. 3.77).

Other characteristic findings are webs, strictures, and rings (Fig. 3.78). These abnormalities can cause severe dysphagia. In one case, severe webs obstructed the upper esophagus, and retrograde endoscopy via a gastrostomy was necessary to evaluate the area (Fig. 3.79). Abnormal peristalsis may also be noted in association with poor acid clearing from the esophagus, leading to changes of reflux esophagitis.

Diagnosis is based on clinical presentation and endoscopic appearance. Biopsies show cellular infiltration and fibrosis which can be distinguished from the fibrosis seen in progressive systemic sclerosis.

Treatment is usually to increase immunosuppressives (e.g., steroids and azathioprine). Esophageal changes often regress with this therapy. Webs, strictures, and rings may require cautious dilation because there is an increased risk of esophageal perforation from dilation in these patients. As bone marrow transplants increase, clinicians will see increasing numbers of patients with the aforementioned esophageal abnormalities. Since the symptoms are severe and the treatments very different, the characteristic presentation, specific diagnostic methods, and differential diagnosis will become increasingly important.

4

Esophagus III: Motor Dysfunction, Vascular Abnormalities, and Trauma

In this chapter we will consider disorders of the esophagus for which endoscopy has a role in diagnosis and therapy. The esophagus has a simple function: to pass food and liquids into the stomach and to keep them there. When the esophagus malfunctions, the disability to the patient may be striking. Among the causes of dysfunction are motor disorders, vascular abnormalities, and injury by a variety of mechanisms.

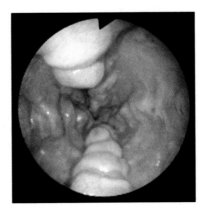

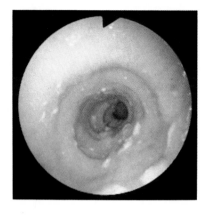

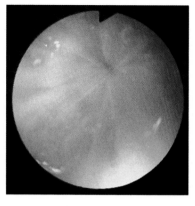

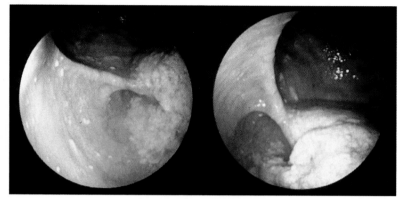

Figure 4.1 Ringlike esophageal contractions caused by diffuse spasm. The overlying mucosa is normal.

Figure 4.2 Diffuse esophageal spasm. Here, the LES is tightly closed.

Figure 4.3 Large epiphrenic diverticulum associated with diffuse esophageal spasm. Note the retained food in the distal esophagus in the picture at left.

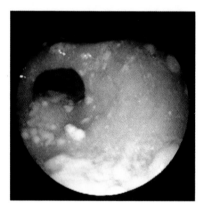

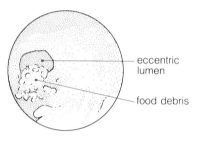

Figure 4.4 In this case of severe diffuse spasm, the lumen appears eccentric with evidence of stagnation and food debris.

contractions of the esophageal musculature occur sporadically in localized segments of the esophagus and may be associated with pain.

DISEASES AFFECTING ESOPHAGEAL MOTILITY

Many disease states can affect the esophagus and its motility. Prominent among these are diffuse esophageal spasm, achalasia, and scleroderma. Endoscopy may be useful for diagnosis of these diseases and their associated complications.

NORMAL ESOPHAGEAL ANATOMY AND FUNCTION

The wall of the esophagus contains striated muscle in the upper one-third and smooth muscle in the lower two-thirds. In its normal resting state the cricopharyngeus sphincter seals the entrance to the esophagus to prevent the negative intrathoracic pressure from drawing air into the esophagus. The lower esophageal sphincter (LES) remains closed at rest to prevent reflux of gastric acid, pepsin, and bile into the esophagus.

At the start of a swallow the hypopharynx generates a high spike of pressure and the cricopharyngeus sphincter temporarily relaxes to allow the bolus of food or liquid to pass. Simultaneously, the LES relaxes until the bolus passes into the stomach. The muscle of the esophageal wall propels the bolus down the esophagus in a process called peristalsis. Primary peristalsis is the normal peristalsis initiated by a swallow. Secondary peristalsis is an orderly peristalsis which occurs in response to distension of the esophagus. For example, when food refluxes from the stomach into the esophagus, a peristaltic wave is initiated to clear this potentially noxious material from the distal esophagus. Tertiary peristalsis is abnormal peristalsis. These random nonorderly

DIFFUSE ESOPHAGEAL SPASM

Diffuse esophageal spasm describes a clinical condition caused by tertiary esophageal contractions. The patient may experience sudden regurgitation of swallowed liquids and may or may not have difficulty swallowing solids. This contrasts with dysphagia caused by organic narrowing, in which symptoms initially are associated with solids and gradually progress to liquids as the lumen narrows. Symptoms of esophageal spasm may be intermittent, may be brought on by hot or cold liquids, and may be relieved by a Valsalva-type maneuver. The spasm may produce severe chest pain radiating to the back, resembling pain of coronary artery disease. Therefore coronary angiography and investigations of the esophagus may be necessary to make the diagnosis.

ENDOSCOPIC EXAMINATION

Esophageal motility is difficult to evaluate endoscopically; one may observe a peristaltic contraction and have the general impression that it is moving distally but the movement is difficult to confirm. Tertiary esophageal contractions appear as contractions of the esophageal wall with transient narrowing of the lumen. The mucosa is normal (Fig. 4.1). Spasm of the LES is an associated finding (Fig. 4.2), and diverticula may be present (Fig. 4.3). The esophageal lumen

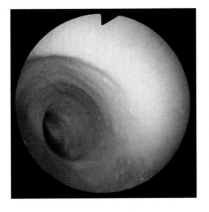

Figure 4.5 Achalasia. The esophageal mucosa appears white.

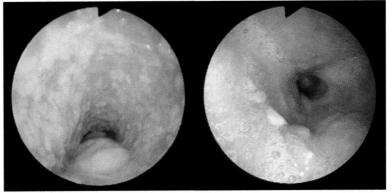

Figure 4.6 Achalasia. *Left,* The esophageal lumen is wide, and food residue from long-standing obstruction can be noted. *Right,* An aperistaltic esophagus with food stagnation.

may appear eccentric, especially distally, and retained food debris may be noted (Fig. 4.4).

Better methods of evaluating esophageal motor function include fluoroscopic studies and manometry. Using fluoroscopy, a radiologist can watch a column of barium pass through the hypopharynx, cricopharyngeus, and into the esophagus. This process can be filmed and later reviewed. The radiologist can then determine whether hypopharyngeal coordination is normal, whether pulmonary aspiration occurs, and whether normal peristalsis is present. Tertiary contractions can be diagnosed, and the function of the LES can be evaluated. A tertiary contraction observed by fluoroscopy and associated with chest pain supports the diagnosis of esophageal spasm.

Manometry is the other commonly used diagnostic method for motility problems. An esophageal catheter with single or multiple pressure transducers is used. Peristalsis can be recorded, the height and duration of the wave determined, the relationship of the peristaltic wave to a swallow studied, and the progression of the contraction down the esophagus evaluated. The LES can be studied with regard to baseline pressure, whether it relaxes normally with swallowing, etc. These probes can be combined with pH-sensitive transducers to simultaneously determine whether reflux is present and whether it triggers the esophageal contractions and symptoms. Technology is available to permit 24-hour pH and pressure monitoring.

ACHALASIA

Achalasia is a disease in which a usually hypertensive LES fails to relax adequately with swallowing. The smooth muscle portion of the esophagus is aperistaltic. Contractions may occur but not in an orderly manner. The esophagus eventually dilates because of the combination of poor propulsion and the hypertensive LES.

The cause of achalasia is not known. However, in most cases the number of Auerbach's ganglia in the body of the esophagus is reduced, with inflammatory cells surrounding the remaining cells. In the LES area there may be normal or reduced numbers of ganglia.

A column of fluid may be present in the dilated esophagus, which is seen on routine chest X-ray as an air-fluid level in the esophagus. A barium esophagram is performed next and suggests the diagnosis of achalasia. Barium empties slowly only after a tall column of barium forms. The barium column has a "beaklike" appearance at the LES. The diagnosis of achalasia is supported by esophageal manometry. Aperistalsis of the smooth muscle portion of the esophagus is seen; the LES has an elevated resting pressure and doesn't relax with swallowing. In most cases the diagnosis is confirmed by endoscopy which rules out a neoplasm as a cause of the patient's symptoms.

Symptomatic relief is obtained by reducing LES pressure. This is accomplished using balloon-dilation catheters. If this technique fails, surgical myotomy may be necessary. Early treatment halts the progression of the symptoms.

ENDOSCOPIC EXAMINATION

Endoscopy is of value in achalasia, both for diagnosis and for evaluation of the complications of the disease. Carcinoma infiltrating the area of the LES may produce symptoms, radiographic findings, and manometry similar to achalasia. Endoscopy is essential to exclude this possibility. Some endoscopists perform endoscopy on any patient who presents with achalasia, but all would endoscope a patient over age 40 whose symptoms are atypical, of rapid onset or progression, or who presents with achalasia-like symptoms since such a patient has an increased chance of cancer.

In achalasia, retained food and liquids in the dilated esophagus may increase the risk of aspiration of esophageal contents during endoscopy. Therefore, in patients with known or suspected achalasia, we routinely empty the esophagus with a large-caliber lavage tube prior to the exam. This also improves the quality of the endoscopic examination.

Endoscopically, the esophagus is dilated and aperistaltic, and the mucosa may have a white appearance (Fig. 4.5). Stasis of food is often noted (Fig. 4.6). The LES appears

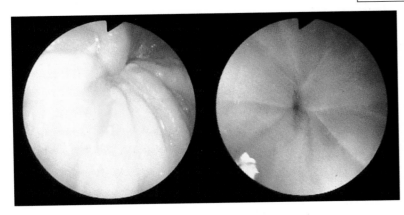
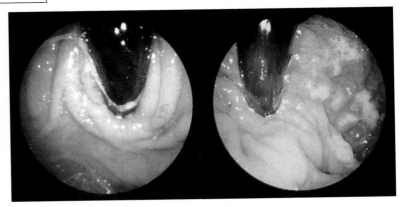

Figure 4.7 Achalasia. *Left,* The LES is closed and remains closed until the tip of the endoscope is ad-vanced against it and into the stom-ach. *Right,* Another example of a tight LES.

Figure 4.8 Two views of the cardia in patients with achalasia *(left)* and vigorous achalasia *(right),* seen with the endoscope retroflexed. In both cases the cardia appears snug around the endoscope.

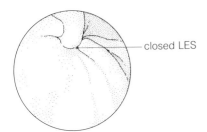

closed LES

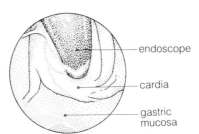

endoscope

cardia

gastric mucosa

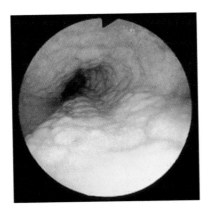
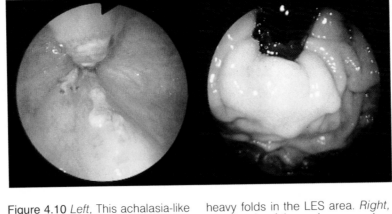
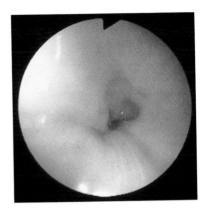

Figure 4.9 A wide lumen and hy-perplastic mucosa are evident in this case of achalasia.

Figure 4.10 *Left,* This achalasia-like appearance was caused by pul-monary cancer surrounding the dis-tal esophagus. The small, white ul-cer-like lesions are the result of previous biopsy several days earlier. There is the suspicion of a mass or heavy folds in the LES area. *Right,* With the tip of the endoscope retro-flexed, a snug mass is seen sur-rounding the endoscope. The mu-cosa over the mass is pale and slightly discolored.

Figure 4.11 Vigorous achalasia. A high-pressure wave contraction is seen as a simultaneous spasm.

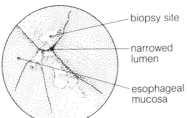

dilated lumen

hyperplastic mucosa

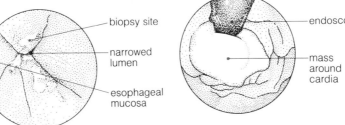

biopsy site

narrowed lumen

esophageal mucosa

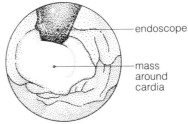

endoscope

mass around cardia

closed (Fig. 4.7), but with gentle pressure on the tip of the endoscope and after a momentary resistance, the endoscope can be passed into the stomach. The mucosa of the LES segment appears normal. The squamocolumnar junction is usually within the level of the LES. The endoscope is then routinely retroflexed to evaluate the cardia of the stomach from below. The cardia appears snug with otherwise nor-mal-appearing gastric mucosa (Fig. 4.8). This maneuver is essential to exclude the possibility of a carcinoma at the gastroesophageal junction. Another mucosal change noted in achalasia is hypertrophy of the esophageal mucosa in re-sponse to the chronic obstruction (Fig. 4.9).

Tumors which can produce an achalasia-like picture in-clude primary gastric carcinoma of the cardia and metastases

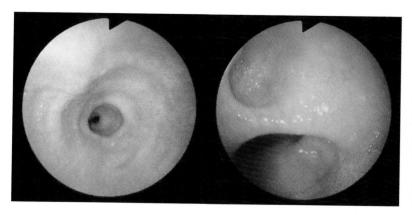

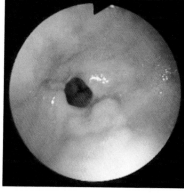

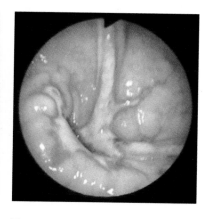

Figure 4.12 *Left,* Pseudodiverticular outpouchings above the closed LES in a patient with achalasia. *Right,* A midesophageal diverticulum in a patient with achalasia.

Figure 4.13 Achalasia treated with pneumatic balloon dilation. Reflux resulted, with erosions and an esophageal stricture.

Figure 4.14 Achalasia treated with a Heller myotomy. Severe reflux resulted, with nonhealing, linear, white-based ulcers.

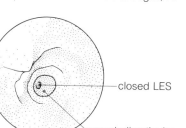

closed LES

pseudodiverticular outpouchings

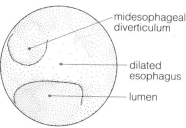

midesophageal diverticulum

dilated esophagus

lumen

erythema

lumen through LES

erosion

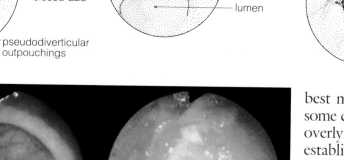

Figure 4.15 Achalasia and a colonic interposition. *Left,* The colonic segment appears normal with haustral folds and normal mucosa. *Right,* The anastomosis of the colon and stomach is narrowed, with evidence of postoperative changes in the form of mucosal deformity and exudates.

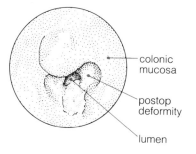

colonic mucosa

postop deformity

lumen

best method for diagnosing this problem (Fig. 4.10). In some cases initial studies may only detect the normal mucosa overlying the tumor, but cytology and biopsy can usually establish the diagnosis.

Some patients with achalasia have high pressure waves in the esophagus which appear as contractions. This is called vigorous achalasia (Fig. 4.11). Small pseudodiverticular outpouchings sometimes occur just above the LES in patients with achalasia (Fig. 4.12). They may complicate treatment of the achalasia with balloon dilation because it may be difficult to position the balloon catheter in the high pressure area.

There is reportedly a slightly increased incidence of squamous-cell carcinoma of the esophagus in achalasia, especially after 10 years of disease. These cancers occur in the distal two-thirds of the esophagus. Cancer may still occur in patients treated adequately with dilation or with surgery to disrupt the hypertensive LES. Therefore, patients with achalasia may benefit from periodic endoscopic screening every few years. Recurrent symptoms of dysphagia, chest pain, or weight loss warrant immediate investigation to exclude another cause such as a stricture or a cancer.

The usual initial therapy for achalasia is to disrupt the hypertensive LES using balloon dilation under fluoroscopic guidance. If balloon dilation fails, a surgical myotomy is often the next treatment. Both of these treatments can result in complications. Chronic gastroesophageal reflux may result from balloon dilation, producing esophagitis with erythema, erosions, linear ulcerations, and strictures (Fig. 4.13). Myotomy can result in incompetence of the LES, producing severe reflux esophagitis and stricture (Fig. 4.14). Other surgical procedures include esophagectomy with an interposed colonic segment (Fig. 4.15).

from another primary center such as lung or breast. If the endoscope will not pass into the stomach, the likelihood of a cancer is increased. This may be a difficult diagnosis because initially the overlying mucosa appears relatively normal. Examination of the gastric cardia from below is the

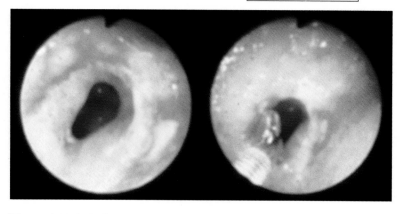 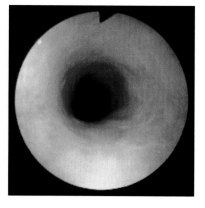

Figure 4.16 *Left,* Scleroderma with evidence of esophageal reflux in the form of erythema and ulceration. A stricture is also present. *Right,* The stricture being biopsied. (Courtesy of Dr. Eric Harder)

Figure 4.17 Scleroderma with an aperistaltic esophagus. The mucosa appears normal.

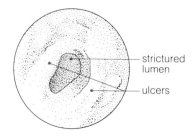

strictured lumen

ulcers

SCLERODERMA

Diseases of connective tissue may affect esophageal function, with the most severe problems seen in scleroderma. In scleroderma, peristalsis is absent or markedly decreased in the lower two-thirds of the esophagus. In addition, the LES has low or absent pressure and fails to function as a sphincter. The combination of aperistalsis and severe reflux of gastric contents into the esophagus severely injures the esophageal mucosa. Fibrosis may occur in the esophageal wall in conjunction with many forms of motor abnormalities. Esophageal dysfunction often progresses even when the cutaneous manifestations of the disease are quiet or regress.

ENDOSCOPIC EXAMINATION

The endoscopic appearance is that of severe reflux with ulceration, erythema, and often tight strictures (Fig. 4.16). The esophagitis may extend into the proximal esophagus. The esophagus may appear aperistaltic (Fig. 4.17), and the LES may appear open without evidence of physiologic narrowing. The main role of endoscopy is in the management of complications. Endoscopy is also indicated to exclude other causes of dysphagia such as concomitant esophageal candidiasis or a carcinoma.

VASCULAR ABNORMALITIES

Several types of esophageal vascular problems are evaluated endoscopically. The most important is esophageal varices. Others include angiodysplastic lesions, phlebectasias, and dysphagia lusoria.

ESOPHAGEAL VARICES

As the result of cirrhosis or other diseases affecting the portal circulation such as thrombosis of the portal vein, increased portal vein pressure causes the portal venous blood to seek collateral pathways to bypass the liver and enter the systemic circulation. Venous collaterals of the anterior abdominal wall, hemorrhoids, and retroperitoneal pathways account for the majority of decompressive flow. However, dilated veins—or varices—in the submucosa of the esophagus also serve as collateral pathways. To reach the systemic circulation, blood flows from the short gastric and coronary veins into the esophageal varices and then to the azygous system. Consequently, varices usually occur in the distal half of the esophagus, but in cases of severe portal hypertension can extend up into the proximal esophagus (Fig. 4.18). There may be associated varices of the cardia and fundus of the stomach.

Esophageal varices cause grave problems clinically. Approximately 10% of patients with upper GI bleeding have bleeding esophageal varices. When these veins bleed there is a substantial risk of death from the bleeding (30 to 40%). There is also a significant risk of rebleeding (approximately 75% over the next 2 years).

Varices may have a characteristic appearance on barium esophagram, but endoscopy is more accurate. Endoscopy is more precise because it can distinguish between folds and vascular structures. In addition, endoscopy allows assessment of gastric varices. Endoscopy can also estimate the risk of rebleeding and enables treatment by injection sclerotherapy.

ENDOSCOPIC EXAMINATION

In most cases the diagnosis of varices can be made endoscopically without difficulty since they have a characteristic

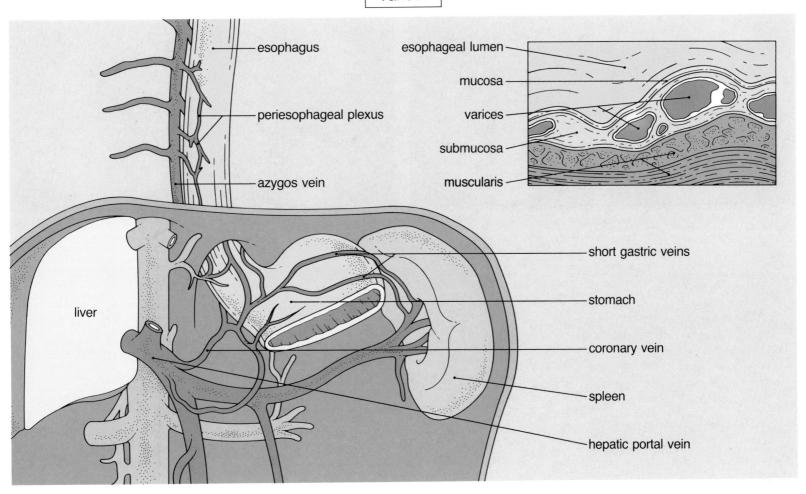

Figure 4.18 Diagram of esophageal varices.

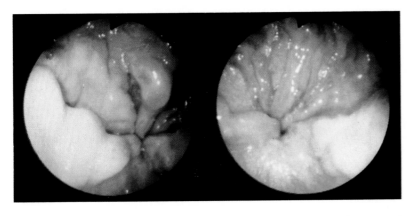

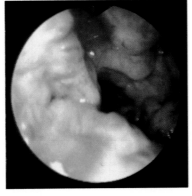

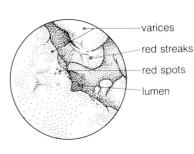

Figure 4.19 Two views of esopha-geal varices. Color variations range from pale covering mucosa to blue. The varices bulge into the lumen and are serpiginous.

Figure 4.20 The red wale sign. Red spots are seen on areas of erythe-ma, and streaks cover the tops of the varices in the background.

endoscopic appearance. The veins appear as irregular, ser-piginous, often bluish structures running longitudinally in the submucosa of the esophageal wall (Fig. 4.19). They are usually most prominent distally. Occasionally it may be dif-ficult to determine if a structure is a fold or a small varix. Clues include the color, tortuosity, and variations with respiration.

Color. Varices are usually blue, although the color in some instances may be white or normal esophageal color, especially if the varices are not bleeding or have been treated.

Neither white nor blue correlates with the risk of bleeding.

In some instances, a portion of the surface of the varix appears red. Termed the red color signs, these findings cor-relate with risk of hemorrhage. There are four subcategories of red signs:

1. The red wale sign: dilated venules appearing like red streaks on the surface of the varix (Fig. 4.20). This has previously been referred to as varices on varices.

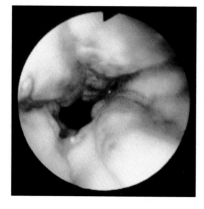

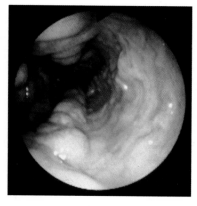

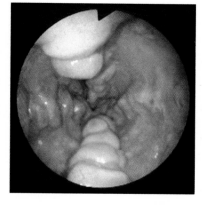

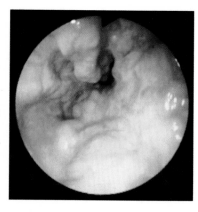

Figure 4.21 Large esophageal varices which presented with an upper GI bleed. The varices are bluish and show evidence of cherry red spots over the surface, suggesting recent active variceal hemorrhage.

Figure 4.22 Large varices with a clear bluish discoloration. Cherry red spots can be noted distally.

Figure 4.23 Varices with positive red signs and, possibly, a hematocystic spot, indicating recent bleeding.

Figure 4.24 Large varices which are relatively straight.

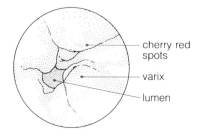

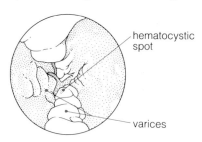

2. Small cherry red dots, less than 2 mm in diameter (Figs. 4.21 and 4.22).
3. A hematocystic spot: a larger, solitary red spot on the varix (Fig. 4.23).
4. A diffuse redness on the area of a varix.

Overall, any red color sign increases the risk of bleeding from 12 to 52%. Of the four signs, diffuse redness and hematocystic spots correlated most highly with the risk of bleeding.

Types of Varices. Varices can be straight (Fig. 4.24), beadlike and markedly large (Fig. 4.25), or nodular and tortuous (Fig. 4.26). Straight varices have only a 7% risk of bleeding whereas the risk with large tortuous varices is as high as 60%. Varices are also graded by extent into the lumen. Grade 1 is less than 1 mm, grade 2 is up to 2 mm, grade 3 is up to 3 mm, and grade 4 is over 3 mm. The largest varices may occupy more than one-third of the lumen and may seem to occlude the lumen; small early varices may simply bulge into the lumen (Fig. 4.27).

Location. The location of the varices is predictive of bleeding risk. Varices are categorized as those above the tracheal bifurcation, those in the middle section, and those in the lower third of the esophagus. Varices which extend proximally have the highest risk of bleeding; the risk with varices in the distal third is lowest. Examining the location of varices is thought to be important because, after injection sclerotherapy, varices first disappear proximally, and this may be a useful marker for successful therapy. Downhill varices may occur in patients with mediastinal disease where esophageal varices bypass a superior vena caval obstruction (Fig. 4.28).

To summarize, the following endoscopic observations of varices connote an increased likelihood of bleeding:

1. Diffuse redness
2. Hematocystic spot
3. Large, tortuous varices
4. Proximal extension
5. Esophagitis

Often, active variceal bleeding can be observed, varying from an ooze to a massive torrential hemorrhage. Active spurting may be seen (Fig. 4.29). Actively bleeding varices are usually in the distal esophagus but may occur in the proximal esophagus, especially in the presence of large varices from high portal pressures. Even if no active bleeding is seen, the presence of the above factors or an adherent clot may indicate that the varices are the likely source of bleeding.

Occasionally it may be difficult to determine if a structure is a varix covered with normal mucosa or an esophageal fold. In this circumstance an endoscopic Doppler probe may be helpful. Another technique is to gradually distend the

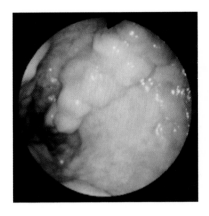

Figure 4.25 A large varix with a beadlike appearance.

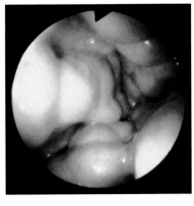

Figure 4.26 Large, nodular, tortuous varices of the esophagus which seem to occlude the lumen.

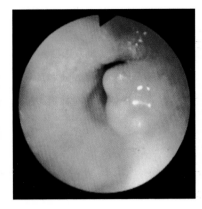

Figure 4.27 A small varix bulging into the lumen.

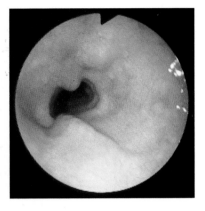

Figure 4.28 Downhill varices in a patient with non-Hodgkin's lymphoma.

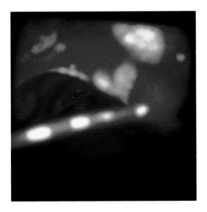

Figure 4.29 An esophageal varix with active, spurting bleeding.

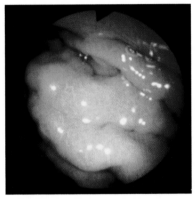

Figure 4.30 Gastric varices in a patient with severe portal hypertension. The covering mucosa is erythema-

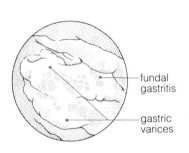

tous from fundal gastritis. Differentiating these varices from gastric folds may be difficult.

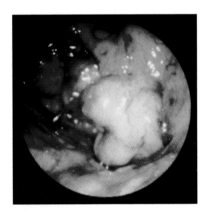

Figure 4.31 Large fundal varices showing evidence of recent bleeding.

esophagus with air while watching endoscopically. A fold tends to flatten and disappear, whereas varices remain visible. Occasionally, as the pressure varies, one may see the varices empty and then refill and distend in a cephalad direction.

Associated gastric varices resemble gastric folds and are more difficult to diagnose (Figs. 4.30 and 4.31). Again, an endoscopic Doppler probe may be helpful for diagnosis.

The entire upper GI tract should be inspected in a patient with upper GI bleeding varices since 30 to 70% of patients with known varices have bleeding from other lesions such as gastritis or ulcers. Diagnosis of the bleeding site is further complicated if blood refluxes from the proximal stomach into the esophagus, leading to a false diagnosis of esophageal bleeding. On occasion this differential diagnosis remains a problem. If the source of bleeding is in doubt but no other lesion is seen other than varices, many feel

that the varices may be assumed to be the source of bleeding. In these circumstances, the presence of endoscopic factors predictive of high bleeding risk such as the red signs are important and increase the likelihood that the source of hemorrhage is the varices.

ENDOSCOPIC SCLEROTHERAPY

All treatments of bleeding esophageal varices have considerable risk, and none have been proved to prolong life. Currently, injection sclerotherapy is the most frequently used therapy for control of the acute hemorrhage. If sclerotherapy fails, most will resort to a decompressive shunt procedure or esophageal transection.

Injection sclerotherapy controls bleeding immediately in about 85 to 90% of patients. Treated patients require fewer blood transfusions and have a reduced incidence of rebleeding. The technique for sclerosing varices is far from stand-

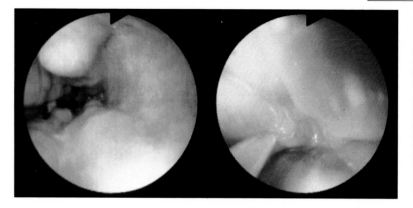

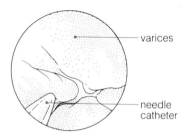

Figure 4.32 *Left,* Large varices of the esophagus. *Right,* An endoscopic injection needle is placed into one of the varices.

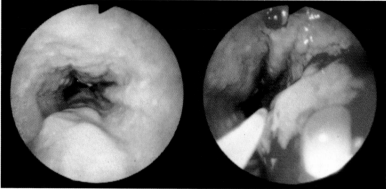

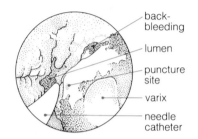

Figure 4.33 *Left,* Large grade 4 esophageal varices. *Right,* After the injection needle is withdrawn from the varix, some back-bleeding occurs. The injected varix is slightly larger than before injection. The puncture site is seen just adjacent to the tip of the needle.

ardized. Rigid and flexible endoscopes are used. Some endoscopists use a balloon at the tip of the endoscope to compress the varix after injection. Some inject into the varix while others inject next to it. There are many variations in the sites injected, the volume of sclerosant injected, types of sclerosing agent used, and the schedule for reinjection. Some use an overtube with a notch to enable a single varix to be isolated and injected.

Once the target varix is selected, an injection catheter is passed down the biopsy channel of the endoscope. A large-caliber endoscope is generally used because the large channel facilitates removal of blood and fluid. The catheter is passed into view and the needle advanced from the tip. The needle is then passed into the wall of esophagus, into or next to the varix (Fig. 4.32). Varices are usually injected initially 1 to 2 cm above the esophagogastric junction. Three injections are made in a ring at this level around the esophagus. In some instances, a second set of injections is made 5 cm more proximally in the esophagus.

After injection of sclerosing agent, the needle is withdrawn. The varix often turns pale or white. There may be some back-bleeding after the needle is removed (Fig. 4.33), which usually stops after several minutes or after reinjection. A volume limit of 15 to 20 ml is usually placed on the amount of sclerosant to be injected.

If bleeding persists, a Sengstaken-Blakemore tube may be required. This tube has a gastric balloon which anchors it in place and an esophageal balloon which, when inflated, compresses the varices and stops the bleeding. Additional lumens are available for suction of the stomach and suction

of the esophagus above the esophageal balloon to remove swallowed saliva and reduce the chance of aspiration. The Sengstaken-Blakemore tube is not always effective and may be associated with complications such as aspiration and laceration of the esophageal wall (Fig. 4.34).

The goal of sclerotherapy is the complete obliteration of the varices. This is accomplished by a series of injections every few days initially and then monthly until the varices have disappeared. After several days, thrombosed varices may appear pale and gradually decrease in diameter as the injections progress. An area of variceal necrosis may be seen. An endoscopic Doppler probe may help in determining whether the varix is thrombosed.

An esophageal ulcer forms at the injection site in more than 30% of patients (Figs. 4.35 to 4.37). The ulcers may be single or multiple, deep or superficial. They are often sharply demarcated and show evidence of recent hemorrhage with a clot at the base. The base may be white with an exudate, or gray with necrotic material. Esophageal ulcers are difficult to treat and are associated with a considerable risk of mortality when they bleed. Esophageal strictures also form after sclerotherapy in approximately 5 to 10% of patients and may require dilation. Esophageal perforation occurs in approximately 1% of patients. Sclerotherapy is usually not effective for controlling bleeding gastric varices.

OTHER THERAPEUTIC PROCEDURES
Surgical treatment of varices includes shunt surgery, esophageal transection, or esophageal resection with a colonic interposition. Shunt surgery should be followed by endo-

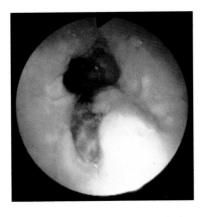 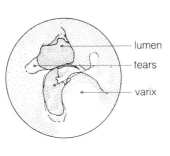

Figure 4.34 Laceration of the esophageal mucosa caused by a Sengstaken-Blakemore tube used to stop bleeding from esophageal varices.

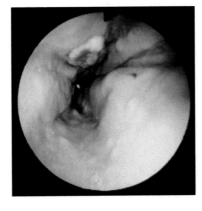 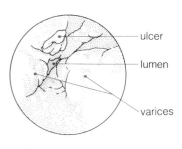

Figure 4.35 An ulcer is seen with overlying necrotic tissue in the distal esophagus 7 days after injection sclerotherapy. In this case varices are still visible.

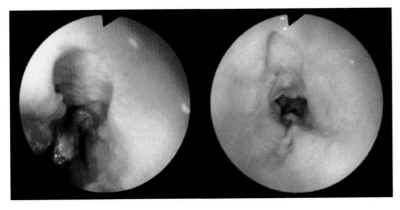

Figure 4.36 *Left,* An acute, deep esophageal ulcer after sclerotherapy. *Right,* Two months later, the ulcer is small but still present. No clear varices are seen.

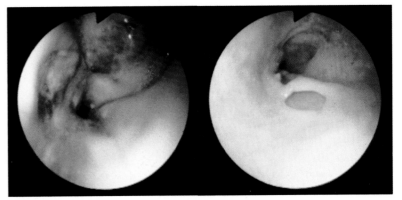

Figure 4.37 *Left,* After sclerotherapy there is a severe inflammatory reaction with mucosal necrosis which led to the ulcerations seen here. *Right,* After healing, an area of mucosal bridging is noted. (Different patients in left and right views.)

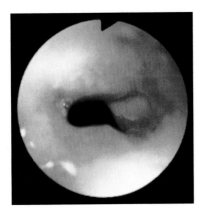 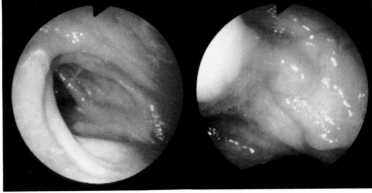 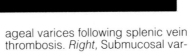

Figure 4.38 A fibrotic ring is seen in the distal esophagus following esophageal transection and insertion of a Boerema button to treat varices.

Figure 4.39 *Left,* Colonic interposition was performed to treat esophageal varices following splenic vein thrombosis. *Right,* Submucosal varices have recurred in the interposed colon.

scopic confirmation that the varices are decompressed. The pressure in the varix may also be estimated using endoscopic methods. Esophageal transection with the placement of a Boerema or Murphy button is a method that disrupts the varices and prevents further bleeding. However, this button may create a visible defect in the esophagus (Fig. 4.38). An interposition of the colon can also be used to interrupt the varices, but because the surgery does not correct the underlying portal hypertension, the varices may recur (Fig. 4.39).

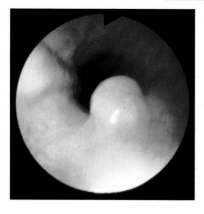

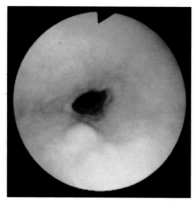

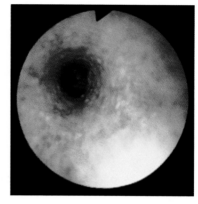

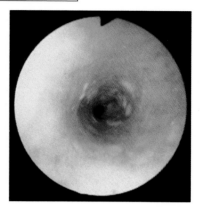

Figure 4.40 This small submucosal bump is vascular in appearance and is presumed to be a small dilated vessel or phlebectasia.

Figure 4.41 This small submucosal lesion in an otherwise normal-appearing distal esophagus was thought to be venous in nature.

Figure 4.42 Acute radiation esophagitis 4 weeks after cessation of radiation therapy. Erythema, punctate hemorrhage, and exudation are evident.

Figure 4.43 Exudative esophagitis 3 weeks after completion of radiation therapy for lung cancer.

OTHER VASCULAR DISORDERS

Angiodysplastic lesions may be noted in the esophagus as part of the spectrum of vascular malformations of the intestine. Phlebectasias are small vascular lesions covered with normal-appearing mucosa which protrude into the esophageal lumen. They appear similar to other submucosal lesions but are small and may have a bluish color suggesting a vascular lesion (Figs. 4.40 and 4.41). Dysphagia lusoria is a condition where an aberrant takeoff of the right subclavian artery crosses behind the esophagus and compresses the esophagus against the trachea, producing dysphagia. Endoscopically, a smooth indentation of the esophageal lumen is seen covered with normal mucosa.

ESOPHAGEAL INJURY

INJURY BY RADIATION

Radiation delivered to neoplasms of the lung or mediastinum may injure the esophageal mucosa at doses as low as 30 Gy. Chemotherapeutic drugs such as Adriamycin potentiate the effect of radiation, causing more severe injury.

ENDOSCOPIC EXAMINATION

Acute radiation injury manifests itself as acute esophagitis. Erythema and exudation are seen in the area maximally exposed to the radiation (Figs. 4.42 and 4.43). Ulceration and necrosis of the tumor may be seen (Figs. 4.44 and 4.45). Later, telangiectasias may be noted in the damaged area (Fig. 4.46). Tight strictures with a peculiar whitish and opalescent color may form and may require dilation to relieve dysphagia (Fig. 4.47). Often the esophagus is dilated proximal to the stricture.

Tracheoesophageal fistula is a serious complication of radiation injury (Figs. 4.48 and 4.49). Lung tissue may be visible at the base of the fistula. When fistulas occur in conjunction with ulceration and stricture, treatment becomes difficult. A guidewire passed endoscopically under fluoroscopic control reduces the chance of esophageal perforation during dilatation and attempts at positioning an endoprosthesis (Fig. 4.50). Strictures and tracheoesophageal fistulas may be caused by recurrent tumor as well as radiation damage. Thoracic computed tomography or endoscopic ultrasonography may be useful to determine whether tumor mass is present in the area of the fistula or stricture.

INJURY BY NOXIOUS AGENTS

Ingestion of substances such as lye or acid may injure the esophagus, causing severe retrosternal pain. The extent of injury may be difficult to judge from examination of the oropharynx or by general examination of the patient. An endoscopist is occasionally called upon to evaluate the extent of injury. In the past, endoscopists were reluctant to endoscope these patients because of the risk of perforating a severely injured gut wall. Now, early endoscopy is recommended using a small-caliber endoscope, often within the first 6 to 12 hours. Endoscopy can determine the extent of injury to the esophagus, stomach, and duodenum, helping to guide management. Endoscopy should not be performed if there is evidence of:

1. Obvious signs of a severe full-thickness esophageal or gastric necrosis with pleural irritation
2. Mediastinal irritation
3. Peritonitis
4. Free air in the abdomen

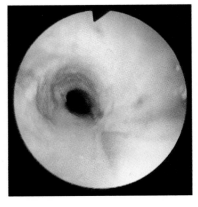
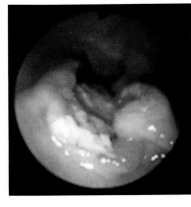
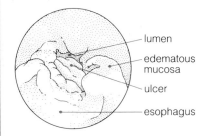

Figure 4.44 Circumferential necrosis 4 weeks after completion of radiation therapy. The entire mucosa is abnormal.

Figure 4.45 Acute radiation esophagitis 3 weeks after radiation therapy. A large deep ulcer is seen in the area of the cardia. The folds surrounding the ulcer are inflamed, red, and swollen.

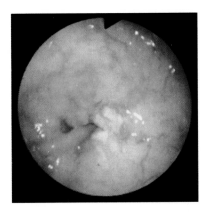
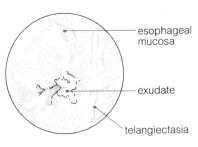
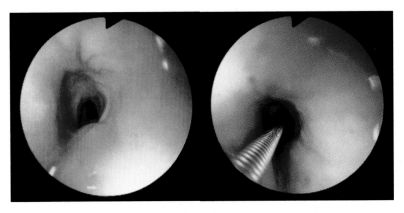

Figure 4.46 Diffuse vascular changes can be noted in the esophageal mucosa following radiation therapy. Telangiectasias and exudates are evident.

Figure 4.47 Left, A stricture appears in the esophagus following radiation therapy. Right, A guidewire is passed endoscopically to assist in dilating the stricture.

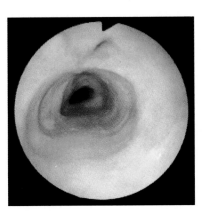
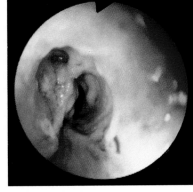
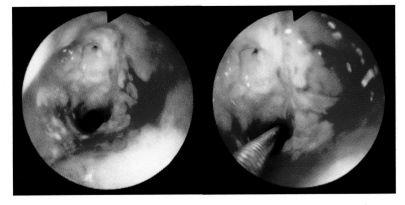

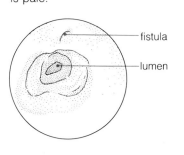
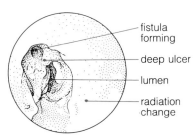
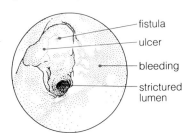

Figure 4.48 After radiation therapy for breast cancer, esophagitis resulted in a tracheoesophageal fistula. The orifice of the fistula is seen here, and the surrounding mucosa is pale.

Figure 4.49 Deep ulceration with an impending tracheoesophageal fistula can be observed in this patient with severe radiation esophagitis.

Figure 4.50 Left, Severe radiation esophagitis, with stricture, ulceration, and early fistula. Right, A guidewire is passed endoscopically through the stricture, reducing the chance of perforation.

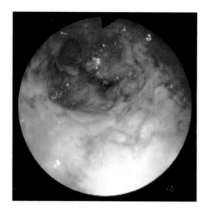

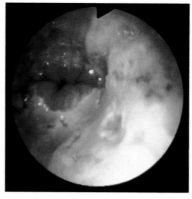

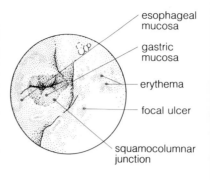

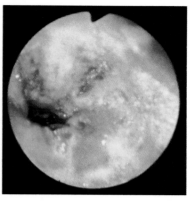

esophageal mucosa

gastric mucosa

erythema

focal ulcer

squamocolumnar junction

Figure 4.51 Stage I–II esophageal injury after caustic ingestion. The patient presented with retrosternal pain and was found to have mild to moderate esophageal damage with erythema.

Figure 4.52 Stage II esophageal injury. Focal ulceration is noted proximal to the esophagogastric junction.

Figure 4.53 Stage III esophageal injury. The mucosa was extensively burned by caustic ingestion and is edematous. The lumen is narrowed.

ENDOSCOPIC EXAMINATION

If exposure is confined to the mouth, the esophagus may appear normal. Stage I injury to the esophagus is mild, with minimal erythema of the mucosa (Fig. 4.51). Stage II is characterized by focal ulceration (Fig. 4.52). In stage III there is extensive necrosis of the mucosa (Fig. 4.53). The more extensive the necrosis, the greater the likelihood of serious sequelae such as stricture formation. Strictures involve the proximal esophagus and may be long and extensive and difficult to dilate. Exposure of the stomach to noxious agents produces an acute gastritis with erythema, exudates, erosions, and ulcerations.

Long-standing strictures produced by lye are thought to be premalignant. Consequently, yearly endoscopy or exfoliative cytology may be beneficial to detect early malignancy. Irregularities of the mucosa should be biopsied and brushed for cytology. Endoscopy should be considered when such patients have a change in symptoms with a worsening of dysphagia.

INJURY BY MEDICINES

Prolonged contact with certain medicines can irritate the esophageal mucosa, causing esophagitis and ulceration. Affected patients often have motility disorders of the esophagus or abnormally narrowed esophageal segments. The problem may occur in normals if medications are ingested with minimal fluid right before lying down. Tetracycline taken chronically for acne is a common offender. These patients often present with severe odynophagia, dysphagia, or chest pain. The injury is often in the proximal esophagus but may be proximal to a physiologic or pathologic narrowing, such as above the impression caused by the left atrium or by an enlarged aorta.

ENDOSCOPIC EXAMINATION

Often, a localized area of irritation is seen associated with exudation and ulceration (Fig. 4.54). In other cases the esophageal mucosa may appear relatively normal, with a cleanly punched-out ulcer or, in some cases, two "kissing" ulcers on opposite sides of the esophageal wall (Fig. 4.55). If the necrosis is severe, the mucosa may slough with bleeding (Fig. 4.56). Subsequently, a stricture may form in the area of the injury (Figs. 4.57 and 4.58). In most of these patients the esophageal mucosa distal to the injury is normal, which helps differentiate this type of injury from reflux injury. In the absence of Barrett's metaplasia, reflux damage is always noted distally, starting just above the squamocolumnar junction.

TRAUMATIC INJURY

Nasogastric tubes, placed postoperatively while the ileus resolves or used therapeutically for conditions such as pancreatitis, are the most common cause of traumatic injury to the esophagus. The tube interferes with swallowing, makes reflux of gastric contents into the distal esophagus more likely, and interferes with the natural acid-clearing mechanism of the distal esophagus. The likelihood of injury increases with time, with the most severe injuries occurring after more than 1 week; however, significant injury may occur after shorter periods of time. Less frequently, endoscopes and Sengstaken-Blakemore tubes used to control bleeding esophageal varices may injure the wall.

Frequent and forceful vomiting may also injure the esophagus. The gastric mucosa may prolapse into the distal esophagus, tearing the esophageal or gastric mucosa. This type of mucosal injury with bleeding is called a Mallory-Weiss tear. A deeper, full-thickness tear is referred to as Boerhave syndrome.

ENDOSCOPIC EXAMINATION

Injury from nasogastric tubes varies from red streaks with rows of submucosal petechiae to severe esophagitis with linear ulcers, erythema, and exudation (Figs. 4.59 to 4.61). If the injury continues, a tight stricture may result. These strictures are often short but may involve more than 10 cm of esophagus. Dilation may be difficult, especially if the

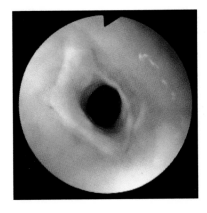

Figure 4.54 Ulceration and stenosis in the proximal esophagus due to pill ingestion.

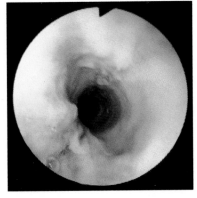

Figure 4.55 "Kissing ulcers" in the proximal esophagus caused by the ingestion of indomethacin.

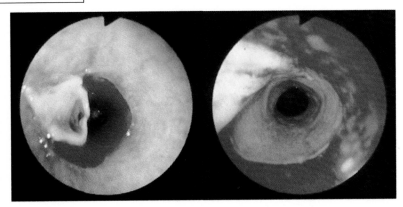

Figure 4.56 *Left,* Severe drug-induced esophageal injury. The narrowed, circumferentially injured esophageal mucosa has pulled away from the wall and is being sloughed. *Right,* A closeup view of the sloughed mucosa reveals raw, bleeding underlying submucosa.

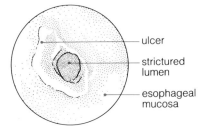

ulcer
strictured lumen
esophageal mucosa

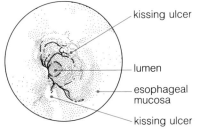

kissing ulcer
lumen
esophageal mucosa
kissing ulcer

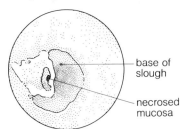

base of slough
necrosed mucosa

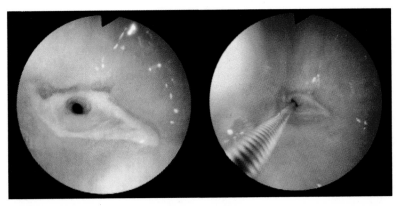

Figure 4.57 *Left,* Proximal esophagitis with a stricture caused by medication ingestion. *Right,* A guidewire is passed endoscopically to facilitate dilation of the stricture.

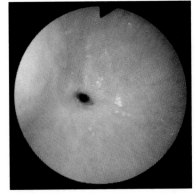

Figure 4.58 This tight esophageal stricture resulted from medication. The mucosa down to the stricture appears normal.

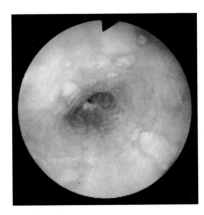

Figure 4.59 Shallow, linear esophageal ulcers caused by prolonged contact with a nasogastric tube.

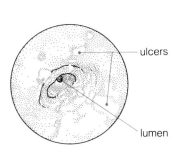

ulcers
lumen

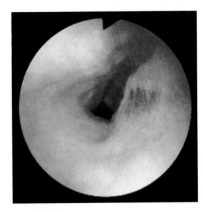

Figure 4.60 Longitudinal erosions and exudates caused by a nasogastric tube.

Figure 4.61 The erythematous patch in the distal esophagus is a submucosal bruise caused by suction from a nasogastric tube.

4.15

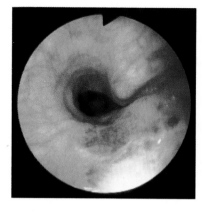

Figure 4.62 Evidence of minimal trauma to the esophagus in the form of scattered petechiae and minimal exudation resulted from endoscopy several days earlier.

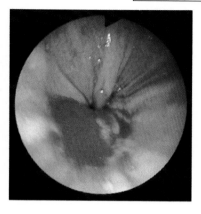

Figure 4.63 An actively bleeding Mallory-Weiss tear just above the esophagogastric junction.

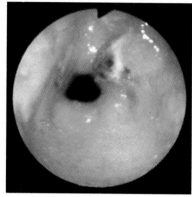

Figure 4.64 A Mallory-Weiss tear on the gastric side of the squamoco-lumnar junction. The bleeding point is seen as a dot on the lesion; no active bleeding is noted.

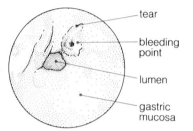

Figure 4.65 A Mallory-Weiss tear in a patient on hemodialysis for renal failure. The patient bled severely. A protruding coagulum is seen at the base of the tear.

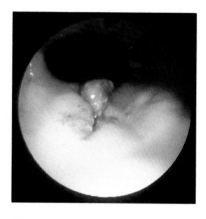

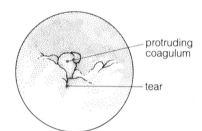

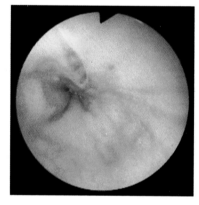

Figure 4.66 Nontransmural laceration of the esophageal mucosa caused by excessive vomiting.

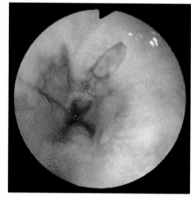

Figure 4.67 Partial Boerhave syndrome with a deep, nontransmural tear of the distal esophageal mucosa caused by vomiting.

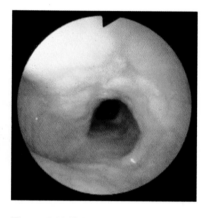

Figure 4.68 This unusual case shows marked hyperkeratotic thickening of the esophageal mucosa which occurred after healing of a massive intramural bleed and subsequent sloughing of the mucosa.

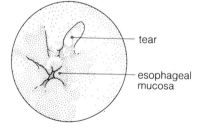

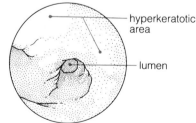

stricture is long. Because of this problem, some physicians favor the placement of percutaneous gastrostomy tubes. Draining the stomach reduces the chance of reflux and obviates the need for a tube through the esophagogastric junction. The tube can be used to feed the patient, sometimes in conjunction with feeding jejunostomy tubes.

Injury from an endoscopic procedure has a characteristic appearance of erythema with a few scattered petechiae in a linear pattern (Fig. 4.62).

Mallory-Weiss tears cause upper GI bleeding, and may occur in the esophagus (Fig. 4.63) or in the stomach (Fig. 4.64). At endoscopy, they may appear to be actively bleeding, show signs

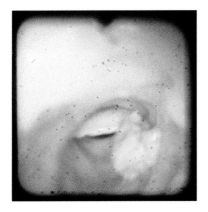

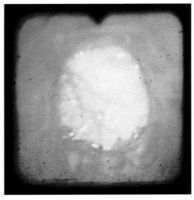

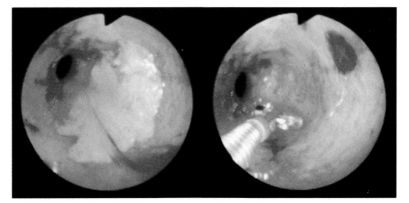

Figure 4.69 A bone is seen implanted in the distal esophagus.

Figure 4.70 A bolus of food is impacted in the distal esophagus just above a web. (Courtesy of Dr. Michael Schuffler)

Figure 4.71 *Left,* A food bezoar above a tight esophageal stricture. *Right,* Biopsy of mucosa at the stricture site. (Courtesy of Dr. Eric Harder)

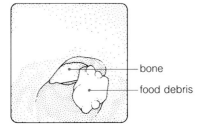

of recent hemorrhage with an adherent clot, or show no evidence of recent bleeding. In some cases a protruding clot may be noted (Fig. 4.65). The tears in the mucosa may be superficial (Fig. 4.66), or deep (Fig. 4.67), although not transmural. Patients with full-thickness tears usually show clinical signs of a perforated esophagus, and endoscopy is contraindicated. Unusual situations may be encountered, as in the patient with massive intramural esophageal bleeding which resulted in an extensive slough of mucosa and a hyperkeratotic response during healing (Fig. 4.68).

FOREIGN BODIES

A variety of foreign objects may become lodged in the esophagus. This may occur proximal to an abnormal narrowing of the esophagus, such as a ring, stricture, or carcinoma. Foreign bodies may also impact in the esophagus of a patient with a motor disorder such as achalasia. The object should be removed, broken up, or dissolved but not pushed down into the stomach. Blindly pushing the object past the obstruction could result in a tear or a perforation.

The exact location of a foreign body can usually be determined by X-ray of the chest and neck. Objects located in the esophagus must be removed to prevent ulceration, perforation, or bleeding. Most objects in the stomach may be observed for several days or weeks if they are not sharp and do not cause symptoms. An exception is miniature batteries which pose a danger because of their chemicals.

ENDOSCOPIC EXAMINATION
Endoscopy in connection with foreign body ingestion is not simple. The technique must be gentle to avoid injuring the esophageal wall, especially if the object is sharp or an edge is embedded in the mucosa (Fig. 4.69). Initially, one may only see the top of the foreign body (Fig. 4.70). Once the foreign object is removed, the cause of the obstruction, such as a stricture, may become apparent (Fig. 4.71). Sometimes the cause of the obstruction may be disrupted while removing the foreign body. In some cases, general anesthesia is required; the endotracheal tube protects the airway from aspiration as the endoscope is removed while grasping the foreign body.

REMOVAL WITH THE FLEXIBLE ENDOSCOPE
Objects lodged in the esophagus can be removed using either a flexible or rigid endoscope. Each has advantages and disadvantages. The flexible endoscope passes more easily, does not require anesthesia, and permits good visualization of the area. An accessory such as a snare can be passed through the endoscope biopsy channel to grasp the object. The object can then be removed as the endoscope is removed. There are several disadvantages to the fiber-endoscopic method. The small biopsy channel may limit the size and ability of the accessory forceps to firmly grasp the object. The object could be dropped in the hypopharynx, causing aspiration. A sharp object can injure the esophageal wall as it is removed. The object may need to be removed in pieces, requiring several passes of the endoscope, which is uncomfortable for the patient.

REMOVAL WITH THE RIGID ENDOSCOPE
The rigid endoscope has a large central lumen through which large-caliber strong grasping forceps can be passed. The foreign body can occasionally be removed via the lumen of the endoscope with the endoscope left in place. Thus the airway is protected and there is no chance of a sharp object injuring

4.17

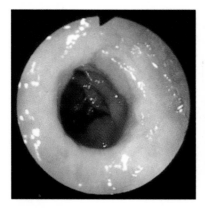

Figure 4.72 Normal esophagojejunal anastomosis after a total gastrectomy for Menetrier's disease.

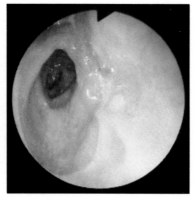

Figure 4.73 Normal esophagojejunal anastomosis. The slightly retracted anastomotic line is a surgical deformity.

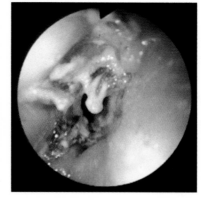

Figure 4.74 Esophagojejunal anastomosis after total gastrectomy. The blue suture is surrounded by a granuloma.

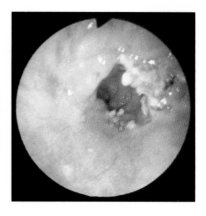

Figure 4.75 Inflammation in the distal esophagus after a distal esophagectomy for leiomyosarcoma. The suture material is clearly visible.

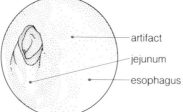

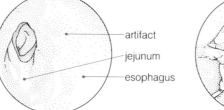

artifact
jejunum
esophagus

suture
inflammation
esophageal mucosa
suture

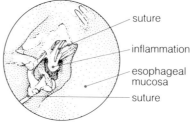

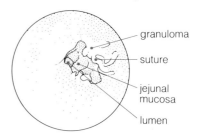

granuloma
suture
jejunal mucosa
lumen

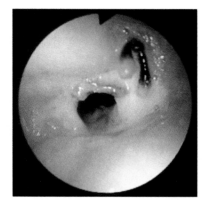

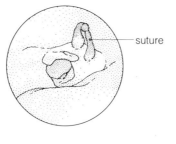

suture

Figure 4.76 A suture is seen with surrounding ulceration at the anas-tomotic site after esophagogastrectomy.

object is grasped by the endoscopic forceps or snare, both the endoscope and foreign body can be removed through the lumen of the overtube. The overtube protects the mucosa of the esophagus against injury, protects the airway, and allows the endoscope to be rapidly placed back into the esophagus with no additional discomfort to the patient.

A variety of forceps have been developed to enable the endoscopist to grasp and hold the foreign body. Snares and baskets can also be used. Firm grip and extreme attention to detail are essential to prevent dropping the object in the hypopharynx and causing aspiration. It is often useful to practice with a similar foreign body to be certain the object can be grasped firmly with the device.

the esophagus. Repeated extraction of fragments of the foreign body can be done without having to reinsert the endoscope. A disadvantage is that general anesthesia is required.

Use of the rigid endoscope is especially helpful for foreign bodies impacted in the proximal or cervical esophagus because the endoscopist can see the esophageal lumen as the endoscope is passed. With flexible endoscopes, initial passage is often blind and the proximal esophagus is not well seen. If a flexible endoscope is used, the endoscopist should use constant inspection to minimize the risk of blind intubation and to avoid pushing into the foreign body and injuring the esophageal wall.

USE OF AN OVERTUBE

Use of an overtube over a flexible endoscope combines the advantages of rigid endoscopes with the convenience of the flexible type. Once the tip of the endoscope is in the esophagus, the overtube is passed over it. Then, when the foreign

POSTOPERATIVE APPEARANCES

Another source of abnormal findings in the esophagus is postoperative states. If the distal esophagus has been removed and a segment of jejunum or colon positioned, it may be possible for the endoscopist to inspect the interposed segment and the anastomosis. This area may appear normal (Figs. 4.72 and 4.73), or granulomas from the sutures may be noted (Fig. 4.74). The sutures themselves can sometimes be seen (Figs. 4.75 and 4.76). If a segment of colon is interposed, one can usually enter this segment, visualize the normal colonic appearance and, in most cases, enter the stomach through the anastomosis of the colon and stomach. If the colonic segment is placed anteriorly, subcutaneously, or retrosternally, the anastomosis between the proximal esophagus and the colon may be at an acute angle. Intubation of this colonic segment may be difficult or impossible because of the angulation and patient discomfort.

5

Stomach I: Gastric Ulcers, Anatomic and Vascular Abnormalities, and Postoperative Evaluation

Gastric ulcers are a frequently encountered problem in clinical medicine in general and in gastroenterology in particular. In this first of three stomach chapters we will describe the appearance of the benign gastric ulcer, the correct endoscopic diagnostic approach to this lesion, and the method of distinguishing a benign gastric ulcer from a neoplasm of the stomach. Later in this chapter we will consider anatomic changes of the stomach, including diverticula, ectopic pancreas, prolapse, and tears, as well as vascular abnormalities, foreign bodies, and the postoperative stomach.

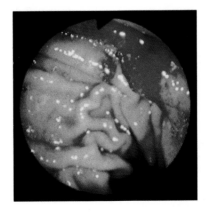

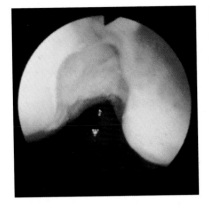

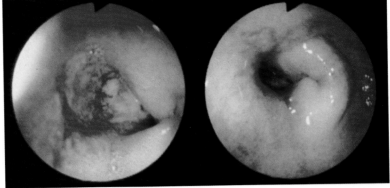

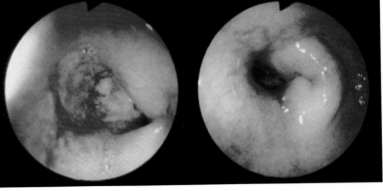

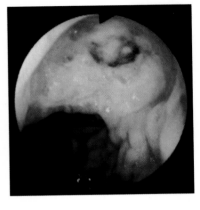

Figure 5.1 Typical benign gastric ulcer at the incisura angularis. Note the characteristic clean white base.

Figure 5.2 *Left,* Prepyloric ulcer with marked erythematous swelling of the margins. *Right,* In this view one can

better appreciate the deformed and narrowed pyloric channel.

Figure 5.3 Large gastric ulcer at the incisura angularis. The black spots are due to a thrombosed dilated artery caused by a pseudoaneurysm.

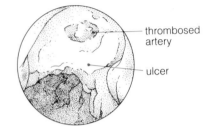

GASTRIC ULCERS

Gastric ulcers are sharply delineated defects in the mucosal lining that penetrate the mucosa and muscularis mucosae into the submucosa and even into the muscularis propria. Most benign gastric ulcers are found in the distal body of the stomach or close to the gastric angle—the incisura angularis (Fig. 5.1). Benign gastric ulcers may also be found elsewhere in the stomach, including along the greater curvature, in the proximal body of the stomach along the lesser curvature, and in the antrum. Ulcers may occur in the prepyloric antrum at the border between the duodenal and antral mucosa (Fig. 5.2). The location of this interface may vary somewhat because duodenal mucosa may extend in a cephalad direction for some distance through the pyloric channel into the distal antrum.

In elderly patients, gastric ulcers tend to occur in the upper portion of the body, fundus, or cardia. This is probably because of the gradual upward migration with age of the junction of the parietal cell mucosa and antral mucosa on the lesser curvature of the stomach toward the cardia. The migration of the mucosal junction seems to occur as the process of chronic atrophic gastritis expands and progresses with age. This mucosal interface, in combination with the atrophic gastritis, provides a focus for gastric ulceration.

Gastric ulcers are usually single. Multiple ulcers are most often the consequence of ulcerogenic drugs such as aspirin or other nonsteroidal anti-inflammatory agents. Occasionally, ulcers are located symmetrically on opposite walls of the stomach ("kissing" ulcers). Most ulcers are 3 cm or less in diameter, with half less than 1 cm. Occasionally a giant gastric ulcer is encountered with a diameter greater than 3 cm.

ENDOSCOPIC APPEARANCE OF THE BENIGN GASTRIC ULCER

The location of the ulcer and the endoscopic appearance of the base and the margins are important clues as to whether a gastric ulcer is benign or malignant.

LOCATION

Benign gastric ulcers are divided into three major types by location. Type 1 ulcers are located at the angularis or above. This is the most common site, corresponding to the border of the antral mucosa and the acid-secreting, parietal-type mucosa. Type 2 ulcers are in the same location, but there is evidence of a duodenal ulcer or a duodenal ulcer scar. Type 3 ulcers are in the prepyloric region, usually within 2.5 cm of the pylorus. The endoscopist should give a detailed description of the features of the base, the margins, and the surrounding folds of any gastric ulcer.

ULCER BASE

The most prominent feature of an ulcer is its white base (see Fig. 5.1). The fibrinous granulation tissue covering the crater has a white or grayish-white appearance. In addition, the base may be stained with blood or hematin. During the acute phase of ulcer formation, the base is typically round or oval and regular, with a smooth, punched-out appearance. Occasionally, a vessel may be visible in the ulcer base (Fig. 5.3). Presence of a visible vessel in a patient bleeding from the upper GI tract suggests an increased risk of rebleeding from the ulcer. For this reason some recommend treatment with endoscopic hemostatic therapy to prevent rebleeding. If the ulcer is exceptionally large, as in drug-induced lesions, the base may

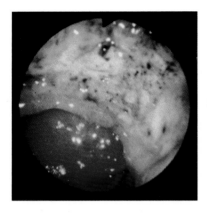

Figure 5.4 This giant gastric ulcer was drug-induced (indomethacin) and involves two-thirds of the stomach circumference. Note the irregular ulcer base.

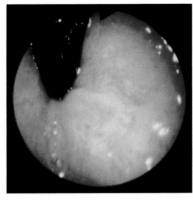

Figure 5.5 Drug-induced ulceration in the cardia viewed with the endoscope retroflexed.

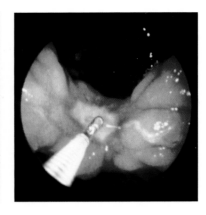

Figure 5.6 Measurement of a gastric ulcer using an open biopsy forceps.

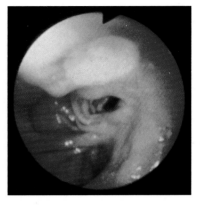

Figure 5.7 Benign gastric ulcer with a smooth, nondistorted margin.

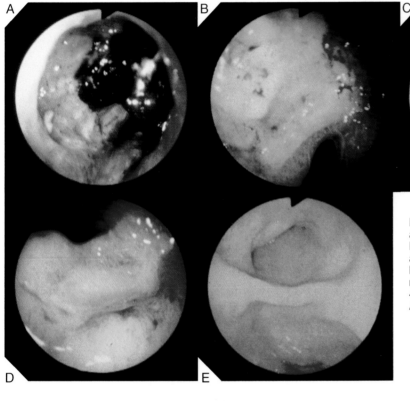

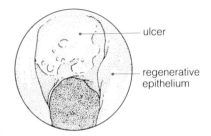

Figure 5.8 Stages of ulcer formation and resolution. **A** A large, benign, NSAID-induced gastric ulcer with adherent clot. **B** One week later, the base is clean. Note erythema at the margin, indicative of healing. **C** After 4 weeks, the ulcer crater is smaller. At the edge, regenerative epithelium spreads over the base. **D** After 8 weeks, we see further regression of the ulcer crater. Erythema remains at the margin. **E** At 12 weeks, healing is complete. Note the severe deformity due to scarring and retraction.

appear irregular due to vascular structures or to nongastric tissue if perforation has occurred (Figs. 5.4 and 5.5). The endoscopist should attempt to estimate the size of the ulcer base by comparing the length and width of the ulcer with the 6- to 9-mm premeasured distance between the cups of an open biopsy forceps (Fig. 5.6).

ULCER MARGIN

A benign gastric ulcer has smooth margins, usually slightly raised in relation to the ulcer base (Fig. 5.7). In early stages the margin is regular without conspicuous erythema. Scarring from previous ulcerations may give the margin a distorted appearance. The folds surrounding a benign gastric ulcer should be inspected to determine if there is tissue separating the folds from the ulcer base. In most cases the folds can be followed right up to the ulcer base. In some cases, however, it may be difficult to appreciate convergence of folds because the ulcer can only be viewed tangentially. In this instance, by placing a forward-viewing endoscope in a retroflexed position, the ulcer margins can be best seen in relation to any surrounding folds. This distinction is more difficult with large ulcers because the swelling at the margin of the ulcer may obscure the fold pattern.

ULCER HEALING

Three stages have been defined endoscopically in the cycle of ulcer formation and resolution: active (A), healing (H), and scarring (S) (Fig. 5.8). During the active phase (A1),

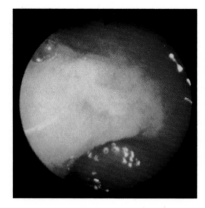

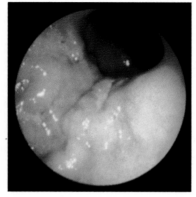

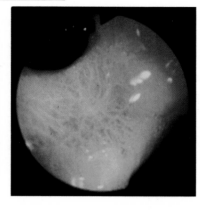

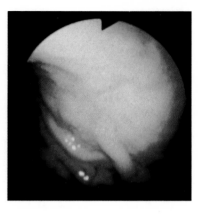

Figure 5.9 Irregular base of a benign antral ulcer during H₂-receptor blockage therapy.

Figure 5.10 Benign gastric ulcer at the greater curvature during the healing stage. The base has become linear, and the heaped-up margin predominates. Note the intact mucosal pattern showing discrete areae gastricae and uniform erythema.

Figure 5.11 The fine red scar represents an almost healed benign ulcer at the incisura angularis.

Figure 5.12 The fine white scar of a subcardial gastric ulcer.

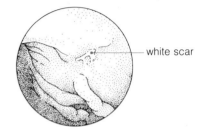

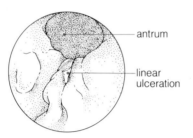

the mucosa surrounding the crater is swollen and edematous, and no regenerating epithelium is seen. Once edema subsides (A2), a small amount of regenerating epithelium becomes visible at the ulcer margin. Converging folds can usually be followed right up to the ulcer margin. A red halo may frequently be seen.

When this erythematous rim surrounding the ulcer base is viewed closely, slightly raised red dots (areae gastricae) are seen interposed between white lines (lineae gastricae). Such inflammatory changes represent the regenerative phase of the healing process.

During healing the ulcer base usually shrinks in a concentric fashion, though occasionally healing occurs linearly. Rarely, the ulcer defect may be divided by a mucosal bridge. In the initial healing stage (H1), the white coating on the base of the ulcer becomes smaller and thinner, and the regenerating epithelium extends into the ulcer base. The ulcer base loses its punched-out appearance, and the base becomes irregular and less well defined (Fig. 5.9). The margin becomes nodular in addition to being erythematous. The gradient between the margin and the ulcer base often flattens even though the ulcer crater is still evident with a relatively sharp margin.

As healing continues (H2), regenerating epithelium cov-ers most of the ulcer floor, the margin predominates, and the white base shrinks, ultimately becoming linear and disappearing altogether (Fig. 5.10). The area of the white coating on the base is approximately one-fourth to one-third of that seen in stage A1. The base fills with granulation tissue.

During the scarring stage (S1), the regenerating epithelium completely covers the floor of the ulcer, replacing the white coating. The regenerating epithelium is initially red due to the presence of many capillaries, hence the term red scar. This area is often characterized by palisade-shaped erythema (Fig. 5.11).

Several months later (S2), the mature epithelium is indistinguishable from the surrounding mucosa, hence the term white-scar or ulcer-scar deformity (Fig. 5.12). The only evidence of a healed ulcer may be gastric folds which converge at the point where the ulcer had been. If the fibrotic process was severe, scarring may produce retraction, a diverticulum-like depression, or an archlike deformity or luminal stenosis (Figs. 5.13 and 5.14). In other instances, mucosa is puckered at the site, or folds radiate outward from the healed ulcer base. Whether gastric ulcers recur may depend on the scarring stage present at the end of medical therapy.

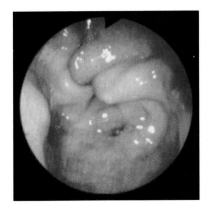

Figure 5.13 Antral deformity due to recurrent ulceration.

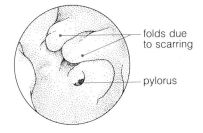

folds due to scarring

pylorus

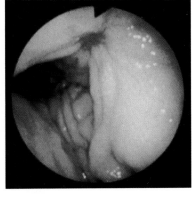

Figure 5.14 Healing ulcer. Note the converging folds running up to the red scar and the archlike deformity.

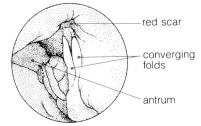

red scar

converging folds

antrum

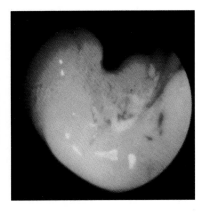

Figure 5.15 Malignant gastric ulcer of the angularis, with irregular ulcer base and irregular erythema of the margins.

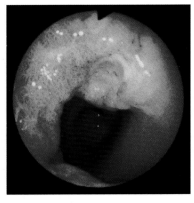

Figure 5.16 This benign-looking gastric ulcer proved to be malignant after multiple biopsies. Note uniform erythema of the surrounding mucosa.

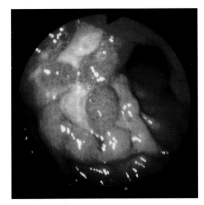

Figure 5.17 Malignant gastric ulcer in the antrum. The nodular heaped-up margins are particularly suggestive of malignancy.

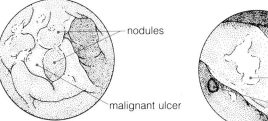

nodules

malignant ulcer

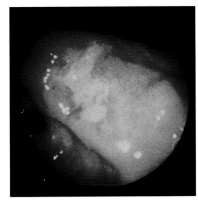

Figure 5.18 This gastric ulcer demonstrates signs of malignancy: a depressed and discolored area, folds that do not merge with the ulcer crater, and irregularity of the crater.

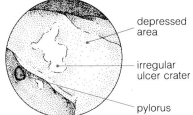

depressed area

irregular ulcer crater

pylorus

ENDOSCOPIC APPEARANCE OF THE MALIGNANT GASTRIC ULCER

In many instances, malignant gastric ulcers can be readily differentiated from benign ones by endoscopic appearance. However, in at least 20% of cases the endoscopist will not be able to confidently designate an ulcer as benign or malignant.

Although the base tends to be irregular in malignant gastric ulcers (Fig. 5.15), there is so much variation as to make this parameter a limited interpretative factor. In early gastric cancer the tumor may be confined to the ulcer margin, leaving the base smooth and regular (Fig. 5.16). Whereas, large benign ulcers may have an irregular and even nodular base.

The appearance of the ulcer margin may be more helpful. This zone, where the normal, smooth, uniform surrounding mucosa meets the ulcer base in a benign ulcer, is a clearly defined interface without nodularity or irregularity. Any pattern other than this normal pattern suggests possible malignancy. Most suggestive of malignancy is the finding of distinct nodules in the ulcer margin (Fig. 5.17) or irregular mucosal coloration without a clear areae and lineae gastricae pattern or lacking a uniform erythematous pattern (Fig. 5.18). The mucosa surrounding a malignant ulcer is often moth-eaten or eroded and the outline irregular.

The surrounding folds of a benign ulcer characteristically terminate at the base or, if the ulcer is very large, merge with the margin. In malignant disease, folds may end a distance from the ulcer base or end with a clubbed or piled-up appearance. An overextended, plateau-like ulcer margin that obliterates the surrounding folds also suggests malignancy. Another finding suggesting malignancy is irregularity of the folds as they approach the ulcer margin. This is caused by depression of the mucosa at the ulcer edge. The mucosa also appears irregular (see Fig. 5.18).

Large ulcers have a somewhat higher likelihood of being malignant. Suggestive findings are a distorted margin and elevated or enlarged edematous folds surrounding the ulcer (see Fig. 5.17). The stages of healing may be atypical.

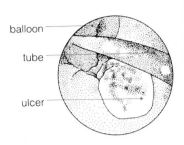
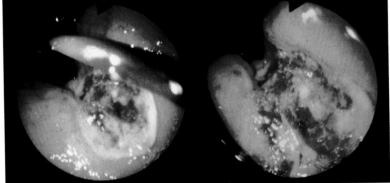

Figure 5.19 *Left*, Large ulceration along the lesser curvature due to pressure necrosis from a gastric balloon inserted for obesity. *Right*, A closeup view.

EXOGENOUS CAUSES OF GASTRIC ULCERS

Mechanical pressure on the gastric mucosa can cause significant gastric ulceration. An example is an ulcer caused by pressure necrosis resulting from an intragastric balloon used as a treatment for obesity (Fig. 5.19). Drugs can also cause gastric ulceration, similar to that noted in the esophagus. These ulcers may occur in the antrum (as is often the case with aspirin) or elsewhere in the stomach, such as the cardia (see Fig. 5.5).

BIOPSY

The early changes of gastric cancer are misdiagnosed as benign disease in approximately 10% of cases. Therefore, many endoscopists feel that multiple biopsies must be obtained from any gastric ulcer. Biopsies should be taken from each quadrant of the lesion, ideally from the inner edge of the margin, and from the ulcer base if it is nodular or abnormal in appearance. Often, only one or two of eight to ten biopsy specimens will reveal a focus of malignancy. Depressed areas at the erythematous margin of an ulcer should be recognized as high-risk areas for a tumor and should be biopsied. Such depressed areas usually appear so red that the differentiation between a neoplasm and regenerating tissue at the margin of a benign peptic ulcer may be difficult.

Healing of a gastric ulcer is no guarantee of its benign nature, because both benign and malignant ulcers may have a healing cycle similar to eachother, and a seemingly healed ulcer may still contain a malignancy. Therefore, several biopsy examinations may be needed, occasionally with biopsies of the ulcer scar, to exclude malignancy.

Provided multiple biopsies are taken, a high accuracy in distinguishing benign from malignant gastric ulcers is probable. Cytologic specimens obtained by brushing or lavage (wash) techniques complement biopsy for diagnosis. Endoscopic brush cytology should be performed before biopsy for maximum diagnostic yield. The salvage cytology technique uses a mucous trap between the endoscope and the suction line. The biopsy channel is aspirated between biopsy specimens and 1 to 5 ml of fluid is collected. The fluid is diluted with alcohol or other suitable fixative and submitted for cytologic examination. This technique salvages malignant cells within the channel that have dropped off the biopsy forceps.

ANATOMIC ABNORMALITIES

GASTRIC DIVERTICULUM

A gastric diverticulum is an outpouching of all of the wall layers. The subcardial region about 2 cm distal from the cardia and 3 cm dorsal to the lesser curvature is most commonly affected (Fig. 5.20). Less common sites are the prepyloric region and, rarely, the fundus or gastric greater curvature. The mouth of the diverticulum is usually round, oval, or slitlike. Radial folds frequently enter the diverticular outpouching. Potential complications are ulceration, hemorrhage, and food impaction, but these are rare.

ECTOPIC PANCREATIC TISSUE

Ectopic masses of pancreatic tissue are usually encountered along the greater curvature of the antrum (Fig. 5.21). Foci of ectopic pancreas generally show characteristic bridging folds (Fig. 5.22). A dimple may be seen on the surface, which represents the opening of the draining ectopic pancreatic tissue.

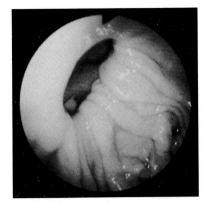

Figure 5.20 Subcardial diverticulum, with folds entering the outpouching.

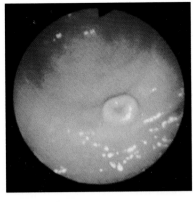

Figure 5.21 Characteristic appearance of ectopic pancreatic tissue. Note the central dimple.

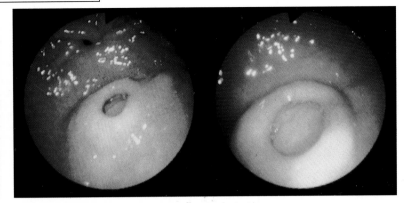

Figure 5.22 *Left,* Ectopic pancreas with bridging folds along the greater curvature. *Right,* A closeup view.

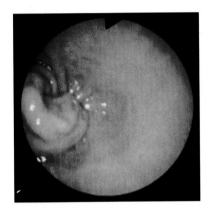

Figure 5.23 Gastroesophageal prolapse. A knuckle of reddened gastric mucosa is visible in the distal esophagus.

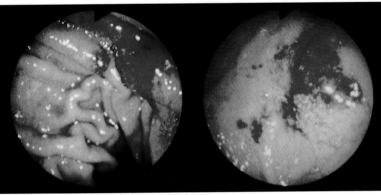
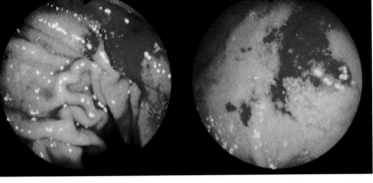

Figure 5.24 *Left,* Damage to the greater curvature area with erythema, intramural petechiae, and hematoma formation due to gastroesophageal prolapse. *Right,* A better view of the hematoma.

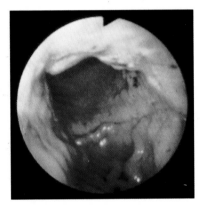

Figure 5.25 Sloughing of the subcardial lesser curvature area after intramural bleeding secondary to prolonged violent retching.

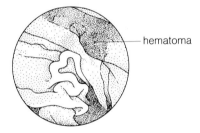

hematoma

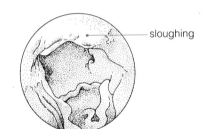

sloughing

GASTROESOPHAGEAL PROLAPSE

Discrete gastroesophageal prolapse may be observed during endoscopy. Violent vomiting or retching during endoscopy may lead to repetitive forceful gastroesophageal prolapse and subsequent traumatization of the gastric mucosa. A major part of the stomach may enter the esophagus, especially when the hiatal ring is patulous. A characteristic endoscopic finding is the presence of a knuckle of inflamed and sometimes bleeding mucosa which repeatedly prolapses into the esophageal lumen during retching (Fig. 5.23) and retracts into the stomach during relaxation. The resulting lesion is usually within 5 cm of the gastroesophageal junction, though not continuous with it. The damaged area is usually a well-defined, relatively small, circular area of inflamed or hemorrhagic mucosa. The edges are usually abrupt, with normal mucosa suddenly changing to erythematous or blotchy, bright red, hyperemic mucosa. The shape and position of the lesion depends on which part of the stomach is forced through the cardiac orifice. Either a ringlike or a disk-type lesion may be produced. As a consequence of prolapse, more extensive intramural bleeding may occur, occasionally leading to sloughing of the underlying mucosa (Figs. 5.24 and 5.25).

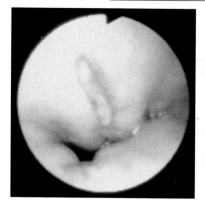

Figure 5.26 Longitudinal necrotic defect due to a Mallory-Weiss tear.

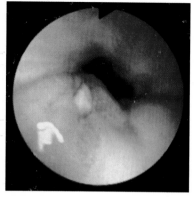

Figure 5.27 Epithelial defect with inflamed edges during the healing stage of a large Mallory-Weiss tear.

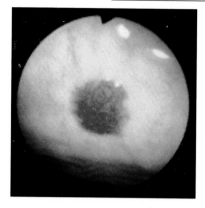

Figure 5.28 An intensely red, slightly raised telangiectatic lesion along the posterior wall of the corpus. Note the starlike contours of the lesion.

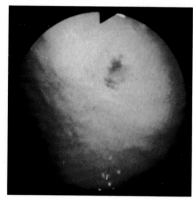

Figure 5.29 A solitary telangiectasia in the proximal stomach. Mild inflammatory changes are visible in the surrounding mucosa.

MALLORY-WEISS TEAR

Mechanical laceration in the area of the gastroesophageal junction, termed a Mallory-Weiss tear, is a common cause of upper GI bleeding. Sudden increase in intra-abdominal pressure during violent retching or vomiting is considered the main cause. Alcoholics or patients on dialysis are most susceptible. The tears are usually linear, longitudinally oriented, and occasionally star-shaped. Tears are usually only a few millimeters wide, but sometimes up to several centimeters long. They often extend into the squamous mucosa, but more commonly involve the columnar cardiac-type mucosa. The tears may be superficial or extend into the submucosa. During the acute phase, oozing or even spurting bleeding may be seen, although most often the lesion is covered with an adherent clot. After sloughing of the clot a superficial necrotic defect remains, covered with a white base (Fig. 5.26). Rapid healing usually occurs (Fig. 5.27).

VASCULAR ABNORMALITIES

GASTRIC TELANGIECTASES

The terminology of vascular lesions in the upper GI tract is confusing. Vascular lesions have been described by many terms such as A-V malformations, angiodysplasia, telangiectasia, hemangioma, telangiopathy, and mucosal vascular abnormalities. While telangiectatic vessels can be seen endoscopically, it is not possible to determine the size or depth of the underlying vascular structures. This may be important when considering endoscopic treatment with a heater probe or laser.

Gastric telangiectases have been associated with von Willebrand's disease, collagen vascular disorders, Turner's syndrome, valvular heart disease, previous radiation therapy, chronic renal failure, and especially the hereditary hemorrhagic telangiectasia syndrome (Osler-Weber-Rendu). The latter disorder is inherited as an autosomal-dominant trait with an incidence of about 5 per 100,000. These patients have telangiectases of mucous membranes, tongue, toes, and fingers. Most bleeding telangiectases in Osler-Weber-Rendu syndrome are located in the cecum, right colon, or the posterior aspect of the gastric corpus. Less commonly involved are the duodenal bulb, the postbulbar duodenum, and the sigmoid colon.

Endoscopically, telangiectases are bright, cherry red, flat or slightly elevated lesions, varying in diameter from pinpoint to 10 mm. They may be single or multiple (Figs. 5.28 to 5.30). Small telangiectatic lesions are limited to the mucosal layer. Larger, slightly elevated, or umbilicated lesions may have extensive submucosal or transmural anastomoses.

The differential diagnosis of small, flat, telangiectatic lesions includes clots or adherent blood, erosion, an endoscopic suction artifact (Fig. 5.31), and, rarely, Kaposi's sarcoma (Fig. 5.32). Petechiae and submucosal hemorrhages related to thrombocytopenia, sepsis, severe coagulopathy, or renal failure are easily distinguished by their appearance and clinical setting. Depressed, angiomatous lesions may be mistaken for ulcers or erosions, particularly if adherent clots are present.

Small, flat, discrete telangiectases measuring less than 5 mm in diameter are the easiest to treat endoscopically, using

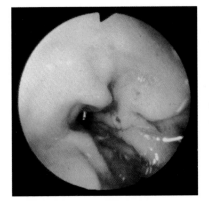

Figure 5.30 Multiple, small, red telangiectasias in a patient with Osler-Weber-Rendu syndrome.

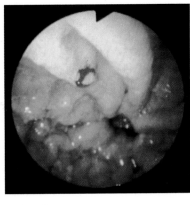

Figure 5.31 Suction artifact in a Billroth II stomach mimics a vascular lesion.

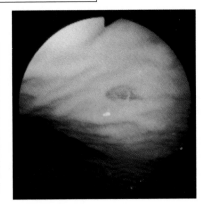

Figure 5.32 This small focus of Kaposi's sarcoma mimics a telangiectatic lesion.

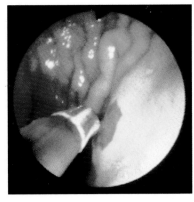

Figure 5.33 Bipolar electrocoagulation probe in close proximity to a telangiectatic lesion.

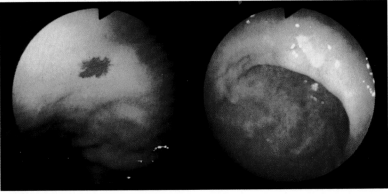

Figure 5.34 *Left,* Gastric angiodysplastic lesion before laser therapy.

Right, A small ulcer remains a few days after laser photocoagulation.

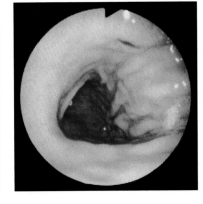

Figure 5.35 Telangiectatic lesion after laser therapy. Inflammatory changes are visible around the slightly hemorrhagic central necrotic spot.

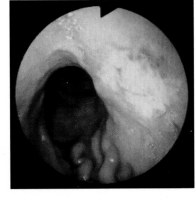

Figure 5.36 Necrotic changes and whitish discoloration 1 day after coagulation of a large hemangioma with a heater probe.

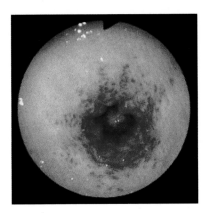

Figure 5.37 Antral telangiectasia. Note the characteristic linear red stripes.

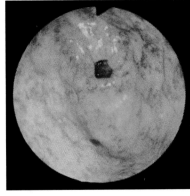

Figure 5.38 Antral telangiectasia, with somewhat convoluted and sacculated columns of vessels.

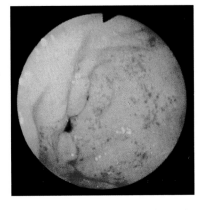

Figure 5.39 Mild antral telangiectasia in a cirrhotic patient. Clusters of red dots simulate petechiae.

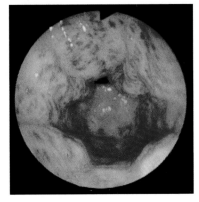

Figure 5.40 Antral telangiectasia, with a peculiar alignment of erythematous dots along ridges of mucosal folds.

electrocoagulation, heater probe, or laser (Figs. 5.33 to 5.36). Larger lesions can also be treated, but they may bleed during therapy. Bleeding can usually be stopped with further endoscopic treatment.

More extensive telangiectatic lesions, especially in the antrum, occur in patients with cirrhosis of the liver. Parallel longitudinal rugal folds are seen traversing the antrum and converging onto the pylorus, each containing a visible convoluted column of vessels. The aggregate appearance resembles the stripes on a watermelon (Figs. 5.37 and 5.38). In addition, round red spots may be observed in the surrounding mucosa (Figs. 5.39 and 5.40). Unlike the ab-

5.9

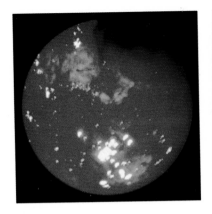

Figure 5.41 Spontaneous or scope-induced bleeding of an antral telangiectasia.

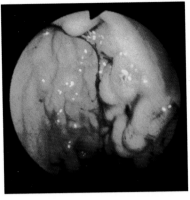

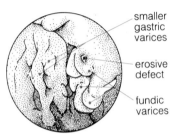

Figure 5.42 A cluster of varices in the gastric fundus, with erythematous spots on top of convex bulges.

smaller gastric varices

erosive defect

fundic varices

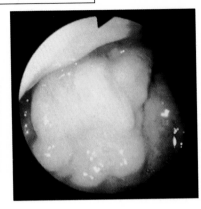

Figure 5.43 A cluster of tortuous fundic varices covered by normal-appearing mucosa, which may be confused with enlarged gastric folds.

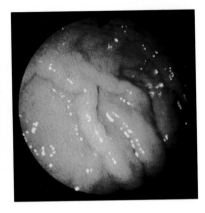

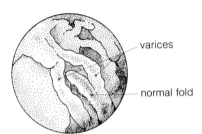

Figure 5.44 Gastric varices mimicking gastric folds. Note the discrete nodularity.

varices

normal fold

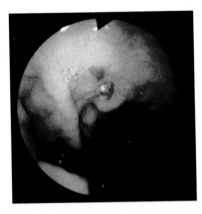

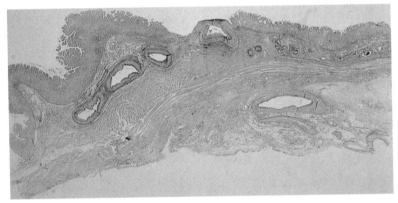

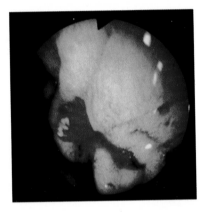

Figure 5.45 *Left,* Dieulafoy lesion covered with an adherent clot. This lesion was responsible for recurrent massive bleeding. *Right,* Corresponding histology of the anomaly.

Figure 5.46 Histologically confirmed vasculitis of the stomach mucosa, with hemorrhagic gastritis and chronic bleeding.

normalities seen in hemorrhagic gastritis, the red, linear streaks in the antrum blanch upon pressure with a biopsy forceps. There is a peculiar tendency for the telangiectatic lesions to cluster along the crest of the longitudinal folds. Spontaneous bleeding as well as bleeding on contact is frequently noted (Fig. 5.41). On careful inspection, some of the red dots have a brownish discoloration suggesting prior bleeding. The mucosa is unusually mobile with a tendency to prolapse into and out of the aborally progressing contraction waves.

Histologically, capillaries are dilated with focal thrombosis and fibromuscular hyperplasia of the lamina propria. The lesion is thought to develop from intramural vascular shunts as a response to portal hypertension. Endoscopic biopsies are inadvisable because such lesions may bleed excessively.

GASTRIC VARICES

Gastric varices are seen as submucosal structures which may have a mottled appearance or even resemble clusters of grapes (Figs. 5.42 to 5.44). The bluish color characteristic of esophageal varices is usually absent in the stomach. Gastric varices may be confused with enlarged folds, except when they run perpendicularly to the axis of the folds. Isolated gastric varices may develop as a consequence of pancreatic disorders that obstruct the splenic vein.

DIEULAFOY LESION

A Dieulafoy lesion is a vascular abnormality usually located along the posterior wall of the corpofundic region. En-

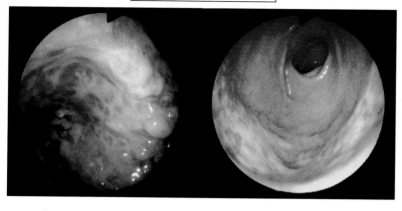

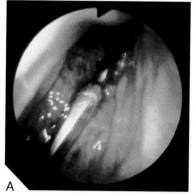 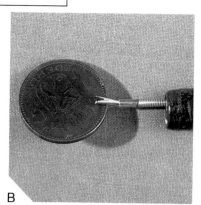

A   B

Figure 5.47 Gastric ischemia. *Left,* Whitish necrotic slough in the proximal stomach. *Right,* In this view we see the sharp transition in the distal stomach between infarcted and noninfarcted mucosa.

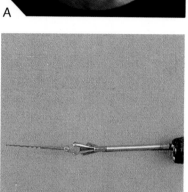 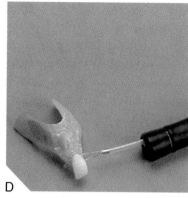

C   D

doscopically, the lesion may not be visible unless there is spurting bleeding or an adherent clot projects from the luminal surface (Fig. 5.45).

VASCULITIS

Vasculitis involving the stomach is rare. The changes are nonspecific and include edema, erythema, and submucosal bleeding spots. The overall appearance resembles hemorrhagic gastritis (Fig. 5.46).

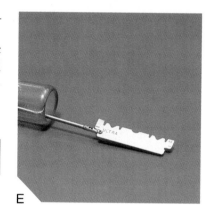

E

Figure 5.48 Foreign bodies in the stomach. **A** A knife. **B** A removed coin. **C** A removed dental drill. **D** A removed dental plate. **E** A removed razor blade. Use of an overtube to safely remove the blade is demonstrated.

OTHER GASTRIC ABNORMALITIES

GASTRIC ISCHEMIA

Rarely, ischemic necrosis of the stomach may occur when the arterial blood supply to the stomach is severely compromised due to obstruction of the celiac trunk and the superior and inferior mesenteric arteries. Ischemic damage is usually characterized by extensive sloughing of the superficial layers of the stomach with sharp transition between the infarcted areas and the normal adjacent mucosa (Fig. 5.47).

FOREIGN BODIES

Foreign bodies such as coins, balls, dental drills, dental plates, blades, and knives may become lodged in the stomach (Fig. 5.48). If the object is sharp, a plastic overtube is recommended to protect the cardia and the esophagus during removal. An overtube also protects against tracheal aspiration as the object is removed. Strong grasping forceps or polypectomy snares are recommended for removal. For objects impacted on both ends against the stomach wall, a lasso may be created around the foreign object using a

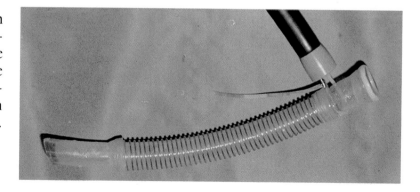

Figure 5.49 This endoprosthesis was removed from the stomach using a double-channel endoscope.

double-channel endoscope. This allows retrieval of the foreign object, provided the object is flexible enough to pass the cardia and upper esophageal sphincter while being held (Fig. 5.49).

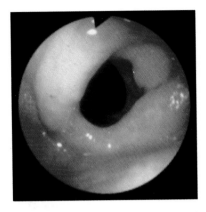

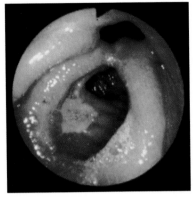

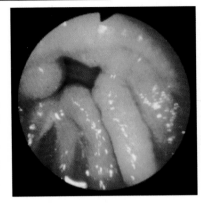

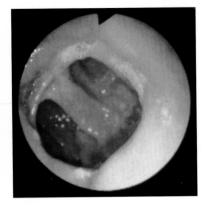

Figure 5.50 Heineke-Mikulicz pyloroplasty, with a gaping pylorus and a concentric second ring.

Figure 5.51 Jaboulay-type pyloroplasty with recurrent ulceration. Note the bridge between the pylorus and the gastroduodenostomy.

Figure 5.52 Billroth I partial gastrectomy produced this anastomosis with a somewhat nodular enlargement of the folds of the stoma. Erythema can also be noted.

Figure 5.53 Billroth II partial gastrectomy produced this anastomosis with a bridging fold separating openings of the afferent and efferent loops.

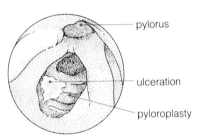

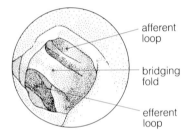

THE POSTOPERATIVE STOMACH

The stomach is a site of various surgical procedures. The endoscopist should be aware of the various features which develop as a consequence of surgical manipulation.

SURGICAL ARTIFACTS

PYLOROPLASTY

After truncal vagotomy, a concomitant pyloroplasty is often carried out. The defect created by a Heineke-Mikulicz procedure is typified by an open pylorus through which another ring may be seen. This type of pyloroplasty can be difficult to examine. The endoscopist must be concerned about the occurrence of an ulcer in the deformed area. Therefore it is important to carefully examine the areas of both rings and the mucosa between the rings (Fig. 5.50). The Jaboulay pyloroplasty is actually an anastomosis between the antrum and the duodenum created adjacent to the stenosed pylorus. When a deep ulcer results in a fistulous tract between the antrum and duodenal bulb, a double pylorus is noted, similar to the defect after a surgical gastroduodenostomy (Fig. 5.51).

PARTIAL GASTRECTOMY

In a Billroth I partial gastrectomy, the rugal folds terminate abruptly and circumferentially around the stoma, occasion-

ally creating a nodular appearance. The mucosa covering these nodules is identical to that surrounding the stoma. The width of the nodules, however, may exceed that of the more proximal rugal folds. Within the stoma, erythematous gastric mucosa joins the grayish-pink flat duodenal mucosa (Fig. 5.52).

In a Billroth II operation, the stoma is usually 15 to 20 cm below the gastroesophageal junction. The transition between the orange-red gastric mucosa and the more yellow-gray jejunal mucosa is easily identified within the stomal opening. Some nodular folding may be observed along the lesser curvature as a result of the surgical procedure. A carina-like structure may be noted just beyond the gastrojejunostomy, on either side of which one may see the efferent and afferent loops (Fig. 5.53). The opening of the efferent loop is generally larger and connects more directly in relation to the gastric lumen than does the afferent loop.

Both loops may be entered and inspected endoscopically. The afferent loop ends proximally at the duodenal bulb closure. The latter can terminate in a characteristic masslike polyp-simulating deformity (Fig. 5.54). The papilla of Vater can often be identified. If retained antral mucosa is suspected, biopsies should be taken of the blind end of this afferent loop. The efferent loop can also be entered and traversed for 30 cm or more. Close apposition of the openings of the afferent and efferent loops at the same level is termed a double-barrel stoma. Both loops communicate di-

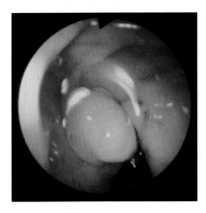

Figure 5.54 Afferent loop with an inverted duodenal bulb suture line, which may simulate a polyp.

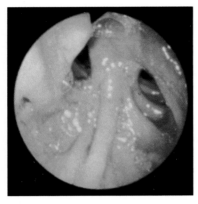

Figure 5.55 Double-barrel stoma. Both loops are seen communicating directly with the gastric remnant.

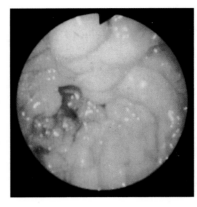

Figure 5.56 This surgical artifact of the lesser curvature area creates the appearance of thick bulging folds covered with normal-appearing mucosa.

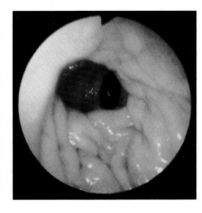

Figure 5.57 Partial gastrectomy with Roux-en-Y anastomosis. Note the normal-appearing remnant and the absence of bile.

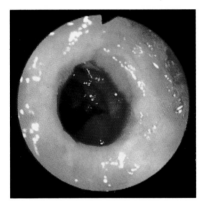

Figure 5.58 Esophagojejunostomy after total gastrectomy. Note the obvious difference in color and fold pattern between the esophagus and the small intestime.

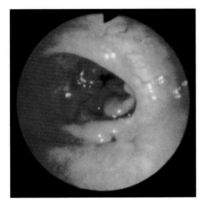

Figure 5.59 Esophagojejunostomy, with development of an endobrachy esophagus due to alkaline biliary reflux.

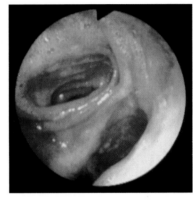

Figure 5.60 Endoscopic view of a Nakayama-type anastomosis with two lumina at the level of the anastomosis of esophagus and small intestine.

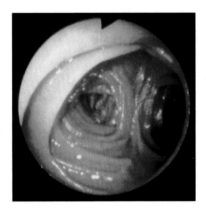

Figure 5.61 Roux-en-Y anastomosis, with duodenal loop entering the jejunum.

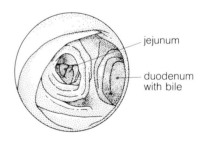

rectly with the gastric remnant (Fig. 5.55). The surgical deformity from a Billroth II may present as abnormal-appearing gastric folds (Fig. 5.56). Presence of only one loop at the stoma suggests a Roux-en-Y anastomosis (Fig. 5.57). If the fluid in the stomach is clear and colorless, this suggests the surgery was a diversion of the Roux-en-Y type which reduces reflux of bile into the stomach.

TOTAL GASTRECTOMY

After total gastrectomy, the esophagus is anastomosed to the small intestine in three ways: end to end, end to side,

or with a Nakayama-type anastomosis (Figs. 5.58 to 5.61). Depending upon the type of anastomosis, bile in the area of the anastomosis may lead to the development of an esophagus with mucosal metaplasia. In the Nakayama-type anastomosis, both limbs create a reservoir pouch that can be entered and examined.

GASTRIC PARTITION

After gastric partition or gastroplasty for obesity, the lower and upper gastric pouches are separated by a lumen that can be passed with a small-caliber endoscope. Occasionally,

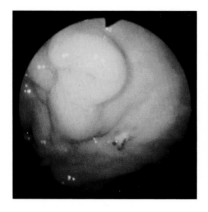
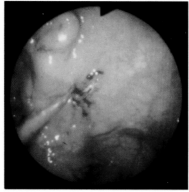
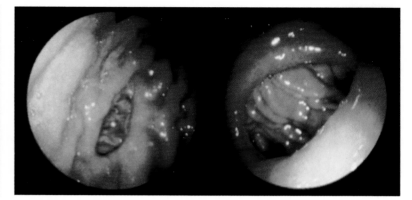

Figure 5.62 Gastric partition, with abnormal folds along the lesser curvature and the narrowed stoma.

Figure 5.63 After gastroplasty, a guidewire is inserted through the narrowed lumen for dilation.

Figure 5.64 *Left,* Gastrojejunostomy. *Right,* A closeup view of the opening.

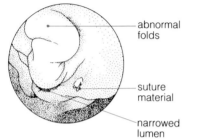

abnormal folds

suture material

narrowed lumen

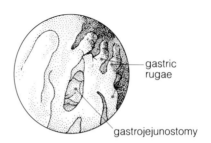

gastric rugae

gastrojejunostomy

this stoma may have to be gently dilated with a dilating bougie, metal olive, or balloon catheter (Figs. 5.62 and 5.63). Care must be taken not to enlarge the stoma much over 1 cm or the purpose of the surgery will be defeated.

GASTROJEJUNOSTOMY

A gastroenterostomy or jejunostomy is recognized endoscopically by the presence of a communication between the stomach and jejunum, usually along the greater curvature of the posterior wall of the distal corpus (Fig. 5.64). The distinction between gastric and small intestinal mucosa is easily recognized. Often, bile mixed with air bubbles refluxes from the small intestine into the stomach. Both the afferent and efferent sides of the anastomosis can usually be entered and examined. Gastrojejunostomy is prone to ulceration in response to copious acid secretion in the stomach.

OTHER SURGICAL PROCEDURES

Rare surgical artifacts in the stomach are the consequence of previous gastrostomy (Fig. 5.65) or prior marsupialization of a pancreatic pseudocyst (Fig. 5.66).

ABNORMALITIES OF THE GASTRIC REMNANT

After partial gastrectomy, several types of abnormalities may be detectable in the gastric remnant. Slight, nonspecific erythema of the stoma is a common finding (Fig. 5.67). Such erythema is made up of innumerable reddish spots, presumably representing the areae gastricae separated by the interconnecting lineae gastricae. Because of the mucosal

capillary ectasia, there often is some degree of mucosal friability as the endoscope passes across the stomal area. Not uncommonly, the stomal area has a somewhat nodular aspect which is usually due to the presence of prominent folds. Nodular deformity may also be due to the presence of polypoid lesions. Such lesions may appear quite erythematous and manifest some superficial erosions (Fig. 5.68).

Protruding sutures may be observed around an area of anastomosis, even years after the previous surgery. Characteristically, retained sutures will present as small suture granulomas. These nodules may appear discolored, and it may be possible to see the actual suture material. Exudation and inflammation may be present (Fig. 5.69). If the inflammation is severe, an ulcer may be found. Suture granulomas are submucosal masses that result from marked inflammation around suture material. They tend to deform the stoma in an asymmetrical fashion and occasionally mimic gastric neoplasm. Sutures rarely cause symptoms and need not be removed. By contrast, suture ulcers may produce symptoms and removal of such sutures may initiate healing. This is done by extracting them with a biopsy forceps or cutting with a suture-cutting forceps (Fig. 5.70).

ALKALINE REFLUX GASTRITIS

Diffuse mucosal erythema and bile staining is common after partial gastrectomy. Termed biliary or alkaline reflux gastritis, this entity produces a burning epigastric pain (mainly postprandially), early satiety after meals, frequent bilious vomiting, nausea, and anorexia. Bile salts and lysolecithin

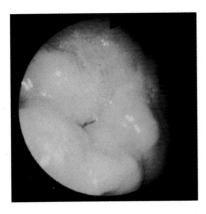

Figure 5.65 An incompletely closed gastrostomy defect created this small fistula.

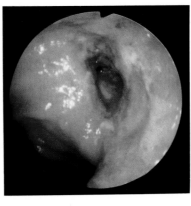

Figure 5.66 A gastric posterior wall defect after marsupialization of a pancreatic pseudocyst.

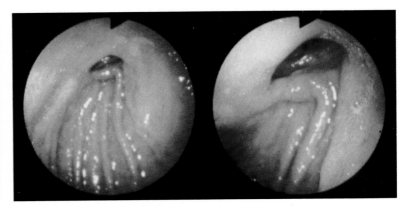

Figure 5.67 *Left,* Billroth II stoma with nonspecific erythema. *Right,* A closeup view of the stoma.

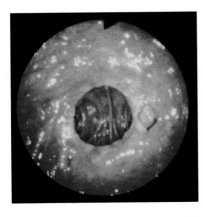

Figure 5.68 Billroth II stoma with small, polypoid excrescence and white discoloration at the anastomotic rim.

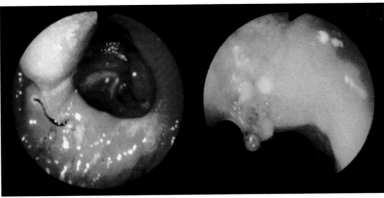
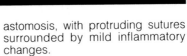

Figure 5.69 Protruding sutures. *Left,* Old Billroth II sutures. Note the stomal erythema. *Right,* Billroth II anastomosis, with protruding sutures surrounded by mild inflammatory changes.

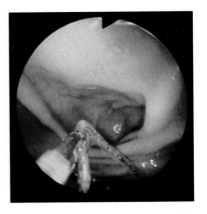

Figure 5.70 A 15-year-old Billroth II anastomosis with persistent suture material being removed with a biopsy forceps because of ongoing ulceration.

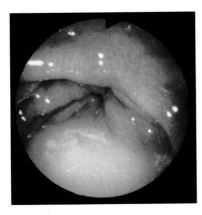

Figure 5.71 Alkaline reflux gastritis, with intense erythema and copious amounts of bile refluxed into the stomach remnant.

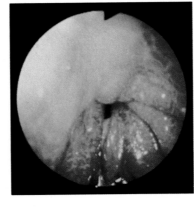

Figure 5.72 Alkaline reflux gastritis, with heavy folds and conspicuous

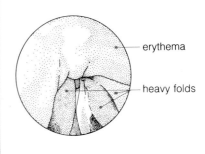

erythematous changes of the mucosa.

are well-known disruptors of the epithelial barrier against acid reflux, causing back-diffusion of acid in the stomach and resulting inflammation.

The characteristic endoscopic appearance is that of severe erythema and swelling of the mucosa stained with refluxed biliary fluid. The intensely red discoloration is usually striking (Fig. 5.71). The folds are markedly swollen (Fig. 5.72), especially in the area of the stoma, and can take on a pseudopolypoid aspect. This erythema may be dramatic in patients with reflux gastritis, and is a clue to the underlying

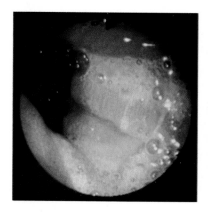

Figure 5.73 Alkaline reflux gastritis, with intense erythema and swollen folds.

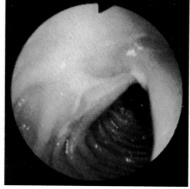

Figure 5.74 Ulcer jejuni pepticum in the efferent loop after a Billroth II partial gastrectomy.

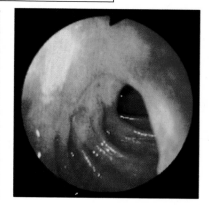

Figure 5.75 Ulceration and erosive changes in the efferent loop.

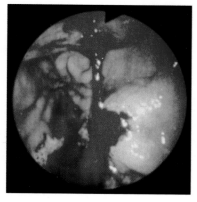

Figure 5.76 Spurt bleeding from an ulcus jejuni pepticum.

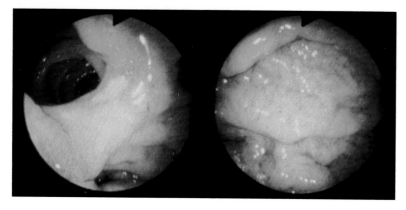

Figure 5.77 *Left,* Ulcer jejuni pepticum located at the barrel between efferent and afferent loops. This ulcer was resistant to H₂-receptor blockade therapy. *Right,* Prominent areae gastricae pattern compatible with acid hypersecretion.

stoma. Mucus on the mucosa may simulate an ulcer; a wash catheter will clarify this issue. Most marginal ulcers occur on the gastric side of the stoma, whereas jejunal ulcers occur opposite the stoma.

A jejunal ulcer is comparable in appearance to a bulbar ulcer, with a fibrinoid, whitish-gray crater and inflamed edges (Figs. 5.74 and 5.75). Occasionally, they may be large. If the ulcer is in the stomach it is considered a gastric ulcer. Bleeding may be a complication (Fig. 5.76). Rarely, a jejunal ulcer may perforate into the colon, creating a gastrojejunal colonic fistula. If the ulcer is entirely within the intestinal mucosa, gastric hypersecretion may be present (Fig. 5.77). Hypergastrinemia must always be excluded with recurrent stomal ulceration.

STOMAL NARROWING

Stomal narrowing or stricturing may be due to surgical technique (peristomal leak or hematoma) or secondary to stomal ulceration. Inability to pass a 10-mm endoscope across the stomal area suggests stenosis, except when the stoma is constructed with an unusual angle. To exclude obstruction confidently, both loops should be inspected for at least 5 cm. The endoscopic appearance is that of a narrowed, fibrotic opening at the stomal area which resists passage of the endoscope. Often there is concomitant evidence of food residue or bezoar formation indicative of gastric stasis (Figs. 5.78 and 5.79).

STOMAL INTUSSUSCEPTION

Stomal intussusception is a rare, serious complication which may involve the efferent or afferent loop, or both. Endoscopically, an erythematous mass made up of jejunal folds is seen projecting through the stoma into the lumen (Fig. 5.80). The mass may prolapse intermittently through the stomal opening into the gastric lumen during episodes of

nature of the patient's illness (Fig. 5.73). There is usually friability, easily noticeable upon endoscopic manipulation. Superficial erosive defects may also be present. Histologically, the erythema usually represents marked capillary dilation. In addition, there may be evidence of nonspecific inflammation with alteration of the epithelial layer and decreased mucus production.

STOMAL ULCER

Stomal ulceration or ulcus jejuni pepticum is common after partial gastrectomy. Erosive or ulcerative defects can best be evaluated endoscopically, although it may require considerable effort to identify ulcerative defects hidden between gastric golds or inside the jejunal edge of the stoma. Stomal ulcers are usually located within 2 cm on either side of the

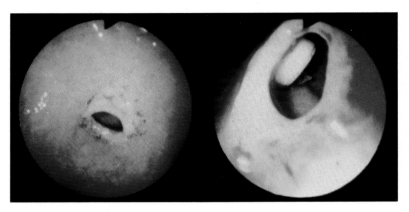

Figure 5.78 *Left,* Billroth I stomach with stomal stricture. *Right,* Retained tablet just beyond the stricture.

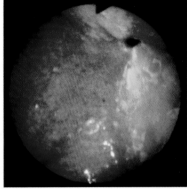

Figure 5.79 Billroth II stomach with stomal stricturing and biliary reflux.

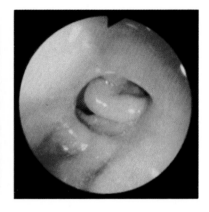

Figure 5.80 Receding intussuscepting folds through a Billroth II stoma.

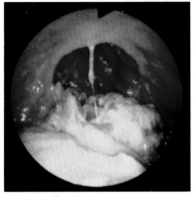

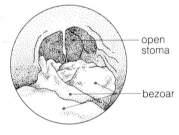

Figure 5.81 Bezoar in a Billroth II stomach. The stoma is wide open.

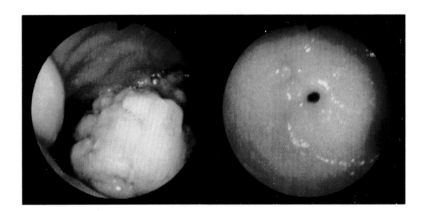

Figure 5.82 *Left,* Bezoar formation due to pyloric stenosis after eso-phageal transection for bleeding varices. *Right,* Pyloric stenosis.

vomiting or retching during endoscopy. Sometimes, only erythematous changes and conspicuous erythema are seen in the upper segment of the efferent or afferent loop, indicating previous intussusception.

BEZOAR FORMATION

A gastric bezoar is a mass of solidified food that persists in the stomach. It is a common complication after surgery for peptic ulcer disease. Bezoars may be a clinical problem in patients who have had a gastrectomy. The cause of the abnormality is not known. Various types of vegetable matter may form a mass which cannot be passed from the stomach (Fig. 5.81). This mass may actually produce obstruction of the gastric outlet. There may be obstruction at the level of the stoma, but usually the stoma is wide open, indicating that bezoar formation is related to dysmotility of the gastric remnant, presumably secondary to damage of the gastric pacemaker area.

Usually a bezoar is loosely constructed and has an irregular appearance. Fragmentation may be attempted endoscopically using a washjet technique. An overtube can be inserted for repeated passage of the endoscope as pieces of the bezoar are removed. The overtube also protects the patient's airway as the objects are removed. Endoscopic removal is followed by a combination of dietary restriction of fiber, instruction in proper mastication, and occasionally the use of an oral preparation of cellulase.

Bezoars may also form in an intact stomach due to motility disturbances or diabetes, and also in postvagotomy pyloric stenosis (Fig. 5.82). In certain geographical areas, persimmon bezoars are the most common form of postoperative phytobezoar. Gastric juice precipitates out the soluble phlobotanin in persimmon, which then acts as a glue binding other substances.

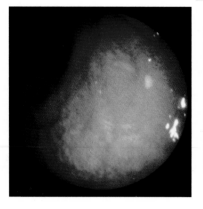

Figure 5.83 Atrophic gastritis in a resected stomach.

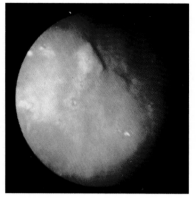

Figure 5.84 Xanthelasma in atrophic Billroth II mucosa.

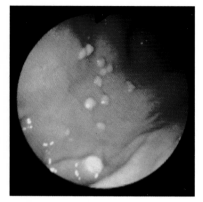

Figure 5.85 Raised xanthoma in an intact stomach.

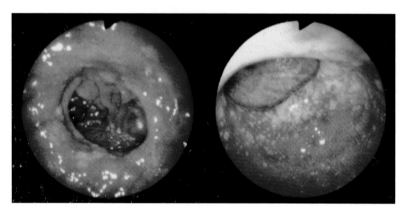

Figure 5.86 *Left,* Whitish discolored areas at the anastomosis due to intestinal metaplasia. *Right,* More extensive intestinal metaplasia.

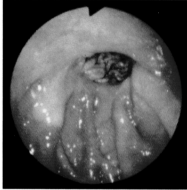

Figure 5.87 Stomal area 20 years after a Billroth II resection shows evidence of severe dysplasia.

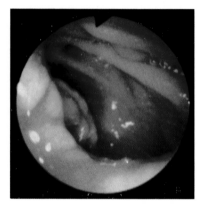

Figure 5.88 Intestinal metaplasia and dysplasia in other areas of stoma.

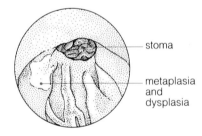

stoma

metaplasia and dysplasia

MUCOSAL ALTERATIONS

Atrophic gastritis and mucosal atrophy are common after partial gastrectomy (Fig. 5.83). Development of xanthelasma or xanthoma is not uncommon in such atrophic mucosa. These xanthelasmas are tiny plaque-like lesions measuring up to a few millimeters in diameter. They are composed of foamy lipid-laden macrophages, may be single or multiple, and are yellow in color (Fig. 5.84). Xanthoma may also develop in the intact stomach in the absence of atrophic gastritis. Such xanthomatous lesions may be flat or raised (Fig. 5.85). Intestinal metaplasia is also common in the resected stomach. This may be seen as tiny, whitish patches usually in the area of the anastomosis (Fig. 5.86).

POSTGASTRECTOMY NEOPLASIA

Patients who have had partial gastrectomies are at a somewhat increased risk of gastric cancer after 10 to 20 years, although this risk varies by geographical region (high in Scandinavia and low in the USA). Before development of invasive cancer, severe dysplasia may be detectable in routine biopsies (Figs. 5.87 and 5.88). Early malignancies are not associated with symptoms and in asymptomatic patients are usually only found upon routine screening. The most common appearance is that of a small polypoid mass or an area of mucosal discoloration or of a minor erosive-ulcerative defect (Fig. 5.89). Such lesions may arise anywhere within the remnant and may be multifocal, but the mucosa with-

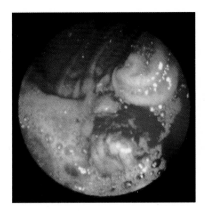 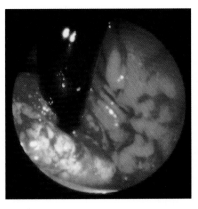 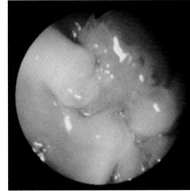 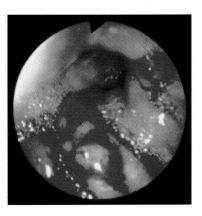

Figure 5.89 A small, polypoid Billroth II stump cancer.

Figure 5.90 Malignancy spreading along the lesser curvature, seen with the endoscope retroflexed.

Figure 5.91 Stump cancer spreading into the distal esophagus.

Figure 5.92 Longstanding Billroth II remnant with alkaline reflux gastritis after biopsy. Note the abundant blood loss.

in 2 cm of the stoma and anastomosis is by far the most common location. The vast majority of the gastric remnant cancers are seen as advanced lesions and look like polypoid masses or infiltrating lesions. Such cancers usually involve the stoma and extend for variable distances into the remnant (Fig. 5.90). Some of these malignancies have a linitis plastica appearance, involving the entire remnant and spreading submucosally above the gastroesophageal junction (Fig. 5.91).

As the prognosis of advanced cancer is dismal, some investigators advocate periodic endoscopic screening of all postgastrectomy patients. When there is evidence of severe dysplasia, more frequent examinations are indicated. Others feel that the risk is too low to justify screening. The decision must be partly based on the incidence of cancer in the specific country. If screening is done, multiple biopsies from all quadrants of the stomal area and of the lesser and greater curve must be obtained because even severe dysplasia may be invisible to the naked eye. Because of the friability and atrophic changes, there is an increased chance of bleeding after multiple biopsies (Fig. 5.92).

6

Stomach II: Tumors and Polyps

In this chapter we will consider the differential diagnosis of gastric lesions including early and advanced adenocarcinoma, less common gastric malignancies, and gastric polyps.

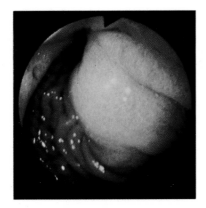

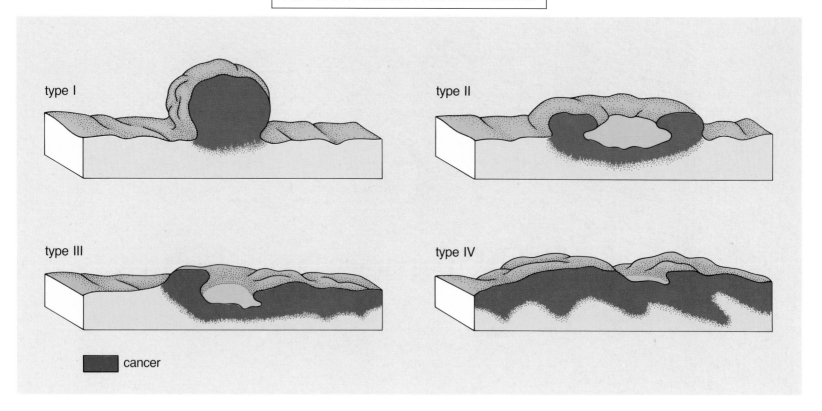

Figure 6.1 Borrmann classification of advanced gastric cancer.

ADENOCARCINOMA

Even though the incidence of gastric carcinoma has decreased over the past several decades, it is still the third most common GI malignancy after colonic and pancreatic cancer. The disease usually occurs in patients over 50 years old. Japan, Chile, Finland, and parts of the USSR and Colombia have especially high incidences of gastric carcinoma. Of the gastric malignant lesions, adenocarcinoma accounts for about 85 to 90%. The cause of gastric adenocarcinoma is not known, but both genetic and environmental factors may be involved. The disease tends to run in some families. There are geographic areas in which the disease is prevalent. People who relocate from these areas reduce their risk by about 25%, and their descendants have a further 25% reduction in risk.

RISK FACTORS

Conditions associated with an increased incidence of gastric cancer include previous gastric surgery, adenomatous gastric polyps, pernicious anemia, and atrophic gastritis with intestinal metaplasia.

The association with gastric surgery was noted several decades ago and reexamined recently. In some countries the incidence of gastric carcinoma 20 years after a Billroth II gastrectomy is as high as 8%. Presence of adenomatous polyps is associated with an increased incidence of cancer of the stomach. The association with atrophic gastritis occurs mainly with gastritis involving the antrum, with focal changes in the rest of the stomach, no parietal cell antibodies, and moderate decrease in acid production.

Survival rates are high if gastric cancer is diagnosed early, with 5-year survival rates of over 90%. In the later stages, 5-year survival is only about 10%. In most countries only 5 to 8% of cases are diagnosed at an early stage, compared to 30% in Japan where endoscopic screening programs are used widely. Screening programs of this type may not be practical in areas where gastric cancer is less prevalent. New diagnostic techniques using tumor markers or endoscopic ultrasound may make screening programs more practical in the future.

SITES OF DISEASE

Although figures vary, approximately 40% of carcinomas occur in the body, 35% in the antrum, 20% in the cardia or fundal area, and 5 to 10% are diffuse. Cardial carcinomas often extend into the distal esophagus, causing dysphagia. A barium esophagram will confirm the diagnosis by show-

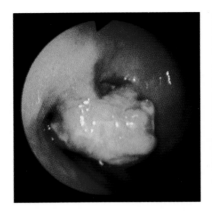

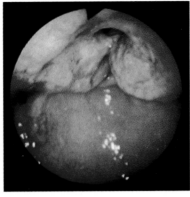

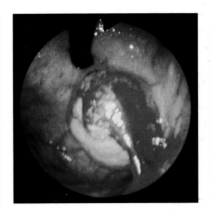

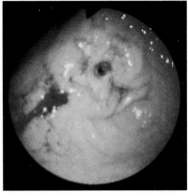

Figure 6.2 Type I adenocarcinoma of body of stomach appears polypoid and pedunculated.

Figure 6.3 Type I adenocarcinoma of the antrum, occluding the gastric outlet.

Figure 6.4 Bleeding polypoid type I adenocarcinoma of the cardia.

Figure 6.5 Type II adenocarcinoma of the distal antrum. A central ulcer is separated from the surrounding mucosa by tumor nodules and infiltrated folds.

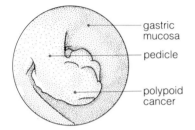

gastric mucosa

pedicle

polypoid cancer

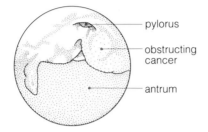

pylorus

obstructing cancer

antrum

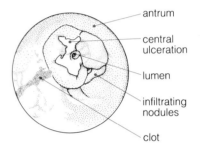

antrum

central ulceration

lumen

infiltrating nodules

clot

ing a narrowed esophagogastric junction. Endoscopy and biopsy are necessary to establish the diagnosis. Occasionally the tumor invades submucosally and can present with an achalasia-like radiographic picture. This may also be found with metastatic lesions to this area.

ADVANCED GASTRIC ADENOCARCINOMA

CLASSIFICATION AND ENDOSCOPIC APPEARANCE
The TNM system is commonly used to classify gastric adenocarcinoma. *T* refers to the extent of tumor invasion (T1 to T4); *N* refers to nodal involvement (N0 to N3); and *M* refers to the presence of metastases (M0 or M1).

The Borrmann method is more applicable to endoscopy. In this classification, advanced gastric cancer is divided into four stages (Fig. 6.1):

Type I: Nonulcerated, exophytic polypoid masses growing into the lumen.

Type II: Circumscribed masses with sharp margins and a central ulceration.

Type III: Less well circumscribed, infiltrating masses, with ulceration. Ulcer margin blends into the surrounding mucosa. The base is infiltrated with cancer.

Type IV: Diffusely infiltrating masses which are mainly submucosal. Local areas of ulceration may occur. Submucosal spread makes endoscopic recognition and histologic verification difficult. Very diffuse tumors, referred to as linitis plastica, characteristically are associated with poor gastric distensibility and little peristalsis.

Type I Carcinoma These represent 3 to 20% of gastric cancers, depending on the series. Of 5-year survivors, 30% have type I carcinomas. The tumors present as polypoid masses without ulceration. They are commonly (60%) located in the gastric body (Fig. 6.2) but also occur in the cardia and antrum (Fig. 6.3). The lesions are well-demarcated from the surrounding mucosa. The surface is irregular and grayish. Since malignant cells are at the surface of the lesion, biopsy is often positive. The mass may be friable and bleed (Fig. 6.4), and may narrow the lumen.

Type II Carcinoma Of gastric carcinomas, 20 to 40% have the configuration of an ulcerated mass. About 60% of 5-year survivors have this type of lesion. The lesion is usually a clear mass, well-demarcated from the surrounding mucosa. Rugal folds terminate at the edge of the mass, separated from the ulcer base by tumor nodules and infiltrated tissue (Fig. 6.5). The base of the ulcerated lesion is necrotic tumor and granulation tissue, often with tumor nodules

6.3

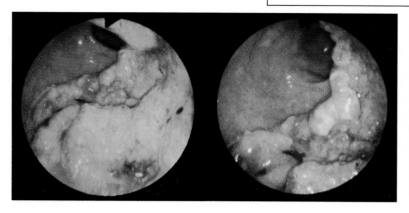

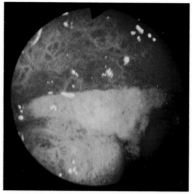

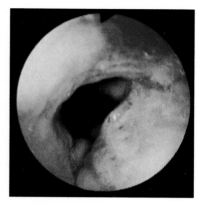

Figure 6.6 *Left,* Type II adenocarcinoma with a large central ulcer. The base of the ulcer is necrotic tumor, granulation tissue, and tumor nodules. *Right,* In this view, tumor nodules can be clearly seen at the distal rim of the ulcer. This would be an appropriate area for biopsy.

Figure 6.7 Erythematous mucosa surrounding the central ulcer of a type II adenocarcinoma.

Figure 6.8 Type III adenocarcinoma. The tumor is diffusely infiltrating with an associated ulcer.

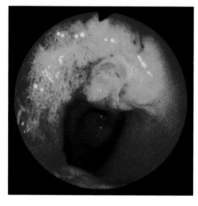

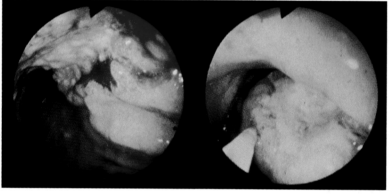

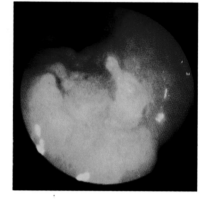

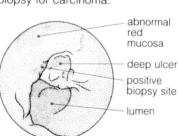

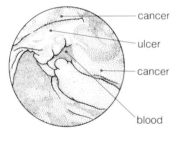

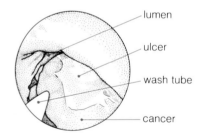

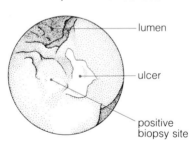

Figure 6.9 This deep ulcer is seen in association with a type III adenocarcinoma. The folds adjacent to the ulcer are indurated and positive on biopsy for carcinoma.

Figure 6.10 Large ulcerations associated with type III gastric cancers. *Left,* The mucosa surrounding the ulcer is infiltrated. *Right,* A wash tube is seen in preparation for obtaining a jet cytology.

Figure 6.11 Although this is a malignant gastric cancer, the surrounding mucosa appears relatively normal. Note, however, that the mucosa to the left of the ulcer is irregular and depressed. Biopsy taken from this area was positive for cancer.

(Fig. 6.6). The tissue over the mass, surrounding the ulcer, is often abnormal with erythema (Fig. 6.7). These lesions are usually easily distinguished from benign gastric ulcers because of the associated mass. Biopsy of the irregular nodular margins or nodules in the base of the ulcer is usually positive for cancer.

Type III Carcinoma This pattern accounts for 10 to 15% of gastric cancers. The lesions may be confused with benign gastric ulcers. Only 10 to 15% of 5-year survivors have type III lesions. There is infiltration of the wall with associated central ulceration. The infiltration of the tumor may appear as heavy folds rather than a clear mass (Figs. 6.8 and 6.9). The central ulceration may be large, often over 3 cm in diameter (Fig. 6.10). Often the ulcer, even if infiltrated, may be surrounded by normal mucosa, making accurate biopsy difficult (Fig. 6.11). Biopsy is most productive if taken at the margin of the ulcer with the surrounding mucosa. Biopsies should also be taken of distorted areas of the base of the ulcer and nodules, or irregular areas at the margin.

Retroflexion of the endoscope may be necessary to view the entire margin of the ulcer to determine whether abnormal mucosa is present, suggesting a gastric cancer (Fig. 6.12). Retroflexion is also frequently necessary to permit biopsy and cytology of the abnormal area. Sometimes the tumor may present as a large, ulcerated, infiltrating lesion with exudation and friability, making iden-

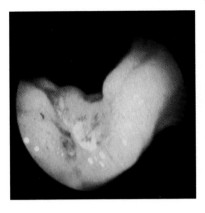

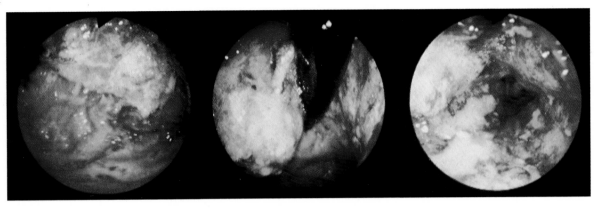

Figure 6.12 Malignant ulcer of the angularis. The tumor can only be visualized, brushed for cytology, and biopsied with the endoscope retroflexed.

Figure 6.13 Examples of large, poorly defined type III adenocarcinomas. Exudation and friability make identification of the margins difficult.

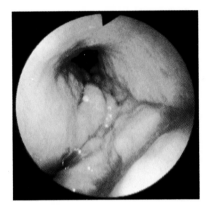

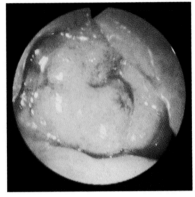

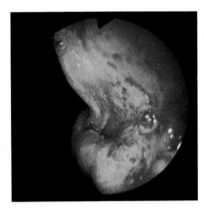

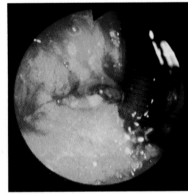

Figure 6.14 Type IV adenocarcinoma (linitis plastica). The mucosa covering the diffusely infiltrating tumor appears normal.

Figure 6.15 Linitis plastica. The mucosa here is slightly erythematous over the indurated, infiltrated folds.

Figure 6.16 Extensive linitis plastica of the corpus and fundus with abnormal erythematous mucosa.

Figure 6.17 The heavy, indurated folds of linitis plastica are covered with abnormal mucosa, seen with the endoscope retroflexed.

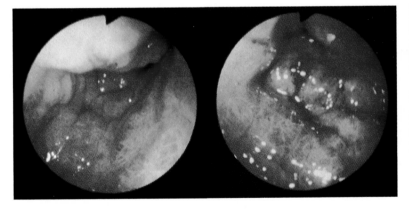

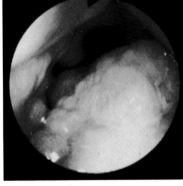

Figure 6.18 *Left,* Linitis plastica mimicking gastritis, with red, inflamed, edematous mucosa. Diagnosis is only possible with a deep biopsy. *Right,* A closeup view of the mucosa reveals edema, erythema, and friability.

Figure 6.19 Nodules in a patient with linitis plastica. The mucosa over the nodules appears relatively normal.

tification of the margins difficult (Fig. 6.13).

Type IV Carcinoma This diffuse infiltrating pattern accounts for 30 to 50% of gastric cancers. People with this pattern do not usually survive 5 years. These tumors may be localized (70%) or diffuse (30%) even to the extent of involving the entire stomach. Many of the localized tumors involve the proximal stomach (cardia or fundus). The diffuse type is called linitis plastica. The tumor growth pattern is submucosal. The covering mucosa may appear relatively normal (Fig. 6.14) or red and inflamed, mimicking gastritis (Figs. 6.15 to 6.18). Visible nodules seen at endoscopy may be covered with normal mucosa (Fig. 6.19) or abnormal

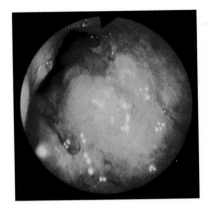

Figure 6.20 Poorly differentiated linitis plastica. The nodules seen here are covered with erythematous mucosa.

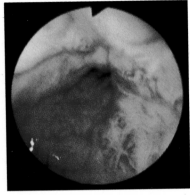

Figure 6.21 Linitis plastica with erythematous mucosa. The lumen is narrowed by the infiltrating tumor. The stellate, red areas may represent tumor breakthrough.

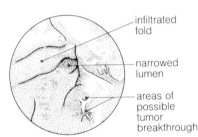

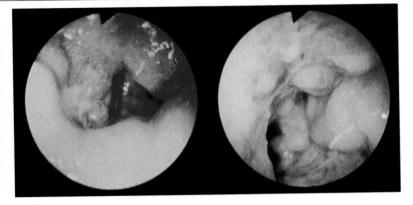

Figure 6.22 Extensive linitis plastica with nodules and ulcerations. These appearances may lead to confusion with type III lesions.

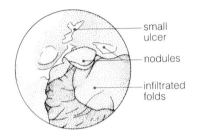

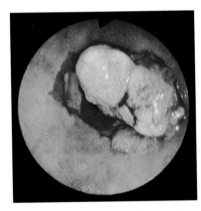

Figure 6.23 Adenocarcinoma of the cardia extending into the distal esophagus.

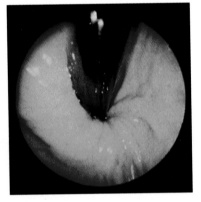

Figure 6.24 Adenocarcinoma of the cardia. The tumor cannot be seen with the endoscope retroflexed, but the indurated mucosa and the impression of a mass surrounding the endoscope can be noted.

erythematous mucosa (Fig. 6.20). Sixty percent of these lesions are reported to have areas of tumor breakthrough. These areas appear red with roughened mucosa and a dull appearance (Fig. 6.21), distinct from the normal appearance of the gastric mucosa. The rugal folds are infiltrated or replaced by tumor. These irregular areas of mucosa should be biopsied to increase the likelihood of sampling malignant tissue. One should also biopsy masses or nodules. Limited areas of ulceration may be noted in association with diffuse inflammation, and these may be difficult to differentiate from a type III lesion (Fig. 6.22).

OTHER ENDOSCOPIC CONSIDERATIONS

Adenocarcinoma of the cardia can be seen as the endoscope is passed down the esophagus (Fig. 6.23) or with a U-turn to retroflex the endoscope tip. If the tumor is mainly infiltrative, the endoscopic appearance may be heavy irregular folds covered with normal mucosa (Fig. 6.24). However, ulceration and obvious tumor breakthrough may be noted.

Especially with infiltrating tumors (types III and IV), the diagnosis may not be easy because the covering mucosa appears relatively normal. Other clues must be used to detect the presence of an abnormal gastric wall. The folds of the stomach may appear rigid and fixed. If the mucosa over these folds is pulled with a forceps out into the lumen, it may not "tent" as it would normally because the mucosa is adherent to the firm, infiltrating tumor underneath. This fixation suggests a tumor, but in some cases tumor may be present without this loss of tenting.

Another clue to the presence of a tumor is an area of abrupt change. At the junction of a tumor and the normal wall adjacent to the tumor, there may be a sharp margin or shelflike effect.

BIOPSY

Many endoscopists favor the use of large particle biopsy forceps which yields a larger tissue specimen compared to routine endoscopic forceps. The number of biopsies taken influences the true-positive rate. If three are taken, the rate of positivity is roughly 60%. If six or more are taken, the

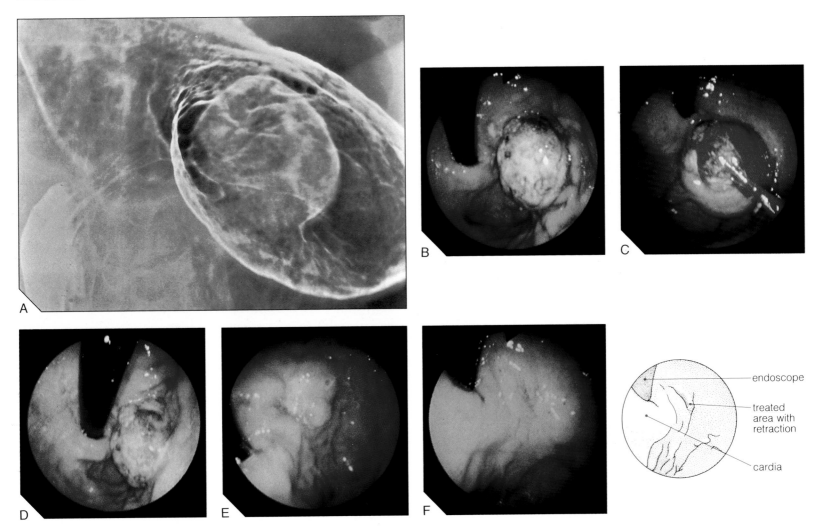

Figure 6.25 Endoscopic laser photocoagulation. A X-ray of gastric carcinoma in an elderly woman who presented with GI bleeding. B Endoscopy revealed a large polypoid cancer in the cardia. The tumor is best seen on retroflexion. C The tumor began to bleed while being inspected endoscopically. D After partial Nd-YAG laser therapy, the tumor is smaller and there is no evidence of bleeding. E Several weeks later after more laser therapy, no cancer is seen. Only a small ulcer is noted in the area of treatment. F Finally, the area is completely healed. Biopsy of the area was negative for residual tumor. The only abnormality is a slight retraction in the treated area.

accuracy is over 90%. Several studies have demonstrated that multiple biopsies are associated with a higher true-positive rate (10 biopsies = 99%).

The location of the biopsy for the optimal yield varies with the classification of the tumor, as shown by the true-positive biopsy rate. Types I and II are easier to biopsy because the malignant tissue is on the surface of an endoscopically visible mass. Types I and II have a true-positive rate with four biopsies of 80 to 90%. The infiltrating tumors (types III and IV) are more difficult to biopsy and obtain positive results. With four biopsies, type III has a true-positive rate of 70%; type IV, 50 to 60%. Directed brush cytology may improve the yield of endoscopy, especially in type IV tumors. Four biopsies and cytology have yielded an 80% positive rate.

NEW DIAGNOSTIC AND THERAPEUTIC TECHNIQUES
New technology may aid in diagnosis. Endoscopic ultrasound may permit high-resolution imaging of the intestinal wall and adjacent structures. Computed tomography and magnetic resonance imaging may also play a role in determining the extent of gastric tumors. Endoscopic laser photocoagulation using the Nd-YAG laser may be useful for tumors which are recurrent or in patients who are not surgical candidates for removal (Fig. 6.25).

EARLY GASTRIC ADENOCARCINOMA

Early endoscopic diagnosis of gastric cancer makes a difference in outcome, since the 5-year survival rate for early cancer is so much better than for advanced cancer. By definition, the lesion involves the mucosa and submucosa but does not extend to the muscularis propria of the stomach wall. In some cases, lesions followed for 2 to 3 years remain localized without evidence of extension into the muscle layer. Some early cancers spread on the gastric mucosa and submucosa without involvement of the muscularis propria. This superficial spreading type may be a variant of early gastric cancer or may be a separate entity.

CLASSIFICATION AND ENDOSCOPIC APPEARANCE
The Japanese Endoscopy Society formulated a widely used classification of this tumor. There are three types and three

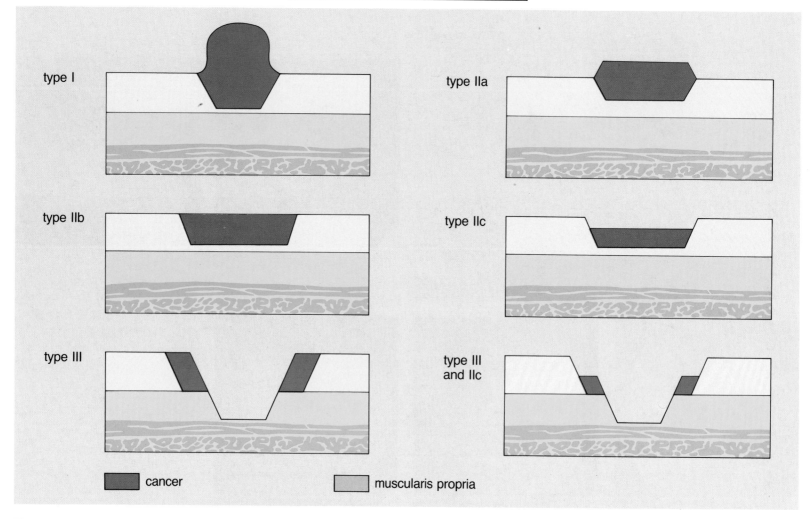

Figure 6.26 Japanese Endoscopy Society classification of early gastric cancer.

subtypes (Fig. 6.26). In addition there are combinations of lesions which incorporate more than one classification. In these combined lesions the predominant pattern is listed first.

Type I: Polypoid lesion of mucosa protruding into lumen.
Type II: Subtle tumors of mucosa. Not as prominent as type I (polyp) or type III (ulcer). Type II is divided into three subtypes:

    IIa: Area of focal mucosal elevation, less marked than in type I.

    IIb: Flat area of abnormal mucosa.

    IIc: Depressed tumor with cancer at base of depression.
Type III: Gastric ulcer with cancer at the margin.

Lesions combining types III and IIc account for about half of all cases of early gastric cancers. About 20% of early cancers are the raised types (I and IIa). The flat or depressed types are found in approximately 30% of cases.

For the most part, symptoms of early gastric cancer are similar to those of advanced cancers. Dyspepsia and epigastric pain occur in both early and advanced cases in 65 to 80% of patients. Hematemesis or melena are seen slightly more often in early than in advanced cancer, and early cancer

has a slightly lower incidence of weight loss. Overall, the diagnosis is made endoscopically. Lesions of early gastric cancer are relatively subtle and in many instances difficult to distinguish from normal mucosa or nonmalignant gastric lesions.

Type I Carcinoma The surface of these polypoid lesions is usually nodular or irregular, more so than is found with typical hyperplastic polyps, adenomatous polyps, and submucosal lesions such as a leiomyoma. The surface may appear erythematous (Fig. 6.27).

Type II Carcinoma In subtype IIa, lesions appear as a slightly raised—but not polypoid—irregular area of gastric mucosa (Fig. 6.28).

Subtype IIb may be difficult to diagnose. The mucosa is neither raised nor depressed. The color may appear abnormal with white or gray areas (Fig. 6.29) or uniformly red, in contrast to the lacy, reticulated, erythematous appearance of regenerative mucosa adjacent to a benign gastric ulcer.

In subtype IIc, lesions are slightly depressed areas of abnormal mucosa (Fig. 6.30).

Subtypes IIb and IIc may have an appearance similar to a healing gastric ulcer. However, benign ulcers have smooth tapered rugal folds which end at the healing area, whereas early cancers have abnormal fold terminations with clubbing

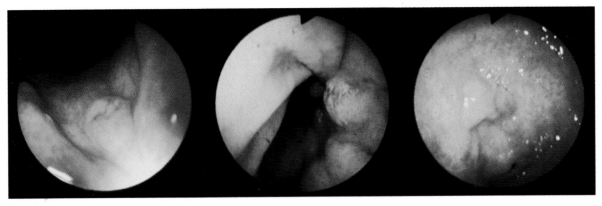
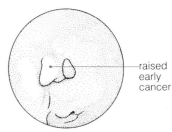

raised early cancer

Figure 6.27 Examples of type I early gastric cancer. Small, polypoid, raised nodules appear in each case, sometimes with signs of erythema.

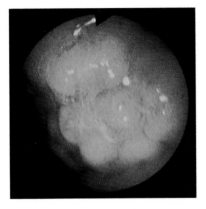
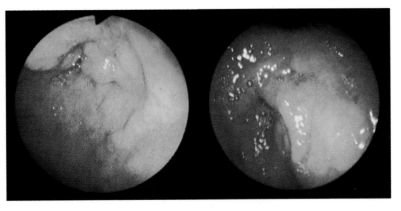

dysplasia

Figure 6.28 Subtype IIa early gastric cancer. The tumor is slightly raised but not polypoid.

Figure 6.29 Examples of subtype IIb early gastric cancer. The mucosa demonstrates subtle changes such as slight discoloration and roughened, irregular appearance.

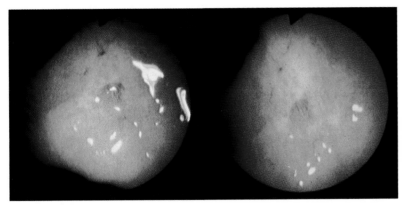
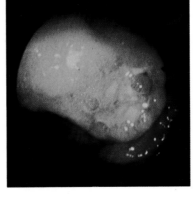
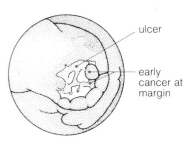

ulcer

early cancer at margin

Figure 6.30 Subtype IIc early gastric cancer. A slightly depressed white area can be noted *(left)*. A different perspective *(right)* allows visualization of the entire lesion.

Figure 6.31 Type III early gastric cancer. Gastric ulceration as well as early cancer at the margin are evident.

or nodules. The color of the mucosa in a healing ulcer has the red lacy appearance of the areae gastricae. In early cancer the mucosa is either intensely red or irregular with red and gray-white areas. These areas are typically sharply demarcated from the surrounding gastric mucosa and, in IIc lesions, slightly depressed.

Type III Carcinoma This lesion is also difficult to diagnose. It may appear adjacent to a benign-appearing gastric ulcer with the tumor in the tissue at the margin of the ulcer crater (Fig. 6.31). The cancer may be in only one quadrant and therefore can be missed if the entire margin of a gastric ulcer is not inspected and biopsied. This inspection may require a retroflexed view of the ulcer. The base of the ulcer may be free of tumor. Signs include depressed and discolored areas. One should also look for abnormalities of the surrounding folds. In the combination lesions (IIC and III

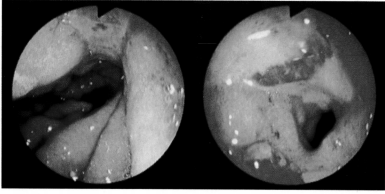
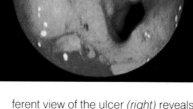
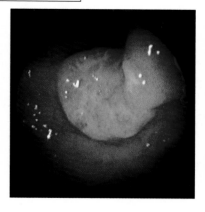
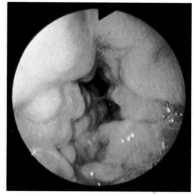

Figure 6.32 A large ulcer in a patient with non-Hodgkin's lymphoma. The folds surrounding the ulcer are indurated and infiltrated (left). A different view of the ulcer (right) reveals friability and narrowing of the lumen caused by the indurated folds.

Figure 6.33 Non-Hodgkin's gastric lymphoma demonstrates a polypoid appearance.

Figure 6.34 In this lymphoma the gastric rugae are infiltrated and may be confused with linitis plastica.

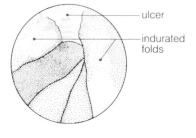

— ulcer

— indurated folds

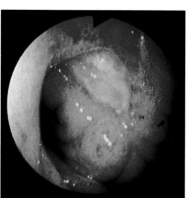

large deep ulcer

Figure 6.35 A large deep ulcer associated with gastric lymphoma.

of the lesion should be sampled. Cytology is not as helpful in early cancer as in other tumors. Brushing for cytology is done under endoscopic guidance and should include the red, irregular, depressed mucosa or the margin of the ulcer in the areas of abnormal mucosa.

OTHER GASTRIC MALIGNANCIES

The next most common tumor after adenocarcinoma is lymphoma, followed by leiomyosarcoma. Other less common tumors are Kaposi's sarcoma and metastatic gastric disease.

GASTRIC LYMPHOMA

About 4 to 8% of gastric tumors are lymphomas. Unlike advanced adenocarcinoma, lymphoma often responds well to therapy, especially if diagnosed at an early stage. Stage I (stomach wall only) has an 80% 5-year survival rate; stage IV (widespread disease) rarely survives 5 years.

Primary gastric lymphoma includes non-Hodgkin's lymphoma and less commonly Hodgkin's lymphoma. For non-Hodgkin's gastric lymphoma, the histiocytic type accounts for 60 to 70%, the lymphocytic type for 30%. The gastric tumors are more often diffuse than nodular. The nodular lymphocytic types have the best 5-year survival rates. Precise diagnosis is essential to guide treatment. Diagnosis of gastric involvement with generalized abdominal lymphoma is important because knowledge of gastric involvement can affect decisions regarding therapy.

or III and IIc, where the first symbol designates the primary morphologic pattern), distinct ulcers are associated with abnormal adjacent mucosa, often with irregular, depressed, and erythematous areas.

BIOPSY
The lesions of early gastric cancer may respond to standard antiulcer therapy and may heal and recur in a cycle similar to benign gastric ulcers. For this reason many endoscopists biopsy all gastric ulcers and do repeat biopsies until the lesion is completely healed. If at least two biopsies are taken from each of the four quadrants of the ulcer (total eight), there is better than a 90% chance of detecting cancer if it is present. For ulcers, the margin of each quadrant is biopsied; the base is less productive. For polyps and for flat and depressed areas (types I, IIa, IIb, and IIc), the base or center

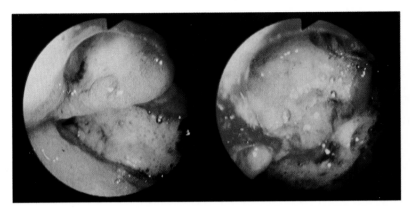

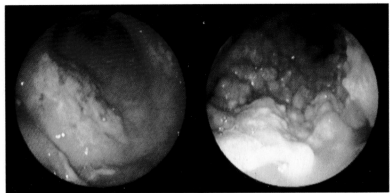

Figure 6.36 *Left,* Recurrent, diffuse non-Hodgkin's lymphoma involving an extensive area of the stomach. The ulcer is large, and the surrounding mucosa is friable, nodular, and clearly infiltrated. *Right,* In this view the nodularity at the ulcer margin is seen.

Figure 6.37 *Left,* Extensive non-Hodgkin's lymphoma with nodular involvement of the gastric wall. This lesion was associated with protein-losing enteropathy. *Right,* The diffuse nodular involvement is better seen in this slightly different view.

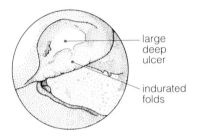

large deep ulcer

indurated folds

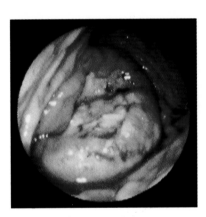

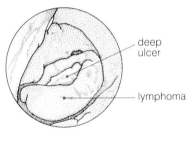

deep ulcer

lymphoma

Figure 6.38 Burkitt's lymphoma of the gastric body, with a central ulceration. (Courtesy of Dr. Michael Priebe)

ENDOSCOPIC APPEARANCE

Gastric lymphoma may be difficult to differentiate from adenocarcinoma or a benign ulcer. Endoscopy in gastric lymphoma is associated with visual diagnosis of a suspected neoplasm in 75% of cases; in the rest, a diagnosis of a benign ulcer or other disease is suspected. Biopsies are always necessary to distinguish between benign disease and tumor.

Characteristically, gastric lymphoma presents as an infiltrating lesion of the gastric mucosa, often associated with ulceration (Fig. 6.32). There may also be polypoid aspects to the tumor's appearance (Fig. 6.33). Occasionally it may resemble an infiltrative adenocarcinoma (linitis plastica) (Fig. 6.34). Single or multiple ulcers may be seen in association with the infiltration. A single ulcer may be deep with a raised margin (Fig. 6.35). This "volcano" appearance is felt by some to be characteristic of histiocytic lymphoma. The ul-

cers may also have an irregular margin which increases the suspicion of a tumor being present. The appearance is often that of infiltrated folds with diffuse ulceration and a very irregular nodular margin (Fig. 6.36). The tumor may be anywhere in the stomach, but often occurs in the body or antrum and may narrow the lumen.

Lymphomas of the stomach may also appear as single or multiple mass lesions. They are often firm and covered with relatively normal-appearing mucosa. Lesions may be large, sessile, polypoid masses or smaller lesions (as small as 1 to 2 cm). Large lesions may be associated with protein-losing enteropathy (Fig. 6.37). Burkitt's lymphoma may appear as a polypoid mass with a deep central ulceration (Fig. 6.38).

BIOPSY AND OTHER DIAGNOSTIC TECHNIQUES

Diagnosis of lymphoma of the stomach is accomplished with endoscopic examination, biopsy, and cytology. The yield of biopsy in this lesion is 70 to 80% and may be as high as 90%. This is slightly better than is seen with infiltrating adenocarcinoma, perhaps because the tumor is more accessible due to the diffuse associated ulceration. Lymphoma is not as often totally submucosal as is adenocarcinoma; however, it it still important to biopsy areas with the highest potential yield of positivity (i.e., ulcers, nodules, and areas of abnormal mucosa) and to perform multiple biopsies. Some recommend 10 to 15 biopsies if lymphoma is suspected. Endoscopically guided sheathed brush cytology may help in the diagnosis. In some instances lymphocytes in the brushing provide a clue. Sometimes deeper biopsies may be necessary, either using endoscopic techniques or at surgery.

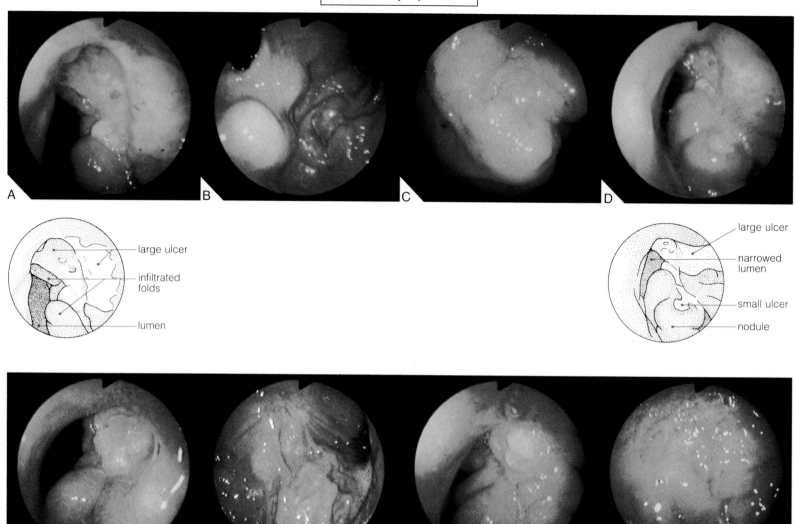

Figure 6.39 Radiation therapy. **A** A large, irregular ulcer in the body of the stomach, caused by gastric lymphoma. **B** With the endoscope retroflexed, large nodules can be seen in the fundus. **C** In the area of the junction of the corpus and fundus the mucosa appears abnormal with nodules and an irregular, coarse fold pattern caused by the infiltration of the lymphoma. **D** Multiple lymphomatous ulcers of varying sizes can be seen in the midcorpus. **E** Two weeks after radiation therapy, the small ulcers are gone, the folds converge, and the large ulcer is somewhat smaller. The mucosa is still abnormal, with indurated folds and erythematous mucosa surrounding the ulcer. **F** Five weeks after radiation therapy, the nodules and coarse folds are returning to normal. Abnormal vessels can still be seen on the mucosa. **G** Five weeks after radiation therapy, the small ulcers are gone, the folds are smaller, and the large ulcer is smaller. Biopsy of the ulcer was negative for tumor. **H** Still 5 weeks after therapy, the fundus is more normal with a less nodular appearance and nearly normal folds.

Endoscopy may also be useful to monitor the effect of radiation therapy (Fig. 6.39) or chemotherapy (Fig. 6.40). Ulcers resolve and the thickened, infiltrated mucosa returns to normal.

Cross-sectional imaging techniques such as computed tomography may help in the diagnosis by demonstrating a mass, a thickened gastric wall, or involvement of adjacent lymph nodes. An excellent new method to diagnose the depth of wall invasion and involvement of adjacent organs is the ultrasonic endoscope (Fig. 6.41). High-resolution ultrasound can also be used to follow the response to therapy, seen as a reduction in the size of the mass and the thickness of the wall.

GASTRIC SARCOMA

Sarcomas account for approximately 2% of gastric malignancies. These mesenchymal lesions are characteristically large masses (4 to 5 cm) with primarily submucosal extension (Fig. 6.42). The mass frequently extends outside of the stomach. In approximately 20% of patients there is a central depression in the surface of the mass caused by necrosis (Figs. 6.43 and 6.44). These lesions may cause GI bleeding (Fig. 6.45). Smaller lesions may appear similar to leiomyomas (submucosal polyps). Leiomyosarcoma is the most common tumor of this type. The differential diagnosis may be a problem even with tissue obtained at biopsy. His-

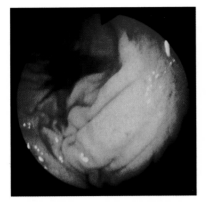

Figure 6.40 Chemotherapy. This patient had been treated with chemotherapy for gastric lymphoma. The stomach now appears normal except for the suggestion of slightly heavy folds.

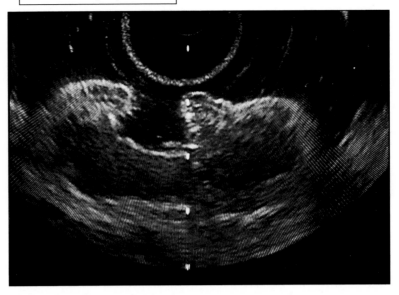

Figure 6.41 Ultrasonic endoscopic image shows a deep ulcer with a tumor mass at the base and margin. This mass proved to be a lymphoma.

Gastric Sarcoma

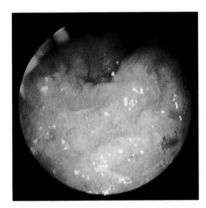

Figure 6.42 Generalized lymphosarcoma involving the stomach with multiple enlarged folds and superficial ulcers. The submucosal nature of the tumor is suggested by the diffuse nodularity.

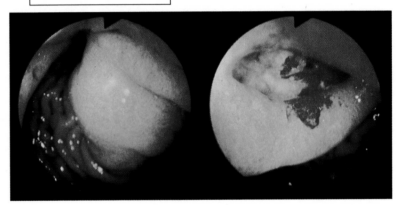

Figure 6.43 *Left,* A large mesenchymal tumor is protruding into the proximal gastric lumen. *Right,* With further insertion of the endoscope it is possible to see the necrosis in the center of the mass, presenting as a deep depression or ulcer. The ulcer is friable.

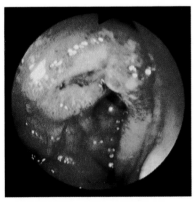

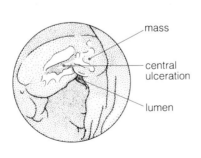

Figure 6.44 Leiomyosarcoma of the stomach, covered with abnormal mucosa and having a central ulceration.

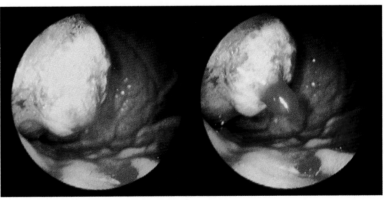

Figure 6.45 *Left,* Sarcoma of the gastric fundus protruding into the lumen. *Right,* While being observed, the tumor began to bleed.

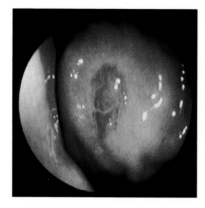

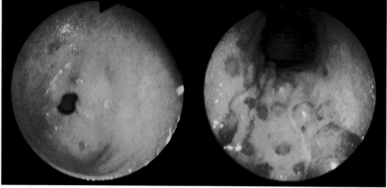

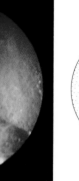

Figure 6.46 Example of a single, intensely red lesion of Kaposi's sarcoma in a patient with AIDS.

Figure 6.47 Examples of multiple lesions of Kaposi's sarcoma in two patients with AIDS. *Left,* Small early lesions. *Right,* Larger later lesions.

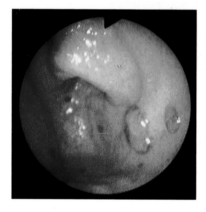

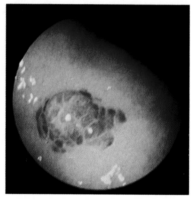

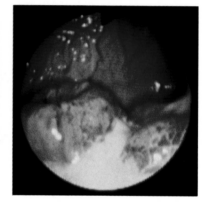

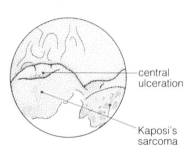

Figure 6.48 Several sessile polypoid lesions in a patient with Kaposi's sarcoma involving the stomach.

Figure 6.49 Lesion of Kaposi's sarcoma in a patient with AIDS. The lesion could be confused with a polyp, but the covering mucosa has the characteristic striking red appearance.

Figure 6.50 Central ulceration in the larger of two Kaposi's sarcoma lesions in a patient with AIDS. (Courtesy of Dr. Fred Weinstein)

tologic examination by biopsy is not as often positive as with other tumors because of the largely submucosal growth pattern. Cytology is of little use in these tumors. The characteristic finding on biopsy is spindle cells with evidence of increased mitotic activity. Less commonly seen sarcomas include liposarcomas, rhabdomyosarcoma, and other spindle-cell sarcomas. The different types of sarcoma cannot be distinguished endoscopically.

KAPOSI'S SARCOMA

This is a systemic disease which involves the skin (especially the soles of the feet and the nose) and may involve the GI tract, especially the stomach and colon. Typically the lesion is seen in patients with acquired immune deficiency syndrome (AIDS) and rarely in the elderly. About half of patients with AIDS and cutaneous Kaposi's sarcoma have involvement of the GI tract.

There are three endoscopic appearances of this tumor: single (Fig. 6.46) or multiple (Fig. 6.47) maculopapular lesions, polypoid lesions (Fig. 6.48), and ulcerating lesions.

Characteristically the lesions are intensely red because of the underlying histopathology which is that of a capillary hemangiosarcoma with endothelial proliferation. One may see a sessile polyp with red mucosa (Fig. 6.49) and occasionally an ulcerated center (Fig. 6.50). Biopsy is usually diagnostic because the tumor is on the surface of the lesion. Characteristic findings at biopsy are a mesenchymal-type tissue with vascular spaces and endothelial cells among spindle cells.

METASTATIC GASTRIC DISEASE

Cancer of the lung and breast and melanoma may metastasize to the stomach. More rarely, tumors of the pancreas, testis, thyroid, and female genital tract may metastasize to the stomach. The finding of a gastric lesion may be the first indication of metastatic spread. These patients may present with pain or bleeding and are then diagnosed at endoscopy to have lesions suggestive of metastases.

These lesions may present as small (1 to 2 cm), multiple submucosal lesions (Fig. 6.51) or as tumors which project

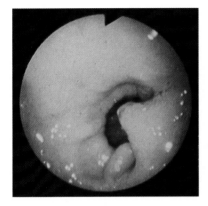

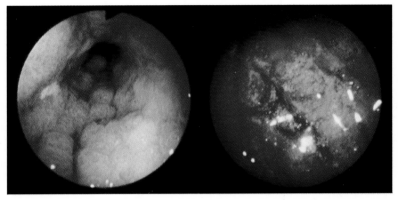

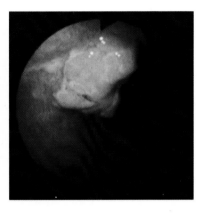

Figure 6.51 Intramural metastasis in the antral wall of the stomach in a patient with squamous-cell carcinoma of the esophagus.

Figure 6.52 Metastatic lesion to the stomach from breast carcinoma. *Left*, The gastric mucosa appears nodular and friable. The tumor infiltrated diffusely. Biopsy was positive for breast carcinoma. *Right*, In other areas, the mucosa appears very bizarre and resembles inflammation with its red, friable appearance. Biopsy is needed to differentiate tumor from gastritis.

Figure 6.53 Intragastric metastasis of carcinoma of the breast. The lesion appears sessile and polypoid, covered with irregular, nodular mucosa.

into the lumen with a central ulceration thought to result from outgrowth of its blood supply. This ulceration may be the cause of a presenting symptom of GI hemorrhage. Characteristic pigmentation may be noted in melanoma although larger lesions may be amelanotic or contain limited pigment. Other cancers, such as metastatic breast cancer, may appear as diffuse infiltrative growths (Fig. 6.52) or sessile, polypoid masses (Fig. 6.53).

GASTRIC POLYPS

Gastric polyps are detected in 2 to 3% of upper GI endoscopic examinations, often incidentally. They are usually small, with a diameter of less than 1 to 2 cm. Occasionally a polyp is seen on barium X-ray and is the reason for a referral for endoscopy. With larger polyps, patients may complain of vague abdominal discomfort and bleeding, and rarely a prolapsing antral polyp may obstruct the gastric outlet.

Polyps may be neoplastic or nonneoplastic. Neoplastic lesions which may present as polyps of the stomach include adenoma (relatively rare), carcinoma (the most common polypoid neoplastic lesion), and some unusual lesions such as carcinoids. Any gastric neoplasm may present as a polyp. Gastric adenocarcinomas presenting as polyps are discussed earlier in this chapter.

About 80 to 90% of gastric polyps are nonneoplastic. They can be divided into epithelial and nonepithelial types. The epithelial lesions include hyperplastic polyps (the most common polyp seen in the stomach) and polyps seen with a variety of polyposis conditions of the GI tract including juvenile polyposis, Peutz-Jeghers syndrome, and Cronkhite-Canada syndrome. These three types of polyps can be difficult to distinguish histologically with the exception of the Peutz-Jeghers polyp which can be differentiated if the entire polyp is available for examination. Endoscopically, these polyps may also appear similar with the exception that the

Peutz-Jeghers polyp is usually larger than the others. All three of these polyps are characteristically larger than the typical hyperplastic polyp (3 to 4 cm compared with 1 to 2 cm).

The other type of epithelial polyp in the stomach is the fundal gland polyp seen in patients with and without familial polyposis coli (FPC) syndrome. These fundal gland polyps consist of dilated foveolae and glandular structures. Patients with FPC have an increased incidence of both adenomas of the stomach and fundal gland polyps. Adenomatous polyps are considered a risk factor for the development of gastric carcinoma; fundal gland polyps are not. Patients with Gardner's syndrome may also develop multiple adenomas.

Patients may present with multiple gastric polyps. If the polyps are adenomatous there is considered to be an increased risk of maliganancy. If the polyps are hyperplastic there is no risk of the polyps themselves becoming malignant, but the surrounding atrophic gastritis may be a fertile soil for the development of malignancy. The fundal gland polyps are not considered to be premalignant.

Nonneoplastic nonepithelial polyps of mesenchymal origin include leiomyomas, adenomyomas, hamartomas, and lipomas. They will be discussed separately under Submucosal Masses at the end of this chapter.

NEOPLASTIC POLYPS

ADENOMATOUS POLYPS
Adenomas are uncommon, accounting for only 5 to 10% of polypoid lesions in the stomach. Up to 40% contain a focus of carcinoma, especially the larger villous lesions (greater than 1 to 2 cm). These polyps may become malignant with time. The risk of cancer in the adjacent stomach tissue may be as high as 30%. These polyps are usually larger than hyperplastic polyps when first detected (over 1 cm in two-thirds of patients). In the US the average size of gastric adenomas is 3 to 4 cm. These polyps are associated with chronic atrophic gastritis and FPC. When adenomas occur

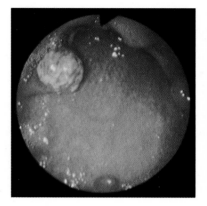

Figure 6.54 Adenoma of the antrum. The surface is covered with exudate.

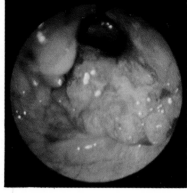

Figure 6.55 Adenoma of the stomach. The polyp is multilobed.

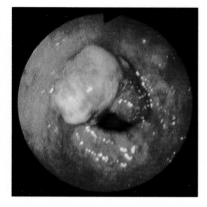

Figure 6.56 Adenoma of the antrum with a surface which is eroded and covered with exudate.

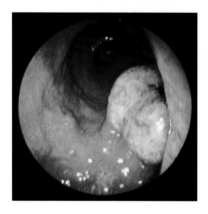

Figure 6.57 Adenomatous polyp of the antrum. The surface is slightly atypical and eroded. In fact, this was associated with a diffuse gastric adenocarcinoma proximally.

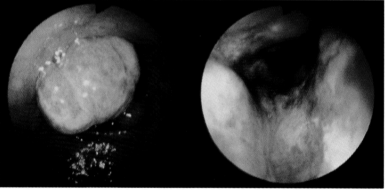
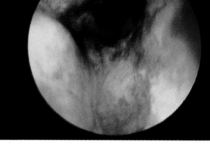

Figure 6.58 Adenomatous polyp with superficial erosion and exudation *(left)*. Histologically, atypia was noted. Circumferential cancer was found to be present along the entire proximal stomach *(right)*.

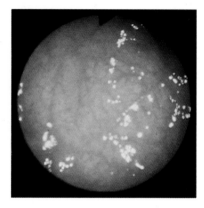

Figure 6.59 Atrophic gastric mucosa in a patient with an adenomatous polyp. Blood vessels are visible through the mucosa. The polyp is not visible.

in FPC, there is disagreement as to the risk of gastric cancer. This risk of malignant degeneration may vary with the country studied.

Adenomas of the stomach have three histologic configurations, similar to adenomas of the colon: tubular, villous, and mixed or tubulovillous. The latter two are associated with the highest risk of developing cancer in the polyp. Villous tumors are often large, antral, sessile, superficially eroded, associated with blood loss, and may obstruct the gastric outlet.

There is disagreement about whether hyperplastic polyps can develop into adenomatous polyps of the stomach. The confusion stems from the rare case in which a polyp contains elements of both adenoma and hyperplastic polyp.

Endoscopic Appearance Adenomatous polyps are red, often with a multilobed surface (Figs. 6.54 and 6.55). The surface may be smooth or superficially eroded (Fig. 6.56). The presence of erosion or ulceration is thought to correlate with an increased risk of cancer in the polyp. Similarly, superficial erosion and atypia may increase the likelihood of a gastric cancer being present (Figs. 6.57 and 6.58). Ad-

enomatous polyps are usually sessile but may have a pedicle similar to a hyperplastic polyp. They occur in the antrum and, less frequently, in the body of the stomach. Adenomas occur singly in 60% of cases. The surrounding mucosa often shows atrophic changes (Fig. 6.59).

NONNEOPLASTIC EPITHELIAL POLYPS

HYPERPLASTIC POLYPS

These are the most common polypoid lesions of the stomach, far more common than adenomatous polyps. They do not seem to enlarge with time as do adenomatous polyps. Rarely, hyperplastic polyps are associated with a carcinoma or an adenoma in the same lesion. The histology is that of hyperplasia of foveolar elements. These polyps may be seen in the stump after gastrectomy.

Hyperplastic polyps and adenomas are both associated with chronic gastritis. The likelihood that hyperplastic polyps are associated with atrophic gastritis is proportional to the number of polyps. If there are more than 10 polyps,

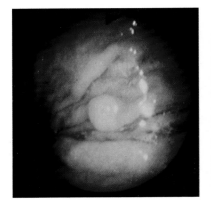
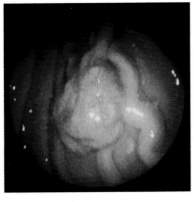
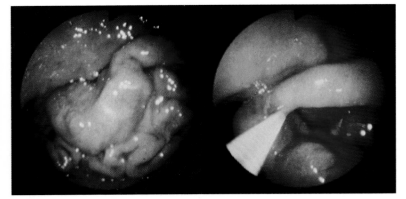

Figure 6.60 A small gastric hyperplastic polyp in a patient with atrophic gastritis.

Figure 6.61 Sessile hyperplastic polyp in the stomach.

Figure 6.62 Hyperplastic polyps in the stomach. With manipulation, the long stalk of the polyp can be seen.

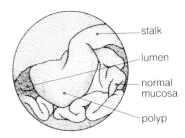

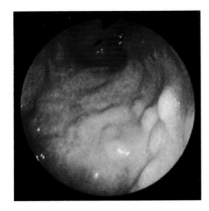
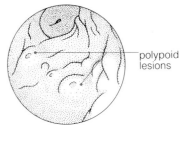
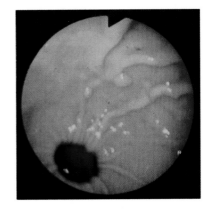
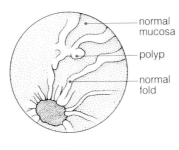

Figure 6.63 Varioliform gastritis in the antrum of a patient with gastric cancer (relationship between gastritis and cancer unknown). Typical polypoidlike lesions with a central dimple are seen.

Figure 6.64 Hyperplastic polyp in the antrum. The surrounding mucosa is normal. This polyp differs histologically from the lesion in varioliform gastritis.

the chance of associated atrophic gastritis is as high as 30%. These polyps probably never become a cancer, but there is a slightly increased risk of cancer elsewhere in the stomach.

Endoscopic Appearance Hyperplastic polyps can occur throughout the stomach. They are usually less than 1.5 cm in diameter (Fig. 6.60), may be single or multiple, and may be sessile (Fig. 6.61) or pedunculated. A long stalk may be seen (Fig. 6.62). The mucosa covering a small polyp may appear normal. With larger polyps, the overlying mucosa is often red and friable, and there may be a small erosion or ulceration on the tip of the polyp. The mucosa in which these polyps occur may be atrophic or show evidence of gastritis. The 10 to 20% of polyps that are larger than 2 cm may be confused with adenomatous or carcinomatous lesions.

The lesions seen in chronic erosive gastritis (varioliform gastritis) may resemble hyperplastic polyps histologically because both represent a response of the gastric mucosa to injury. In chronic erosive gastritis, the injury induces an erosion with hyperplasia of the surrounding mucosa (Fig. 6.63), whereas with a hyperplastic polyp there is hyperplasia without an erosion in most cases (Fig. 6.64).

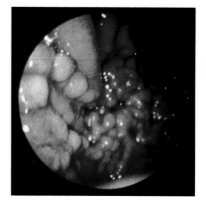

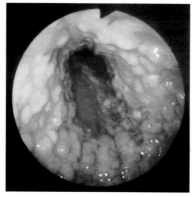

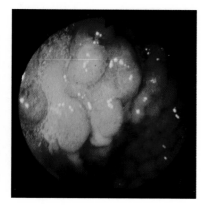

Figure 6.65 Multiple, small fundal gland polyps of the cystic glandularis type in a patient with FPC.

Figure 6.66 A carpet of cystic-type fundal gland polyps in a patient with FPC.

Figure 6.67 Cystic gastric polyposis in a patient without FPC.

FUNDAL GLAND POLYPS

These lesions are seen as single, multiple, or as a carpet of polyps in the gastric fundus (Figs. 6.65 to 6.67). The polyps are bumps with dilated gastric fundal glands and foveolar cells. They occur in patients with and without FPC. These lesions are normally not associated with gastric cancer either in the polyp or in the rest of the stomach.

MANAGEMENT OF POLYPS

Neoplastic and nonneoplastic polyps cannot be distinguished endoscopically. Forceps biopsy alone is not sufficient, as the entire polyp is often needed to establish histologic type. In many instances the polyp can be removed using standard polypectomy techniques (Fig. 6.68). However, there is a risk of hemorrhage especially after removal of large polyps. For polyps larger than 1 or 2 cm, the safest course is to snare off a piece of use a large biopsy forceps rather than attempt total snare resection. If the polyp proves to be hyperplastic it need not be removed, but periodic endoscopic surveillance is recommended because of the risk of carcinoma elsewhere in the stomach. If the polyp is an adenoma, especially if it is sessile, large, and villous or mixed tubulovillous, resection should be considered. Endoscopic snare techniques can be used (Fig. 6.69). Surgical resection may be required in some cases with large, sessile polyps. These patients should also be surveyed periodically for the development of additional polyps and cancer in the stomach. There is a 2 to 3% risk of developing cancer in the stomach after removal of an adenoma.

SUBMUCOSAL MASSES

There are a variety of lesions in the stomach which are occasionally symptomatic (bleeding) but usually found incidentally at endoscopy. These include carcinoids, pancreatic rests, leiomyomas, adenomyomas, hamartomas, and lipomas. As a group these lesions are small and difficult to distinguish from hyperplastic or adenomatous polyps. A common finding is a central depression surrounded by normal mucosa. This contrasts with the typical erosion seen on adenomatous or hyperplastic polyps in which the erosion often covers the surface of the polyp. With a submucosal mass the ulcer is usually sharply delineated from the surrounding normal mucosa. The cause of the depression may be necrosis caused by the tumor outgrowing its blood supply. Because of the submucosal location of these masses, there are often bridging folds on either side of the mass.

Histologic diagnosis is made using a polypectomy specimen or by performing repeated biopsies in the same area to sample progressively deeper tissue. Pedunculated lesions may be safely removed with a snare. Sessile submucosal lesions are either left or removed surgically. Once this type of lesion is recognized, patients are usually just followed. If the tumor is large or bleeding, it may be necessary to surgically remove it.

CARCINOIDS

These lesions are rarely encountered in the stomach: The incidence is 1 or 2% of gastric polyps. The tumor is usually sessile with a small ulcer at the tip. They frequently occur in the cardial area and in the antrum. The lesions may be multiple with small polyps or may appear as flat, occasionally ulcerated lesions. Few patients experience symptoms of the carcinoid syndrome, but the tumor is malignant in approximately 25% of cases. Small lesions are occasionally removed endoscopically, but large sessile lesions and malignant lesions should be removed surgically. After removal, periodic surveillance is indicated to detect the occurrence of new lesions.

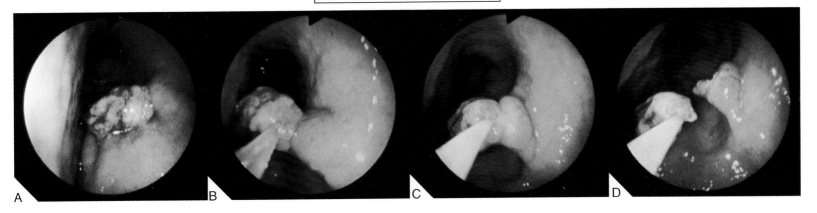

Figure 6.68 Polypectomy. A This patient presented with an adenomatous gastric polyp. The surface is friable, and there is a stalk that is not well seen here. B The polyp is snared. C The stalk turns white as the wire is closed and electrosurgical coagulating current is applied. D The polyp is resected.

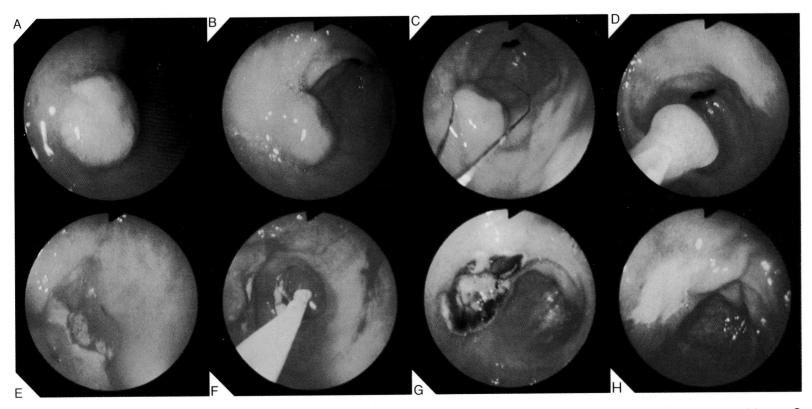

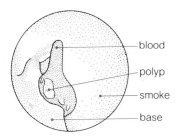

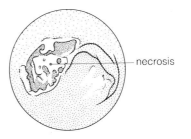

Figure 6.69 Endoscopic snare technique. A A patient with pernicious anemia presented with this sessile polyp which was dysplastic on biopsy and had an unusual surface color. A decision was made to remove the polyp endoscopically. B The polyp is seen in profile. C A snare is placed over the polyp. D The snare is closed. E Smoke is noted as the snare is pulled through the base of the lesion with coagulating electrosurgical current. The polyp is stuck to the base, and a small amount of blood is seen. This picture was taken just after the excision occurred. The snare catheter has been pulled into the endoscope and is not visible. F The polyp is snared again for removal and is now free of the coagulated base. G Twenty-four hours after the procedure, the base is necrotic. H One week after the procedure, the defect where the polyp was attached is healing.

6.19

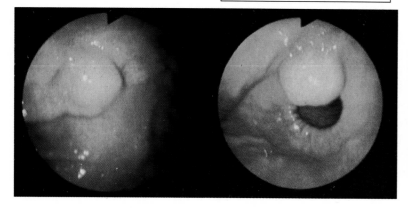
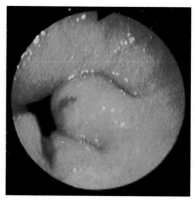

Figure 6.70 *Left,* Small submucosal tumor, typical of a leiomyoma. *Right,* On closer inspection, there is a suggestion of bridging folds.

Figure 6.71 Leiomyoma of the gastric fundus. Note a small dimple on the tip of the mass.

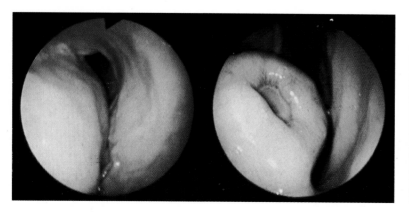
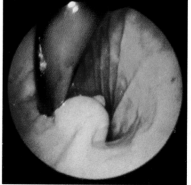

Figure 6.72 *Left,* A large submucosal leiomyoma is seen bulging into the lumen. This patient has presented with GI bleeding. *Right,* With repositioning of the endoscope, an ulcer can be seen at the tip of the mass.

Figure 6.73 A gastric leiomyoma of the fundus with bridging folds.

LEIOMYOMAS

This is one of the more common submucosal tumors. They are usually small (less than 1 to 2 cm) (Fig. 6.70), proximal in the stomach (Fig. 6.71), and are attached firmly to the underlying gastric wall. Rarely, these tumors may be 15 to 20 cm and extend outside the gastric wall and into the gastric lumen (Fig. 6.72). The surface mucosa is not attached to the tumor and may be smooth or have a central depression, especially in large lesions (see Figs. 6.71 and 6.72). This depression may actually be an ulcer which can bleed. Bridging folds may be observed (Fig. 6.73). Histologically, the tissue consists of spindle-shaped cells. The differential diagnosis includes leiomyoblastoma, a similar-appearing tumor with a higher degree of mitotic activity and an increased risk of malignancy compared to leiomyomas.

ADENOMYOMAS AND HAMARTOMAS

These lesions cannot be distinguished endoscopically from other types of gastric polyps. They are the typical size for gastric polyps (1 to 2 cm), sessile or pedunculated, and the covering mucosa may be normal or show superficial erosion. Lesions which at histologic examination contain pancreatic ductal tissue and smooth muscle are called adenomyomas. These rarely contain acinar tissue as do pancreatic rests. They are located in the antrum on the greater curvature side, in the same area of the stomach as are pancreatic rests. Without the pancreatic component to the tissue, they are called hamartomas. Hamartomas occur in patients with Peutz-Jeghers syndrome. Some gastric polyps in juvenile polyposis are hamartomas. These are not premalignant nor is there an increased risk of cancer in the residual stomach.

OTHER TUMORS

Several other types of tumors involve the gastric wall, such as vascular tumors, lipomas, and neurofibromas. Firm lesions are characteristically vascular tumors of the glomus type, gastric fibromas, and neurofibromas. Lipomas are typically yellow, are often associated with lipomas elsewhere in the GI tract, and may be pedunculated or sessile. They are occasionally very large and seem soft when touched with a biopsy forceps. Eosinophilic granuloma is also in the differential diagnosis of a polyp. This lesion has a characteristic histology which includes infiltration by many eosinophilic leukocytes in addition to fibroblasts and histiocytes.

Stomach III: Gastritis and Upper Gastrointestinal Bleeding

In this chapter we will consider a variety of inflammatory lesions of the gastric mucosa referred to as gastritis. We will review the general aspects of gastritis, acute and chronic gastritis, atrophic gastritis, erosive gastritis, drug-induced gastritis, hemorrhagic gastritis, stress-induced gastritis, and gastritis associated with giant folds and radiation. We will also consider gastric manifestations of Crohn's disease and caustic gastric injury. A brief review of endoscopic techniques in the diagnosis of upper gastrointestinal bleeding will be presented.

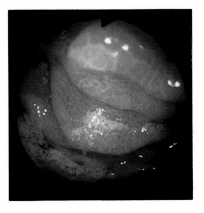

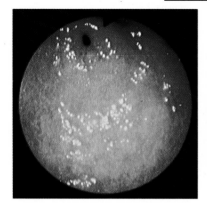

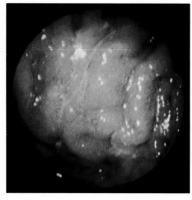

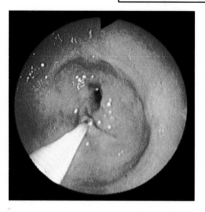

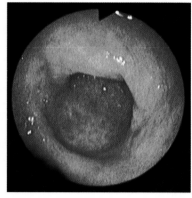

Figure 7.1 Endoscopic features of gastritis. Antrum with mild inflammatory changes shows patchy reddening and discrete unevenness, as evidenced by irregular highlighting.

Figure 7.2 Endoscopic features of gastritis. Mucosa covered with mucus-like material. Rugae are slightly enlarged and show an irregular pattern.

Figure 7.3 Mild nonspecific gastritis with reddened patches. These foci may be related to damage caused by Campylobacter-like organisms. A biopsy is being taken.

Figure 7.4 More obvious gastric changes in the antrum and corpus. Irregular erythema and areas of paler discoloration are evident.

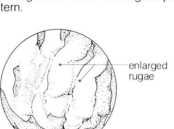

enlarged rugae

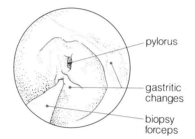

pylorus

gastritic changes

biopsy forceps

GASTRITIS

Normal gastric mucosa is smooth and has a brownish-red shiny appearance. The folds are regular and easily disappear upon insufflation. In gastritis, inflammatory changes take place that may be difficult to interpret because of their variability.

Several diagnostic features are characteristic of gastritis. Mucosal reddening or erythema probably reflects superficial mucosal hyperemia, which is often undetectable histologically. Patches of focal mucosal thickening and whitish discoloration are seen between reddish areas, especially in the antrum. The mucosa may look dull and granular (Fig. 7.1), and the areae gastricae pattern may be especially pronounced and irregular. Mucosal folds can be either reduced or excessively pronounced and tortuous. The mucosa may be covered with excessive amounts of mucus-like gray-yellow, brown, or green material (Fig. 7.2). There may be excessive bile staining the gastric juice or smearing the mucosa. The vascular pattern, especially of the submucosa, may become visible. There may be punctate intramucosal or submucosal hemorrhages (petechiae) or larger hemorrhagic spots. Necrosis of the epithelial layer is visible as flat or raised erosive defects. The severity and distribution of these changes may vary in different parts of the stomach. In general, there is poor correlation between endoscopic findings and underlying histologic changes.

ACUTE GASTRITIS

Patients with acute gastritis experience sudden upper gastric pain, nausea, and vomiting. Many episodes are associated with excessive food or alcohol intake, but in other cases no cause of the gastritis is found. Symptoms are fleeting, which explains why only a few such patients are examined endoscopically.

There are three types of acute gastritis. Type 1 is the mildest form and is characterized by generalized mucosal edema, narrowing of the antrum, and a velvet-like appearance of the mucosa without erosions or other changes. Type 2, the hemorrhagic type, is characterized by swollen folds and diminished distensibility with diffuse hemorrhagic spots and erosive defects. Type 3, the ulcerative type, is characterized by extensive erosions or ulcers accompanied by hemorrhage. After the bleeding stops, irregularly shaped ulcers may become more distinct, especially on the posterior wall of the antrum.

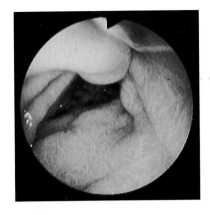

Figure 7.5 Erythematous nonspecific gastritic changes in the corpus and fundus in a patient with renal insufficiency.

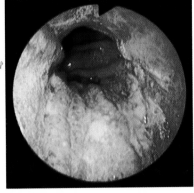

Figure 7.6 Severe swelling and erythema of the corpus and fundus. These changes are presumably due to portal vein thrombosis in a patient diagnosed with severe ulcerative colitis.

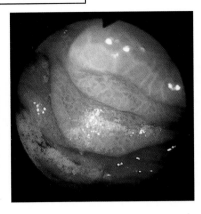

Figure 7.7 More severe, nonspecific gastritis with marked erythema, swelling, and coarsening of fold pattern.

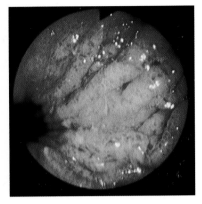

Figure 7.8 Severe nonspecific gastritis of the corpus and fundus. Coarsening of fold pattern, erythema, and mucus accumulation may be noted.

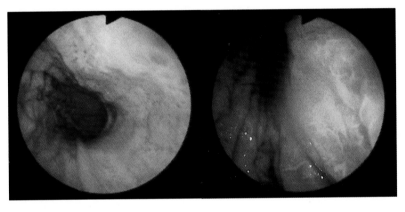

Figure 7.9 Nonspecific gastritic changes of the corpus and fundus areas include erythema and accentuation of the areae gastricae. This condition is commonly seen in cirrhotics with esophageal varices, presumably due to portal hypertension.

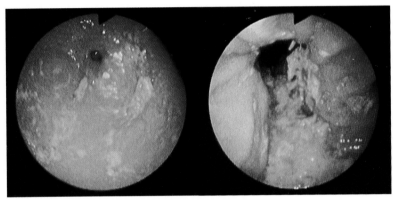

Figure 7.10 Diabetic gastroparesis causing food stagnation and nonspecific gastric changes in the corpus. These changes are commonly observed in patients with gastric stasis.

NONSPECIFIC (CHRONIC) GASTRITIS

Nonspecific erythema of the gastric mucosa is the principal endoscopic finding in chronic gastritis. The mucosa may be involved diffusely, focally, or in a linear fashion (Figs. 7.1, 7.3 and 7.4). The changes may be noted in the body, antrum, or both, and characteristically are found along the crests of the gastric folds. In addition to erythema, patchy edematous areas and, occasionally, some coarsening of the fold pattern may be noted (Figs. 7.5 to 7.8). Accentuation and irregularity of the areae gastricae pattern are also common (Fig. 7.9). In the antrum, patchy opalescent areas may be visible between foci of more reddened mucosa. There may be a granular unevenness to the mucosa and a loss of shininess. Occasionally, reddish streaks in the antrum that run radially toward the pylorus are seen; these may be secondary to damage from duodenal gastric reflux. Nonspecific gastric changes with edema and erythema are commonly observed in patients with gastric stasis (stagnant gastritis), as in diabetic gastroenteropathy (Fig. 7.10).

Histologic findings in nonspecific gastritis are variable. Most commonly, capillaries are dilated. There is also evidence of epithelial mucin depletion. Evidence of superficial or atrophic gastritis is commonly encountered histologically. This superficial gastritis is primarily located in the antrum and less commonly presents diffusely over the stomach or in isolated areas of the corpus or fundus.

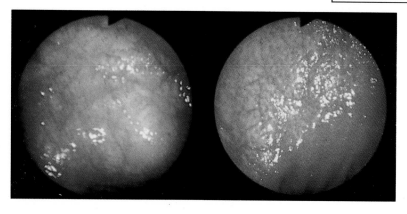

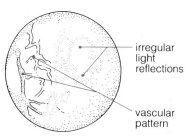

irregular light reflections

vascular pattern

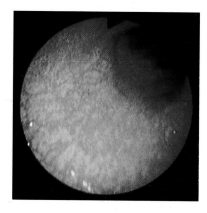

Figure 7.11 *Left,* Early atrophic changes in the corpus mucosa. Note the appearance of a delicate vascular pattern. *Right,* More pronounced atrophic gastritis with a conspicuous vascular pattern and irregularities of light reflections, indicative of mucosal unevenness.

Figure 7.12 Severe atrophic gastritis with marked visibility of vascular pattern. Usually, vessels are visible only with distension of the stomach by air.

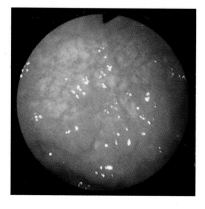

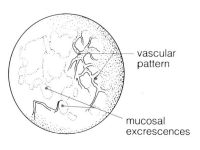

vascular pattern

mucosal excrescences

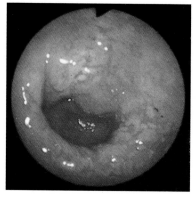

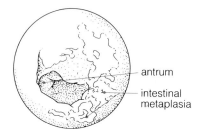

antrum

intestinal metaplasia

Figure 7.13 Tiny mucosal excrescences contrast with slightly depressed areas of atrophy. Visible vascular ramifications are also evident.

Figure 7.14 View of distal stomach with gray-white areas of intestinal metaplasia. This condition, which may occur in conjunction with atrophic gastritis, may be a precursor of gastric adenocarcinoma.

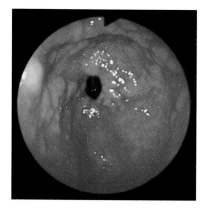

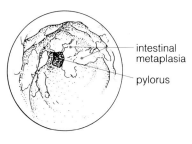

intestinal metaplasia

pylorus

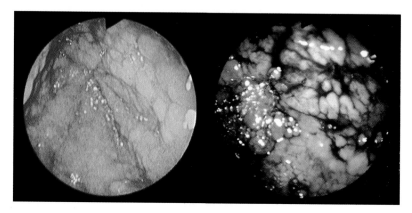

Figure 7.15 Extensive distal antral intestinal metaplasia. The white zones are slightly raised and extend into the pyloric channel, contrasting with reddened areas of surrounding mucosa.

Figure 7.16 Areas of pronounced, slightly raised intestinal metaplasia in the antrum (*left*) are accentuated after methylene blue dye-spraying (*right*).

ATROPHIC GASTRITIS

When the normal stomach is fully distended with air, vessels are typically visible through the mucosa, especially in the fundic region. In atrophic gastritis, mucosal and submucosal capillaries and vessels are visible without distension by air because of marked atrophy and thinning of mucosa (Figs. 7.11 and 7.12). In addition to the blood vessels being visible, other abnormalities in atrophic gastritis include a decrease in the rugal fold prominence, and a smooth mucosa with small mucosal protrusions (Fig. 7.13) or larger hyperplastic or adenomatous polyps.

There are two types of atrophic gastritis. Type A is characterized by mucosal atrophy in the fundus and corpus re-

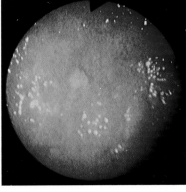

Figure 7.17 Atrophic gastritis with xanthelasma. Note the yellowish appearance of this defect.

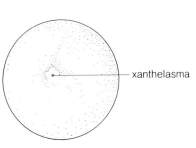

Figure 7.18 Adenomatous polyp in the antrum was found in a patient with atrophic gastritis and pernicious anemia.

Erosive Gastritis

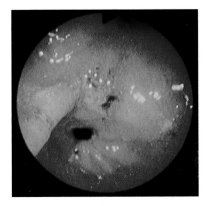

Figure 7.19 A small, flat erosion in the antrum, characterized as a whitish patch in otherwise unremarkable mucosa.

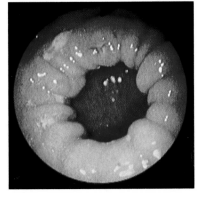

Figure 7.20 Flat superficial or incomplete erosion on top of a peristaltic wave. A minute amount of bleeding is observable. Surrounding patches of whitish mucoid material

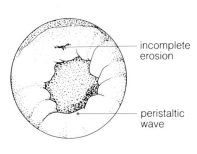

are easily distinguished from erosions. Advantage should be taken of the peristaltic activity to visualize all of the mucosa in detail.

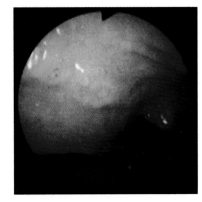

Figure 7.21 Three flat superficial erosions in a row. Each is surrounded by a delicate red halo.

gion. The mucosa of the antrum is normal or shows only evidence of mild gastritis. In type B, the inflammation occurs mainly in the antrum.

Intestinal metaplasia may occur in conjunction with atrophic gastritis; this is seen endoscopically as gray-white patches with a villus-like appearance and slight opalescence (Fig. 7.14). Such areas may be either slightly raised or depressed, and may be more readily identified with dye-spraying techniques, such as with a 0.5% solution of methylene blue (Figs. 7.15 and 7.16). Not uncommonly, xanthelasma with a peculiar yellowish appearance may be seen in atrophic gastritis (Fig. 7.17). Intestinal metaplasia may be a precursor of gastric adenocarcinoma of the intestinal type. Moreover, gastric adenoma, which carries a risk of cancerous degeneration, is commonly found in intestinal metaplasia and may occur in patients with atrophic gastritis and pernicious anemia (Fig. 7.18). There also seems to be an increased prevalence of hyperplasia of endocrine-like cells in the corpus and fundus mucosa and of gastric carcinoids.

Atrophic gastric mucosa and achlorhydria are found in association with pernicious anemia. Because of the increased

risk of cancer, some physicians recommend regular gastroscopic screening of patients with atrophic gastritis and achlorhydria, with or without pernicious anemia. Others feel that the risk is too low to justify regular screening.

Benign gastric ulcers often occur in association with antral and corpus atrophic mucosa. Such patients are often hypochlorhydric and are thought to develop gastric ulcers because of a reduction in mucosal defenses rather than because of hypersecretion.

EROSIVE GASTRITIS

These necrotic lesions of the mucosal lining are limited to the muscularis mucosae. Endoscopically, a distinction is made between incomplete (type 2) and complete (type 1) erosions.

Flat lesions are called superficial erosions (Figs. 7.19 and 7.20). Typically they have a white or yellowish base surrounded by a narrow zone of erythema. These erosions may be multiple (Fig. 7.21) and vary in size. The erosions are

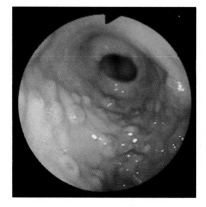

Figure 7.22 Numerous complete or varioliform erosions scattered over the corpus region of the stomach. Note the central depression revealing whitish or reddish discoloration.

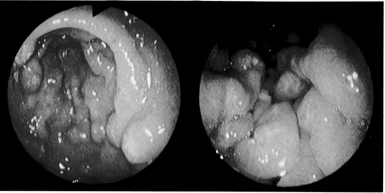 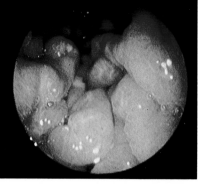

Figure 7.23 *Left,* Multiple complete erosions in the antrum. Note a whitish-gray patch of fibrinous exudate in the center of the nodular elevation. *Right,* Corpus and fundus of the same patient. Diffuse inflammatory changes with swelling, reddening, and coarsening of the rugae are apparent.

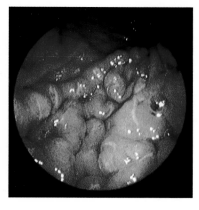

Figure 7.24 Complete erosions. These discrete nodular bulges aligned along the fold show central erosive patches.

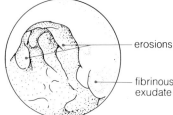 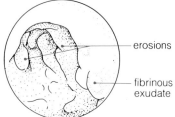

erosions

fibrinous exudate

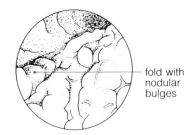

fold with nodular bulges

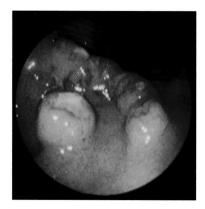

Figure 7.25 Large, complete varioliform erosions with deep central defects covered by a white fibrinous exudate. Some endoscopists suspect that such nodules may lead to formation of hyperplastic polyps.

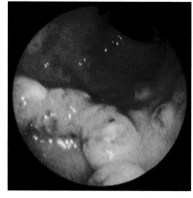

Figure 7.26 Early partial healing of complete erosions. Proximally, erosions still manifest a white necrotic slough. Distally, the erosive defect has healed, as indicated by the appearance of an intensely red fleck in the center of the nodule.

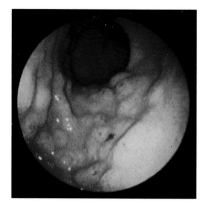

Figure 7.27 More complete healing of complete erosions. A reddish dot remains in center of the nodule, indicative of regenerating epithelium.

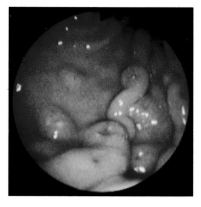

Figure 7.28 Complete erosions during follow-up. Necrotic central depressions become smaller, to be exchanged with a reddish fleck.

fairly simple to detect endoscopically because of the sharp distinction between the exudate over the base and the surrounding erythematous mucosa. They often occur over the crests of gastric folds, especially just proximal to the pylorus. These lesions often heal within days but may persist longer.

Complete or varioliform erosions have an elevated, inflamed border surrounding a small depressed central necrotic patch (Fig. 7.22). The center may be initially hemorrhagic, but after 1 or 2 days it turns yellow-gray as a patch of fibrinous exudate forms (Fig. 7.23). These nodular elevations usually measure between 5 and 10 mm. Complete erosions are usually multiple and develop in the antrum, although they are also found in the corpus and fundus (see Fig. 7.23, *right*). Quite often, complete erosions are aligned along a fold directed toward the pylorus (Fig. 7.24). Endoscopically, these erosive areas have a specific appearance. They often present as a series of nodules or bulges on the crests of the folds, characteristically in the antrum. The distinguishing characteristic, apparent on both endoscopic and radiographic appearance, is a central depression or erosion.

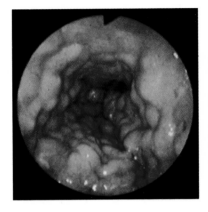

Figure 7.29 Final healing stage of complete erosions. Only the nodular elevations remain, giving the mucosa a coarsely nodular aspect. Epithelial defects have disappeared.

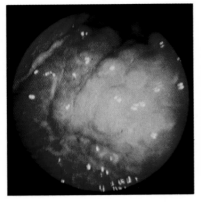

Figure 7.30 Detail of coarsely nodular cobblestone-like deformity developed after healing of complete erosions.

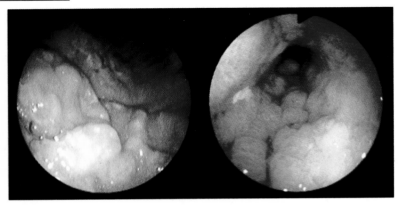

Figure 7.31 Certain malignant diseases in the stomach may mimic complete erosions. *Left,* Non-Hodgkin's lymphoma. *Right,* Metastatic breast cancer.

When not healed, they often are covered with a white or brown exudate. When they heal, the depression in the center is covered with normal-appearing mucosa. Interestingly, although these lesions usually heal in a few days, they may persist for months or years.

Complete erosions may evolve into hyperplastic polyps, presumably due to foveolar hyperplasia in the borders surrounding the central crater (Fig. 7.25). Some feel that this progression is substantiated by the appearance of the tip of the polyp, suggesting a healed erosion (Figs. 7.26 to 7.30). Some investigators do not accept this hypothesis and feel that complete erosions and hyperplastic polyps are different types of responses to injury.

Lymphomatous or metastatic lesions in the stomach occasionally mimic the appearance of complete erosions (Fig. 7.31). An atypical appearance of a lesion should alert the endoscopist that multiple biopsies are needed.

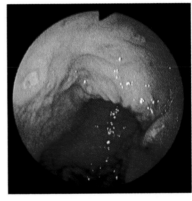
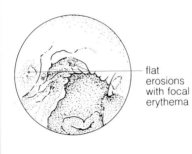

flat erosions with focal erythema

Figure 7.32 Multiple, flat, drug-induced erosions in the antrum. Focal erythema is apparent around the white-based lesions.

DRUG-INDUCED GASTRITIS

The gastric mucosa is vulnerable to injury by drugs, especially aspirin and other nonsteroidal anti-inflammatory drugs (NSAID). Endoscopically identifiable lesions develop in virtually all patients at the start of aspirin therapy, whereas only 20 to 50% of patients on long-term aspirin therapy (several months) have evidence of mucosal injury. Although there are systemic effects from the absorbed agent, the injury may be largely caused by topical or local irritation brought on by the drug in contact with the mucosa.

When aspirin injures the stomach, the location of the injury varies depending where the tablet rests while it dissolves. The lower body of the stomach and antrum are characteristically involved; however, acute gastritis can also involve other areas of the stomach. The lesions often radiate from the pylorus, ranging from a red, hemorrhagic dot to a confluence of dots, merging into a streak or a small erosion with a white center and surrounding erythema (Fig. 7.32). These lesions may progress to larger erosions and eventually to ulceration.

Aspirin or other NSAIDs may also induce the formation of large ulcers (over 1.5 cm in diameter). These ulcers often occur without endoscopic evidence of erosions or erythema in the surrounding mucosa. Usually no evidence of chronic gastritis is seen on biopsy of the surrounding mucosa, as may be seen with non-medication–associated gastric ulcers.

Erosive drug-induced lesions may heal after several days, even with continued ingestion of anti-inflammatory drugs. Large ulcers associated with anti-inflammatory agents heal completely once the offending drug is stopped. These erosions and ulcers may also heal if the patient is placed on H$_2$ receptor blockers while aspirin or NSAID therapy is continued.

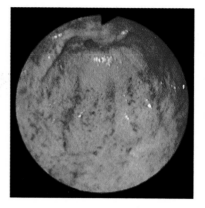

Figure 7.33 View of aspirin-induced gastritis in the antrum. Hemorrhages appear as linear petechial streaks.

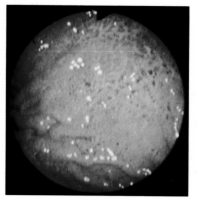

Figure 7.34 In this view, hemorrhagic gastritis is characterized by brownish-black flecks in a sharply delineated area.

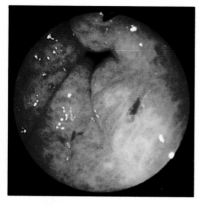

Figure 7.35 Antral telangiectasia in a patient with liver cirrhosis may simulate hemorrhagic gastritis.

HEMORRHAGIC GASTRITIS

Hemorrhagic gastritis is often drug-induced, particularly by aspirin or related compounds. Mucosal or submucosal hemorrhagic spots are the predominant lesions in this type of gastritis. Endoscopically, these spots are reddish or brownish-black, of variable size, and usually sharply delineated (Figs. 7.33 and 7.34). Occasionally they may be indistinguishable from focally dilated vascular structures (Fig. 7.35). Necrotic erosive areas may also be present.

Four grades are commonly used to describe hemorrhagic gastritis. In grade 1, one spot or area of mucosal hemorrhage is visible. Grade 2A has at least two areas of mucosal hemorrhage but they are not numerous or widespread. In grade 2B, two or more mucosal hemorrhages are associated with edema. In grade 3, there are numerous areas of mucosal hemorrhage. In grade 4, there is a large area of mucosal hemorrhage with active bleeding or widespread involvement of the stomach. (The term mucosal hemorrhages refers to both mucosal and submucosal hemorrhagic spots.)

STRESS-INDUCED GASTRITIS

Stress-related gastritis is usually associated with severe trauma, hypotension, sepsis, jaundice, renal failure, respiratory failure, surgical procedures, major burns (Curling's ulcer), and neurosurgery (Cushing's ulcer). Acute stress-related mucosal damage is usually preceded by shock, which decreases gastric mucosal blood flow. Once the primary disease is successfully treated, mucosal regeneration usually occurs, and the integrity of the gastric mucosa is restored. Lesions also occur after intracranial trauma and are often more deeply penetrating than those associated with other causes. Acute stress-related lesions begin minutes or hours after the trauma as shallow erosions in the fundic region of the stomach. In the next 24 hours, petechiae and multiple shallow red-based erosions may be observed in the fundic area. By 48 hours, the erosions deepen and may look black-based with raised upper margins. The erosions may spread to involve the entire corpus and antrum. Extension of the necrotic process to the submucosal layer leads to ulceration. Because major blood vessels may be present in the submucosa, these deep lesions are more likely associated with severe hemorrhage.

Such patients are examined because of upper GI bleeding. Typically, they are hospitalized in intensive care units, often intubated and on assisted ventilation when examined. Some experience is necessary to insert even a small-caliber endoscope past an endotracheal tube in the posterior pharynx. Inspection with a laryngoscope may assist the passage of the endoscope through the cricopharyngeus sphincter.

GASTRITIS OR GASTROPATHY WITH GIANT FOLDS

Gastric rugae are considered enlarged when the folds are wider than 8 to 10 mm (Fig. 7.36). True enlarged or giant folds do not flatten during maximum insufflation. When the folds reveal caliber changes or polypoid irregularities, an inflammatory or infiltrative process seems likely. Giant folds may be spread out over the stomach but are usually present only in the corpus-fundus area. Areas of fold enlargement may begin abruptly or gradually (Fig. 7.37).

Biopsy with a standard biopsy forceps is insufficiently deep to demonstrate foveolar and glandular hyperplasia;

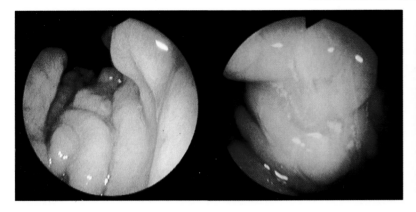
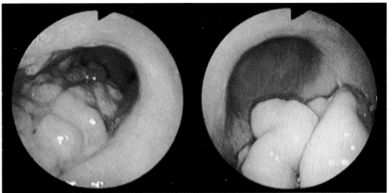

Figure 7.36 Ménétrier's disease. *Left,* These are true giant folds in the corpus area, as evidenced by their persistence despite maximum insufflation. *Right,* A detailed view of the giant folds with adherent mucus strands.

Figure 7.37 Ménétrier's disease. *Left,* A cluster of enlarged folds are seen along the greater curve and persist despite maximum air insufflation. Note the mucus strands. *Right,* The abrupt onset of enlarged folds is obvious in this view.

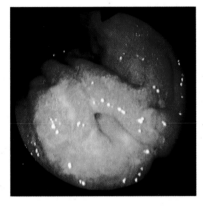
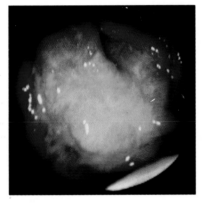
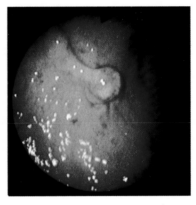
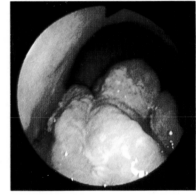

Figure 7.38 Ménétrier's disease. Thickened folds and abundant accumulation of mucus are characteristic.

Figure 7.39 In this patient, Ménétrier-like changes of the greater curve occurred after a pancreatic cystogastrostomy.

Figure 7.40 Antral polypoid lesion in Ménétrier's disease. Giant folds can occur in the antrum but are less often seen than are polyps.

Figure 7.41 Ménétrier's disease. Giant folds here simulate malignancy.

therefore, use of a large-caliber biopsy forceps is recommended. Alternatively, macroparticle biopsy taken with a polypectomy diathermy snare yields specimens 1 to 3 mm in depth, extending into the submucosal layer and averaging about 10 mm in diameter. After ensnaring a large fold, the electrosurgical snare is tightened and the gastric fold is lifted up and away from the gastric wall during the excision to limit depth of damage. The sample is then grasped with the snare and retrieved. This biopsy technique has a higher complication rate than the large-caliber forceps biopsy technique.

The most common causes of enlarged gastric folds are Ménétrier's disease, hypertrophic (hypersecretory) gastritis or gastropathy, Zollinger-Ellison syndrome, lymphoma, carcinoma, peptic ulcer disease, postoperative stomach, granulomatous disease, and gastric varices.

Ménétrier's disease is characterized by impressive foveolar elongation with hyperplasia of mucus-producing cells. This leads to cystic dilation of gastric glands with regression of the glandular tubules. Parietal and chief cells are decreased in number, resulting in acid hyposecretion. The most characteristic appearance endoscopically is that of significantly enlarged giant folds, especially in the corpus area, which do not flatten upon maximum insufflation (see Fig. 7.36). The folds may be convoluted and occasionally appear reddish. Focal variations in caliber are common. There is a conspicuous increase in mucus secretion resulting in strands of mucus covering the folds (Figs. 7.38 and 7.39). Enlarged folds may also occur in the antrum, but polypoid structures are more common there (Fig. 7.40). The question of eventual malignant degeneration has been raised. The appearance of the folds may simulate malignancy (Fig. 7.41).

Hypertrophic (hypersecretory) gastritis or gastropathy has a similar endoscopic appearance to Ménétrier's disease

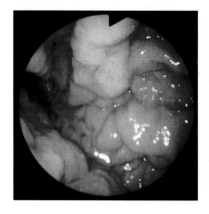

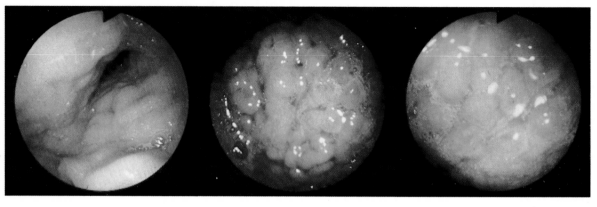

Figure 7.42 Hypertrophic gastritis with coarsely enlarged fold pattern.

Figure 7.43 Hypertrophic gastritis. *Left,* Narrowing of the lumen with coarse nodular deformity and broadening of the fold pattern. *Center,* Detail of coarse nodular deformity. *Right,* Closeup view shows mucus strands between the cobblestone-like deformity of the broadened folds.

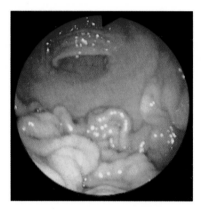

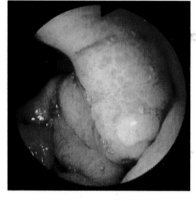

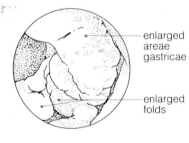

Figure 7.44 Zollinger-Ellison syndrome, marked by an enlarged fold pattern.

Figure 7.45 Zollinger-Ellison syndrome. Massive enlargement of fold pattern and marked accentuation of areae gastricae pattern are evident.

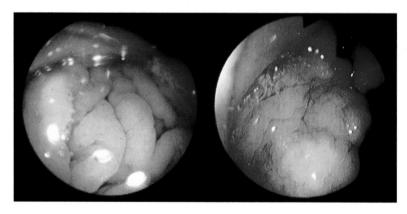

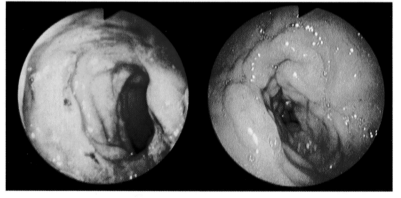

Figure 7.46 *Left,* This patient presented with ulcer jejuni pepticum. After a partial resection (Billroth II), a Zollinger-Ellison-like pattern of accentuated folds developed. *Right,* Accentuation of areae gastricae can be seen.

Figure 7.47 *Left,* Zollinger-Ellison syndrome with extensive bulbo-duodenitis. *Right,* Healing of bulbo-duodenitis after 3 weeks of omeprazole therapy.

and is characterized by hypertrophy of the glandular and foveolar layers (Figs. 7.42 and 7.43).

In Zollinger-Ellison syndrome, the glandular hyperplasia is caused by the trophic action of gastrin from a gastrinoma. The mucosal thickness may be increased to 2 to 3 mm (Fig. 7.44). In most patients the folds are only slightly enlarged and covered with copious amounts of clear, very acidic fluid. Occasionally, the folds are slightly irregular or finely nod-

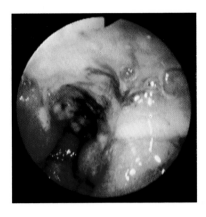

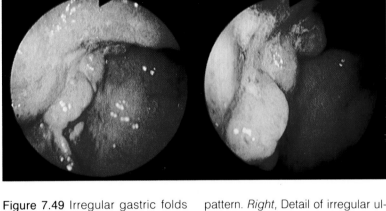

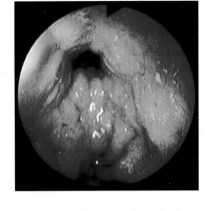

Figure 7.48 Zollinger-Ellison syndrome. Extensive ulceration of the second part of the duodenum is due to acid hypersecretion.

Figure 7.49 Irregular gastric folds due to lymphoma. *Left,* Coarse, enlarged, nodular deformity of fold pattern. *Right,* Detail of irregular ulceration in the center of enlarged folds.

Figure 7.50 Abnormal folds in linitis plastica. This appearance is most often seen as a manifestation of adenocarcinoma, but can also appear in benign conditions such as gastric syphilis.

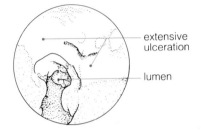

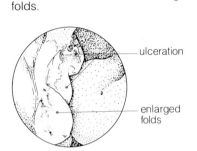

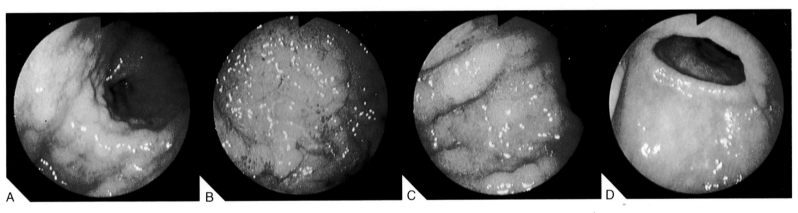

Figure 7.51 Gastric pseudolymphoma. **A** Coarse cobblestone-like deformity of the fold pattern. **B** Coarsely nodular deformity of the rugal pattern. **C** Closeup of the nodular fold deformity and of inflammatory changes. **D** A gaping, immobile pyloric sphincter area in this same patient.

ular. There may also be a conspicuous increase in the size of the areae gastricae (Figs. 7.45 and 7.46). Concomitant gastric ulceration is rare except when there is stasis associated with delayed gastric emptying because of peptic ulcer disease or scarring in the duodenal bulb or postbulbar duodenum. Diffuse inflammation with erosive defects may also be found in the bulb and descending duodenum (Fig. 7.47). Large deep ulcers may be present in the bulb or in the postbulbar duodenum up to the duodenal jejunal flexure (Fig. 7.48).

Irregular gastric folds may also occur in lymphoreticular malignancies. They are usually seen in combination with erosive or bizarrely shaped ulcerative defects (Figs. 7.49 and 7.50).

Enlarged gastric folds may also occur in pseudolymphoma of the stomach, also called benign lymphatic hyperplasia. Occasionally, concomitant superficial or deep and irregular epithelial defects may be present in addition to irregular enlargement of the fold pattern. Cobblestone-like deformity of the mucosal surface may occasionally be seen, especially in the antrum and corpus (Fig. 7.51). The characteristic histologic finding in this condition is the presence of mature lymph follicles with germinal centers; the inflammatory infiltrate has a polyclonal character.

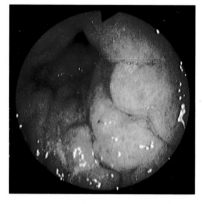 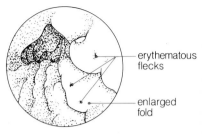

Figure 7.52 Postradiotherapy gastritic changes show enlarged folds and erythematous flecks.

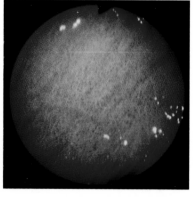 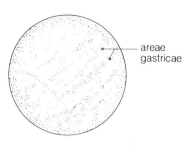

Figure 7.53 Mild radiation damage. Numerous red islands of areae gas- tricae are separated by connecting, pale, linear areas of lineae gastricae.

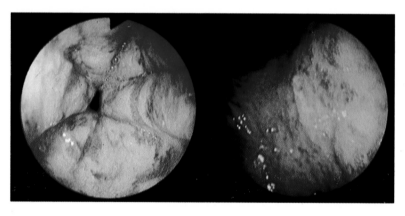

Figure 7.54 Radiation gastritis. *Left,* In the antrum, conspicuous telangiectasia and antral narrowing are apparent. *Right,* Corresponding radiation-induced telangiectatic changes in the corpus-fundus region.

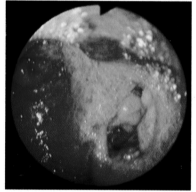

Figure 7.55 Severe radiation damage with pronounced erythema and friability. A gastrojejunostomy was necessary because of gastric outlet obstruction, due to marked antral narrowing.

RADIATION-INDUCED GASTRITIS

Radiation therapy delivered to the upper abdomen may damage the gastric mucosa, producing varying degrees of erythema and friability and prominent gastric folds with diminished pliability (Fig. 7.52). This injury varies in form. The initial injury is characteristically acute inflammation with erythema (Fig. 7.53). If the injury progresses, shallow or deep ulcers may occur and perforate. As they heal, scarring may occur with marked retraction of the lumen. Scar formation can obstruct the gastric outlet. Another finding characteristic of the gastric injury, also noted in colonic injury, is the formation of telangiectasia. Several of these characteristic findings may be noted in a patient (Figs. 7.54 and 7.55).

Differentiation between radiation damage and recurrent malignancy is sometimes difficult. Prominent ulcerative folds of a rubbery consistency with poor tenting of the mucosa are common both to radiation damage and to tumors such as recurrent lymphoma. Multiple biopsies are necessary to make a diagnosis of lymphomatous invasion. Endosonography may also help in the diagnosis of diffuse tumor invasion.

GRANULOMATOUS LESIONS

Several conditions affect the stomach, producing lesions characterized by granulomas. These include granulomatous gastritis, Crohn's disease, and sarcoidosis.

Primary idiopathic granulomatous gastritis affects the elderly and usually involves the more proximal stomach. Endoscopic findings are nonspecific, ranging from normal mucosa, to scattered areas of erythema, to fine or coarse granularity of the mucosa, to obvious irregular nodular deformity of the folds (Figs. 7.56 and 7.57).

In Crohn's disease, involvement of the upper GI tract nearly always occurs in conjunction with involvement elsewhere in the bowel. The frequency of gastric involvement is variable, and the lesions are indistinguishable from those due to causes such as drugs. The diagnosis is nearly impossible to make without involvement of other areas of the bowel. Overall, the endoscopic findings include erythema, mucosal nodularity, aphthoid erosions, and linear or serpiginous ulcers. The prepyloric antrum is a commonly involved site. Typically, aphthoid erosions are seen focally in the prepyloric antrum with the intervening mucosa uninvolved (Fig.7.58). In other cases, the mucosa between the

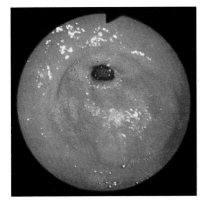

Figure 7.56 Granulomatous gastritis in the antrum. Patchy areas of erythema are apparent.

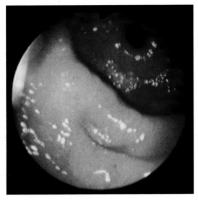

Figure 7.57 Granulomatous gastritis in the corpus with a small punched-out ulcer.

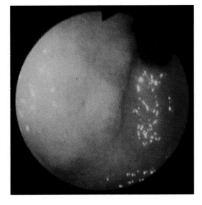

Figure 7.58 Crohn's disease of the stomach. A tiny aphthoid erosion in the antrum is typical.

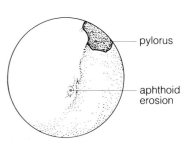

pylorus

aphthoid erosion

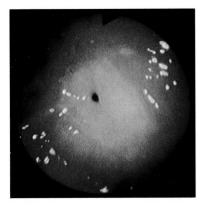

Figure 7.59 Crohn's disease of the stomach, with pinpoint gastric outlet

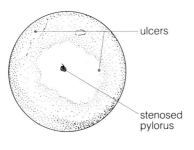

ulcers

stenosed pylorus

obstruction. Note surrounding antral ulceration.

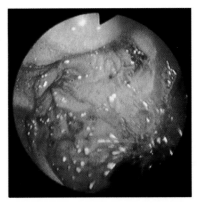

Figure 7.60 Superficial ulcers have developed around a gastroenterostomy in a patient with Crohn's dis-

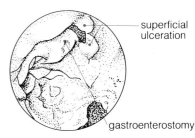

superficial ulceration

gastroenterostomy

ease involving the stomach. The original gastric outlet obstruction was caused by the Crohn's disease.

ulcerations becomes nodular or polypoid, resulting in a cobblestone-like appearance. In addition there may be considerable scarring and deformity of the antrum. If the pyloric channel is narrowed, the stomach may be dilated. Antral peristalsis is diminished, and stricturing may give rise to symptoms of gastric outlet obstruction (Fig. 7.59). Aphthoid erosions and small or large serpiginous ulcers may also occur in the body of the stomach or may develop around a gastrojejunostomy performed for gastric outlet obstruction (Fig. 7.60).

Sarcoidosis may also affect the stomach and should be included in the differential diagnosis of granulomatous lesions. The antrum is commonly involved: the antral folds are prominent, antral deformity occurs, and occasionally there are epithelial destructive lesions. The lack of distensibility and the presence of nodules may mimic an infiltrating malignancy.

Alkaline Reflux Gastritis

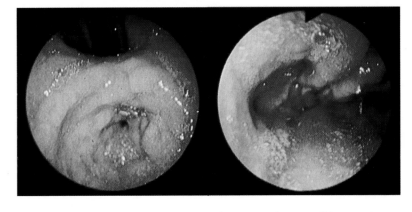

Figure 7.61 Alkaline biliary reflux in the intact stomach. *Left,* The antrum has patchy erythema. *Right,* Corresponding view of the corpus-fundus area shows striking erythema and abundance of bile-stained liquid.

ALKALINE OR BILIARY REFLUX GASTRITIS

Gastritis due to recurrent alkaline or biliary reflux may occur in patients because of an incompetent pylorus. Edema and marked hyperemia are the usual findings (Fig. 7.61). Such changes may also be seen after an episode of prolonged vomiting.

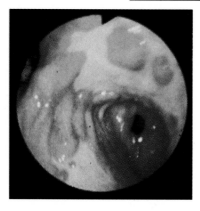

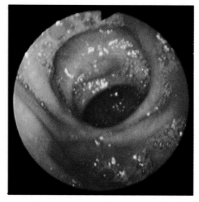

Figure 7.62 Extensive ulceration of the distal stomach after sloughing of necrosis. This damage was caused by ingestion of strong acid.

Figure 7.63 Marked scarring, retraction, and deformity of the greater curvature area due to previous extensive caustic damage.

OTHER MUCOSAL ABNORMALITIES

MASTOCYTOSIS

Gastric and duodenal involvement in mastocytosis may result in erosive, ulcerative defects that tend to bleed. The gastric folds may also appear thick with focal erythema, edema, and flat, round, urticaria-type lesions.

CAUSTIC GASTRIC DAMAGE

Common agents causing caustic gastric damage include sulfuric, acetic, and hydrochloric acids. Less common agents include nitric, formic, and chromic acids. Alkali and lye burns are usually due to caustic soda and bleach. Endoscopy provides information on the extent and severity of the injury. It is a safe procedure in the absence of evidence of perforation or transmural necrosis. The procedure is usually performed with a small-caliber endoscope. Examination of the oropharynx and hypopharynx should always precede endoscopic examination. The presence of an oropharyngeal burn increases the possibility of an esophageal or gastric burn being present. However, as with esophageal injury, there is no correlation between oropharyngeal involvement and presence or severity of lesions in the stomach.

Areas of physiologic narrowing within the esophagus should be carefully examined; damage is often most severe at the lower end. The proximal esophagus may be relatively spared. Involvement of the stomach is usually most severe along the lesser curvature and in the region of the antrum. Concentrated acids or bleach produce isolated gastric damage in a substantial percentage of patients.

Caustic damage or burn to the gastric mucosa may be graded in three stages: mild (grade 1), moderate (grade 2), and severe (grade 3). In grade 1, the only abnormalities are focal or linear streaks of erythema. In grade 2, a few ulcerations are visible in addition to the hyperemia, and there may be slight hemorrhage. The ulcers are usually smaller than 5 mm in diameter, and the focal superficial areas of necrosis are limited to a portion of the esophagus or stomach. In grade 3 there are multiple erosions indicating extensive necrosis of the mucosal lining involving the entire esophagus, stomach, or both, or major parts of the upper digestive tract (Fig. 7.62). In addition to deep ulcerations, there may be massive hemorrhage. The incidence of esophageal and gastric complications after caustic damage is difficult to assess. The most important complications involve esophageal stricture, gastric perforation, scarring (Fig. 7.63), and gastric outlet obstruction.

UPPER GASTROINTESTINAL BLEEDING

Bleeding from the upper gastrointestinal tract is a commonly encountered problem in clinical medicine. The estimated incidence in the United States is about 100 cases per 100,000 per year. The mortality for upper GI bleeding has remained at 10% for the past 40 years, although in view of the aging U.S. population and consequent changes in underlying illnesses, this observation may not be meaningful.

ENDOSCOPIC DIAGNOSIS

Lesions that frequently present with GI bleeding include esophageal varices, gastric ulcers, and duodenal ulcers. When endoscopy is performed within 24 hours of the onset of bleeding, a definitive diagnosis is possible in 80 to 95% of patients. Figure 7.64 summarizes causes of bleeding in a recent series of 2225 cases collected and analyzed by the American Society for Gastrointestinal Endoscopy.

Routine endoscopic evaluation of all patients hospitalized with upper GI bleeding has been criticized on the grounds that a precise diagnosis does not necessarily affect outcome.

Causes of Gastrointestinal Bleeding	
Cause	%
Duodenal ulcer	24.3
Gastric erosions	23.4
Gastric ulcer	21.3
Varices	10.3
Mallory-Weiss tear	7.2
Esophagitis	6.3
Erosive duodenitis	5.8
Neoplasm	2.9
Stomal ulcer	1.8
Esophageal ulcer	1.7
Osler-Weber-Rendu telangiectasia	0.5
Other	6.3

Figure 7.64 Causes of gastrointestinal bleeding. (From the American Society for Gastrointestinal Endoscopy)

In a prospective randomized study of hospitalized patients who were not actively bleeding after the first 6 hours of admission, no difference was found in mortality or morbidity between those who underwent endoscopy and those who had an upper GI X-ray.

The lack of a detectable effect may relate to deficiencies in current treatment of bleeding from specific GI lesions. If effective treatment for GI bleeding becomes available, whether pharmacologic or endoscopic, the outcome for the patient may be dramatically changed by having precise diagnosis made at endoscopy. Ultimately, through clinical trials, we will be able to understand the role that endoscopy will play in the diagnosis and treatment of upper GI bleeding.

THERAPEUTIC TECHNIQUES

Endoscopy now offers not only diagnosis but also therapy. Most endoscopic techniques used to achieve hemostasis use heat to coagulate the bleeding vessels (Fig. 7.65). However they differ substantially in the approach, cost, and ease of use.

LASER PHOTOCOAGULATION

Photocoagulation of a bleeding lesion using an Nd-YAG laser is effective in stopping bleeding. The perforation rate

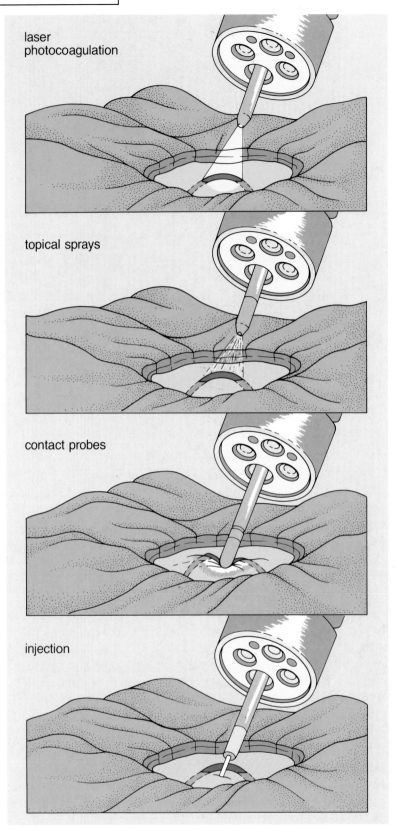

laser photocoagulation

topical sprays

contact probes

injection

Figure 7.65 Endoscopic hemostatic methods.

associated with this technique is 1 to 2%. The laser technique is the most expensive of the hemostatic techniques and is not generally portable; thus, the patient must be taken to the laser therapy area.

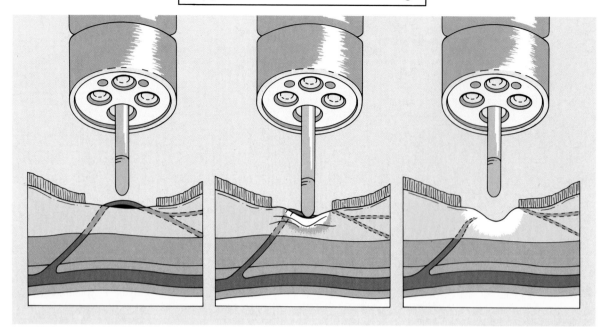

Figure 7.66 Schematic representation of endoscopic hemostasis. A heater probe is pushed against a vessel in the base of a peptic ulcer. A jet of water is used to wash the area prior to heating. If the vessel is me-chanically pressed closed (coapted), bleeding stops. The probe is then activated and the vessel heated and coagulated.

HEATER PROBE

This device is passed down the biopsy channel of an endoscope and pressed against the bleeding lesion. The tip is then rapidly heated to seal the vessel during coaptation (Fig. 7.66). This portable device is relatively inexpensive compared to a laser, and to date has been as safe or safer than the Nd-YAG laser.

ELECTROCOAGULATION

In the monopolar electrocoagulation approach, a radio-frequency current is passed between the active electrode and a broad patient-contact plate. The flow of electrical energy in the small area where the electrode touches the tissue results in heating and coagulation of tissue proteins. The technique is inexpensive and, hemostatically, moderately effective. There have been few studies comparing the hemostatic effectiveness of techniques such as monopolar electrocoagulation with other hemostatic approaches such as the laser. However, monopolar electrocoagulation is reported to be associated with a 1% risk of perforation, and the probe tends to stick to the treated tissue, causing rebleeding when it is removed. The electrohydrothermal approach improves on the monopolar approach by using a continuous flow of liquid at the tip of the electrode. The electrical energy passes through this liquid, preventing sticking and reducing the problem of rebleeding when the probe is removed from the coagulated tissue. The bipolar approach is applied using the BICAP probe. This technique is effective and seems to be safe. Controlled clinical comparisons of the BICAP probe and the heater probe are currently underway.

INJECTION

Alcohol, sclerosants, and vasoconstrictors may be injected into the tissue adjacent to the bleeding vessel to stop hemorrhage. Early reports indicate that this technique is effective and safe. Sclerotherapy is an effective approach to control bleeding esophageal varices.

TECHNICAL ASPECTS

Upper GI endoscopy in patients with bleeding is not a simple procedure and should be performed by experienced endoscopists. Prior to endoscopy the patient is appropriately resuscitated, for example, with insertion of intravenous lines and volume replacement.

The patient's stomach should be emptied of blood and clots as completely as possible. We generally use a large-bore (34 French = 11 mm) tube with extra holes cut in the tip for this procedure. The tube is passed via the mouth with the patient in the left lateral decubitus position and preferably with the head slightly lower than the feet. Suction is available to remove blood or fluid from the oropharynx to prevent aspiration if regurgitation occurs around the orogastric tube (this is also important during endoscopy). Once the tube is in the stomach, the gastric contents are sampled by passive drainage. One should avoid pulling hard on a syringe to remove the contents, as this causes submucosal injury and may confuse the endoscopic interpretation. Water or saline can be gently infused to wash the stomach and remove the blood and clots. An anesthetic spray may be applied to the oropharynx prior to insertion of the endoscope. Use of a spray may slightly increase the chance of aspiration during the procedure but is generally safe. Sedation is optional depending on the general status of the patient. If the patient is hypotensive, administering drugs which could further lower the pressure may be ill-advised.

The endoscope selected varies with the clinical circumstance. If treatment will be attempted, one of the therapeutic endoscopes with a large channel is recommended. The channel helps somewhat with the removal of fluid and clots and with the passage of therapeutic devices.

The endoscope is passed with the patient lying on the left side. Expert endoscopic assistance is essential to reassure the patient and to help protect the patient's airway against aspiration. The esophagus is inspected first to look for signs of esophagitis, ulceration, and varices. The stomach is inspected directly and with the endoscope retroflexed. If a clot is present, the instrument is usually directed above or over the clot to enter the lower gastric body and antrum. In the case of a bleeding duodenal ulcer, blood may be seen refluxing back from the duodenum through the pylorus when this area is inspected from the antral side. The instrument is then advanced to the duodenum. It is important to identify whether a clot or blood vessel is visible in a duodenal or gastric ulcer. With a visible vessel, there is an increased chance of rebleeding, and therefore these lesions may be suitable for endoscopic therapy.

If possible, the endoscope is advanced into the descending duodenum to detect any postbulbar ulcers or lesions. Then, as the endoscope is gradually withdrawn, the descending duodenum, duodenal bulb, pyloric channel, antrum, and stomach are inspected. Retroflexion is essential to detect lesser curve, cardial, and fundal lesions. It may be necessary to reposition the patient, shifting the gastric pool and blood to uncover areas of the gastric mucosa for inspection. If there is active bleeding, a stream of blood can be followed to locate and determine the source. A vortex of blood seen in the pool may be caused by an arterial jet; repositioning the patient may allow this area to be inspected. A decision can then be made regarding use of endoscopic hemostatic therapy. It is essential when repositioning the patient to take steps to prevent vomiting and aspiration. The importance of having well-trained assistants cannot be overemphasized.

In summary, we do recommend endoscopy in patients with significant upper GI bleeding. In the vast majority of these patients, several facts about the bleeding can be established: (1) that the patient is having an upper GI hemorrhage; (2) whether the bleeding is from the esophagus, stomach, or duodenum; (3) exactly what type of lesion is bleeding; and (4) whether the bleeding is ongoing. All this information may be very important to plan therapy for these patients. It is certainly essential for a surgeon who must operate on a patient with torrential bleeding to know the diagnosis preoperatively. Information obtained from endoscopic inspection may help predict the clinical course of the patient in terms of potential rebleeding.

Also, we can now treat patients with upper GI bleeding using endoscopic hemostatic devices. These devices in early clinical trials seem to provide effective hemostasis with a very low risk of complication. Many active bleeders can be stopped permanently. In other cases, the technique may control the bleeding temporarily, converting emergency surgery to elective surgery, with a much lower risk of morbidity and mortality. In the future, pharmacologic agents may be used to control bleeding. Candidates for this approach include H_2 blockers, prostaglandins, and other hormones such as somatostatin. Further clinical trials are necessary to complete the evaluation of both pharmacologic agents and endoscopic hemostatic devices. Hopefully we will be able to demonstrate that some of these approaches safely and effectively benefit patients with upper GI bleeding.

8

Small Bowel

This chapter reviews the endoscopic appearance of the normal pylorus, bulb, and duodenum. Abnormal findings related to extrinsic factors, peptic disease, and nonpeptic disease are presented, as well as vascular abnormalities and tumors of the small bowel.

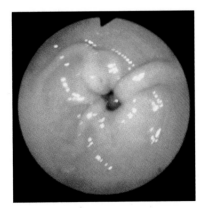

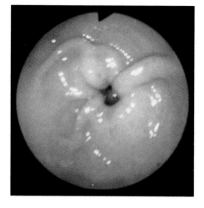

Figure 8.1 Pyloric channel. This view shows the opening with prominent radiating folds.

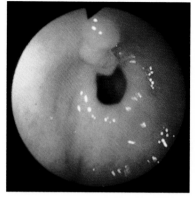

Figure 8.2 Pyloric channel. A prepyloric fold is located at its midpoint.

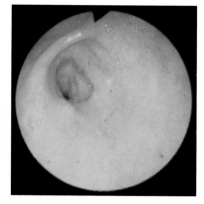

Figure 8.3 This eccentrically located pylorus has a rooflike fold.

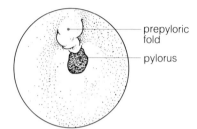

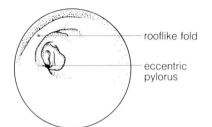

THE PYLORUS

ENDOSCOPIC APPEARANCE OF THE PYLORUS

The pyloric channel is a tubular opening, 5 mm long, which expands to a diameter of 1 to 1.5 cm when relaxed. A larger channel is referred to as patulous. The antrum surrounding the pylorus may show folds radiating from the pylorus or relatively smooth mucosa (Fig. 8.1). Sometimes a prepyloric, rooflike fold lies over the midpoint of the channel; although it may appear distorted, the channel itself is symmetrical (Fig. 8.2). The pyloric channel is usually in the center of the distal antrum, but sometimes lies adjacent to the greater or lesser curve (Fig 8.3). A 13-mm-diameter endoscope usually passes easily through the channel.

ENDOSCOPIC APPEARANCE OF THE DISEASED PYLORUS

Peptic ulcer disease is the most common abnormality of the pyloric channel (Fig. 8.4). If peptic ulcer disease is suspected, several passes of the endoscope are required to examine each quadrant for recessed or otherwise hidden ulcers, especially if the channel is deformed. Ulcers will usually be found between the opening of the channel and a pyloroduodenal junction fold. Wide-caliber instruments do not allow a detailed examination of the channel in one pass; a 9 mm instrument is preferable.

A smooth, perfectly symmetrical prepyloric antrum with intact mucosa in a patient with a narrowed, abnormal pylorus suggests benign ulcer stenosis, whereas an asymmetrical appearance or an ulcer with atypical features suggests malignancy. If pyloric folds are prominent, the margin of a benign pyloric channel ulcer may appear nodular or masslike, especially if the ulcer is deep. A pyloric channel ulcer is indistinguishable from a malignancy if the margins are markedly irregular or heaped-up, and the base does not show a sharp differentiation from the surrounding mucosa. It may be difficult to distinguish heavy folds caused by a benign ulcer from that caused by a malignancy. Clues to a malignancy include indurated, irregular folds with an associated sessile or polypoid mass and either shallow or deep adjacent ulceration (Fig. 8.5). Ultimately, echo endoscopy may distinguish between a wall affected by ulcer scarring from that thickened by a tumor not apparent from the mucosal surface.

Pyloric deformity may result from narrowing of the channel due to scarring from previous ulceration. This scarring may also coincide with a transverse, pyloroduodenal junction fold connecting the anterior wall of the channel with the posterior wall of the bulb (Fig. 8.6), which may accentuate the anterior fornix. Scarring and retraction of bulbar ulceration may also cause pyloric changes, including an eccentric location or keyhole deformity (Fig. 8.7).

A double, or split, pylorus occurs when a fistula forms between the prepyloric antrum and the duodenal bulb as a

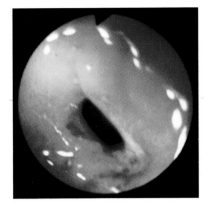

Figure 8.4 Pyloric channel ulcer.

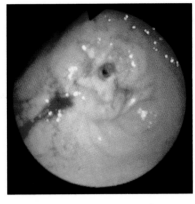

Figure 8.5 Distal antral malignancy is infiltrating and narrowing the pyloric channel.

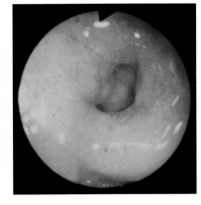

Figure 8.6 Deformity of the pyloric channel. A transverse pyloroduo-

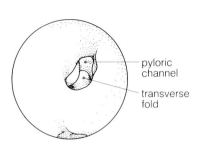

denal junctional fold due to ulcer scarring narrows the channel.

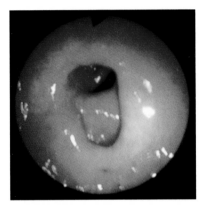

Figure 8.7 Keyhole deformity of pyloric channel. Scarring and retraction due to bulbar ulcer disease have caused these changes.

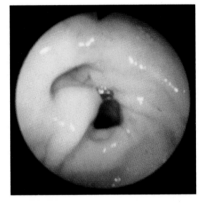

Figure 8.8 Split pylorus. The fistula created above the original pyloric opening is the result of a penetrating ulcer.

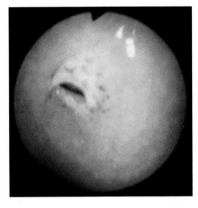

Figure 8.9 Pyloric stenosis. In this patient, the narrowing occurred after pyloroplasty.

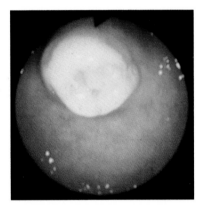

Figure 8.10 Adult-type hypertrophic pyloric stenosis. Thickened pylorus muscle, which can be easily passed by a standard endoscope, bulges into the antrum.

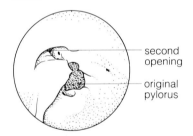

consequence of a penetrating ulcer. Most often this is located above the original pyloric channel (Fig. 8.8). When this fistula heals, the mucosa may appear similar to that of a double pylorus with little evidence of the old inflammation and fistula.

The channel is considered abnormally narrow when it measures less than 1 cm in diameter, has lost its compliance, and does not admit even a 9 mm endoscope. However, failure to pass an endoscope may simply reflect inadequacy of technique in centering or stabilizing the tip. If the channel is less than 6 mm in diameter it is considered pyloric stenosis. Sometimes the pylorus is so small as to become difficult to identify. For practical reasons the pylorus is called stenotic when it is impossible to pass a small-caliber endoscope (9 mm diameter or less)(Fig. 8.9).

Not infrequently pyloric obstruction leads to the formation of gastric bezoars. Occasionally an ulcer located proximal to, within, or just distal to the already compromised pylorus functionally obstructs the channel because of inflammation and edema.

In adult-type hypertrophic pyloric stenosis, the pyloric channel is elongated, extending over 2 cm. In addition, there is extensive circular prepyloric folding which extends into the lumen. The pylorus protrudes into the antrum with a masslike deformity (Fig. 8.10) due to compression of the prepyloric mucosa by the hypertrophic pyloric musculature.

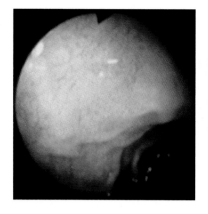

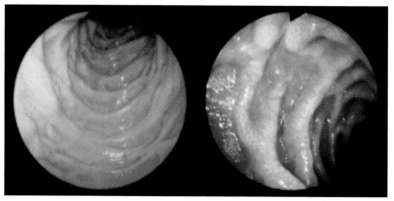

Figure 8.11 Mucosa of the bulb has a villous appearance.

Figure 8.12 *Left,*Whitish discoloration of mucosa due to lipid accumulation in the lamina propria lacteals. *Right,* In a similar case, detailed view of the whitish discoloration of the mucosa covering Kerckring's folds.

THE BULB AND DUODENUM

ENDOSCOPIC APPEARANCE OF THE BULB AND DUODENUM

THE DUODENAL BULB

The duodenal bulb is a small, triangular structure 4 to 6 cm long and 2 to 3 cm wide that bridges the more anterior, intraperitoneal antrum of the stomach with the more posterior, retroperitoneal descending duodenum. The base of the bulbar triangle is demarcated by the angular fornices. From these, the anterior and posterior walls extend to a third triangular terminal point, the apex.

In some patients, when using a small state-of-the-art endoscope, it may be possible to retroflex the endoscope tip inside the bulb and examine the fornices directly.

Because the bulb courses posteriorly, its most distal point (apex) appears first in the 3 o'clock position of the visual field. The superior wall of the bulb is in the 12 o'clock position, and the inferior wall is in the 6 o'clock position.

At the apex of the bulb there is often an abrupt angle at a fold leading into the descending duodenum, often referred to as the superior duodenal angle. Heavy folds may appear at the apex, just proximal to entering the descending portion. Mucosa of the descending duodenum has circular Kerckring's folds that begin just beyond the apex of the duodenal bulb. This sign helps to determine when the tip of the endoscope leaves the smooth mucosa of the bulb and enters the circular folds of the descending portion.

The mucosa of the bulb is somewhat pale and yellowish-gray compared to the orange-pink color of the stomach. When closely inspected, the fine villous texture of the mucosa can be appreciated as a granular appearance with tiny dots of reflected light (Fig. 8.11). The vascular pattern, as seen with air insufflation, consists of tiny interconnecting vascular structures which terminate abruptly after only a short distance.

Because the bulb is small, it can be difficult to examine unless approached in a careful and systematic fashion. A small-caliber instrument is preferred, especially if bulbar pathology is suspected, because of its shorter turning length. Retroflexion is necessary to examine the pylorobulbar junction and the fornices; this is accomplished by upward deflection with continued intubation in the midbulb.

DESCENDING DUODENUM

Several differences separate the descending duodenum from the stomach and the bulb. Bile may be noted as well as considerable luminal motility. When a hypotonic agent like glucagon has been administered, it is easier to inflate and examine the duodenum. Circular folds are seen. Although the papillae are seen occasionally with an end-viewing endoscope, they are better examined with a side-viewing scope. The main papilla of Vater is located on the medial wall in the middescending duodenum. There may be a second or minor papilla of Santorini which is characteristically proximal to the main papilla, smaller and fleshy in appearance.

The descending duodenum has a yellow-orange coloration compared to the yellowish-gray appearance of the bulb. Usually there is no mucosal vascular pattern. Especially in the presence of slow gastric emptying, some whitish discoloration may be present in the mucosa due to lipid in the lamina propria lacteals (Fig. 8.12).

ABNORMALITIES OF THE BULB AND DUODENUM DUE TO EXTRINSIC FACTORS

BULB ABNORMALITIES

Enlargement of adjoining anatomic structures may impinge on the bulbar architecture and alter its shape. Examples include enlargement of the head of the pancreas, which can

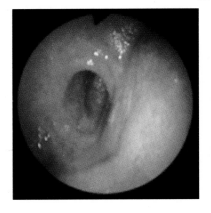

Figure 8.13 Nonspecific compression of the posterior wall of the bulb.

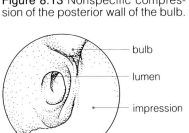

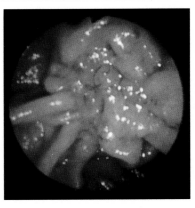

Figure 8.14 Duodenal wall deformity due to infiltrating suprapapillary pancreatic malignancy.

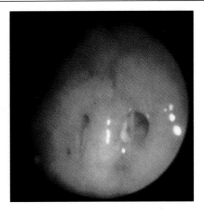

Figure 8.15 Fistulous opening in the duodenal wall, seen after spontaneous breakthrough of a pancreatic abscess.

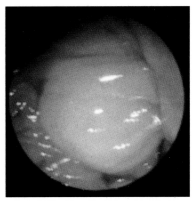

Figure 8.16 The impression on the duodenal wall is associated with a dilated common duct due to pancreatic cancer.

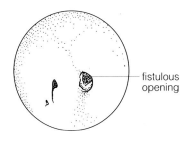

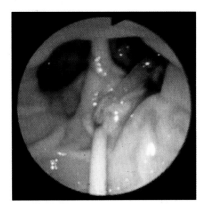

Figure 8.17 Two diverticula adjacent to the papilla. Note the drain projecting from the papillary orifice.

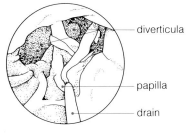

deform the bulb at its apex and along the inferior wall. Massive dilation of the common bile duct may compress the bulb at or just beyond the apex. Gallbladder enlargement may deform the anterior aspect of the bulb. Apical stenotic deformity due to peptic ulcer disease may dilate the bulb, giving the apex a puckered appearance with a pinpoint lumen. Bulbar dilatation may also be seen in association with scleroderma.

Adjacent malignancy usually produces extrinsic compression from the anterior aspect of the duodenal bulb; a masslike deformity can be seen obstructing the lumen at the apex. The bulb proximal to this appears dilated. Sometimes a nonspecific compression of the posterior wall of the bulb may occur; this must be distinguished from an adjacent malignancy (Fig. 8.13).

DUODENAL ABNORMALITIES

Abnormalities of the descending duodenum include changes in the papilla or its immediate surrounding structures. Papillary changes include carcinoma of the papilla, adenoma of the papilla, and a perivaterian diverticulum. Adjacent structures may also impress the descending duodenum. The descending duodenum is retroperitoneal and fixed in position. When compressed by an enlarged adjacent organ, extrinsic pressure distorts the duodenal lumen. Examples include a cyst of the pancreas (either a pseudocyst or a true cyst) or a carcinoma of the head of the pancreas. In these circumstances it may be difficult to identify the duodenal anatomy, and to locate and cannulate the papilla.

Endoscopically, extrinsic compression is commonly seen with carcinoma of the pancreas (Fig. 8.14). Swelling caused by a pancreatic abscess may be seen. The opening of a spontaneous fistula tract draining the abscess into the duodenal lumen is rare (Fig. 8.15). The bile duct runs in the duodenal wall, and if this structure is obstructed by a stone or cancer of the pancreas, papilla or distal bile duct, the duct may bulge into the duodenal lumen. When this is noted, the opening of the papilla is usually seen at the distal end of the bulge (Fig. 8.16).

Penetration of the bile duct through the wall creates a weak spot which may form a diverticulum. For this reason the diverticula of the descending duodenum are usually next to the papilla (Fig. 8.17). An unusual type of diverticulum is an inverted diverticulum in which the orifice appears next

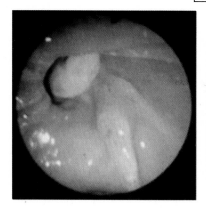

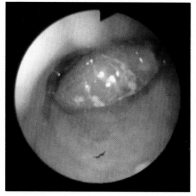

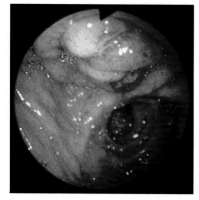

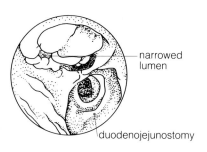

Figure 8.18 Peripapillary diverticulum. A concrement is evident in the papillary orifice.

Figure 8.19 Duodenal diverticulum. Bile-stained concrement fills the diverticulum.

Figure 8.20 Annular pancreas. The duodenal lumen is markedly narrowed by pancreatic tissue. A duo-

denojejunostomy was surgically created to bypass the obstruction.

to the lumen of the descending duodenum. These diverticula may be inflamed or contain food or secretions (Figs. 8.18 and 8.19).

Occasionally, a congenital band or ring of pancreatic tissue surrounds the second portion of the duodenum and constricts it; this anomaly is termed annular pancreas. At endoscopy, a stenotic area may be seen, or there may be complete obstruction, generally beginning within 3 cm of the apex (Fig. 8.20). Just above the stenotic area, extrinsic compression from the lateral wall can be observed. The constricting limb is usually above the major papilla. If ERCP is technically feasible, it can confirm the presence of an annular pancreas with the pancreatic duct circling the duodenum. No other relevant endoscopic abnormalities are seen in most cases.

A congenital duodenal diaphragm or septum is a ringlike focal narrowing 5 to 10 mm wide which may become manifest in adult life (Fig. 8.21). At endoscopy, a characteristic slitlike narrowing is seen in the midportion of the descending duodenum.

Dilatation of the descending duodenum may occur because of mechanical obstruction of the third and fourth portion, due to stricturing malignancy, Crohn's disease, or vascular mesenteric root obstruction. In case of sclerodermatous involvement, the duodenum may dilate up to 7 or more cm, which decreases the size of or entirely effaces Kerckring's folds.

POSTSURGICAL ABNORMALITIES

Postsurgical deformity of the bulb and duodenum is usually due to a choledochoduodenal anastomosis. In the case of a proximal choledochoduodenostomy, the anastomosis is located at the posterior wall of the bulb (Fig. 8.22). At

endoscopy, converging folds are seen on the posterior wall aspect of the apex; often bile drains from this area. In the case of a distal choledochoduodenostomy, a surgically created stomal orifice is seen just proximal and posterior to the normal-looking papilla. Another postsurgical abnormality is a peripapillary fistula (Fig. 8.23). This is often seen just cephalad to the papilla and may result from an injury to the distal common bile duct during biliary surgery.

Catheterization of a choledochoduodenostomy is usually possible. Occasionally, food residue may be seen through the stoma opening. Enlargement of a strictured anastomosis is possible over a distance of not more than 3 to 4 mm using a papillotomy wire or knife. This must be done with utmost care because of the risk of bleeding or perforation. An alternative is to dilate the opening with a balloon catheter.

NONSPECIFIC BULBODUODENITIS

Nonspecific bulboduodenitis may be a manifestation of duodenal ulcer disease. Whether duodenitis is the precursor or the healing state of the bulboduodenal ulcer is unclear. There is little if any relationship between symptoms and presence or severity of duodenitis as assessed endoscopically or histologically. This has contributed to the confusion about the significance of this entity. Based on the available evidence, bulboduodenitis seems to be a stage in the formation of an ulcer.

Patchy or diffuse reddening of the entire bulb is the most common finding. Focal erythematous areas usually measure 0.3 to 1.5 cm. Hypermotility usually accompanies erythema, and puckering folds prolapse back and forth within the bulb (Fig. 8.24). The aspect of reddish patches with intervening pale areas is termed *salt and pepper* appearance.

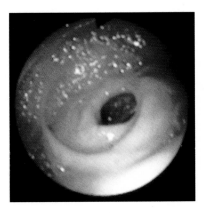

Figure 8.21 Congenital duodenal diaphragm. This abnormality becomes manifest in adulthood.

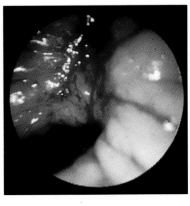

Figure 8.22 Postsurgical deformity caused by a recently performed suprapapillary choledochoduodenostomy. Minor inflammatory changes are also present.

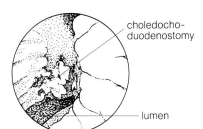

choledocho-duodenostomy

lumen

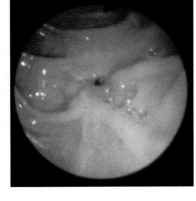

Figure 8.23 Iatrogenic peripapillary fistula. A fistulous opening is seen just above the fistula.

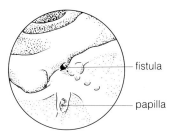

fistula

papilla

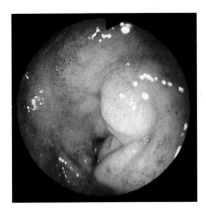

Figure 8.24 Mild bulboduodenitis. Swollen apical folds prolapse back and forth in this patient, previously treated for a duodenal ulcer. Patchy erythema is also discernible.

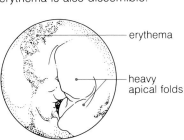

erythema

heavy apical folds

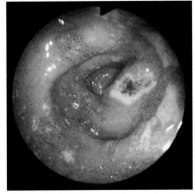

Figure 8.25 Erosive bulboduodenitis. Multiple erosions are seen; one shows stigmata of recent bleeding.

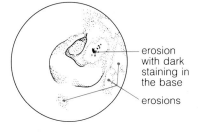

erosion with dark staining in the base

erosions

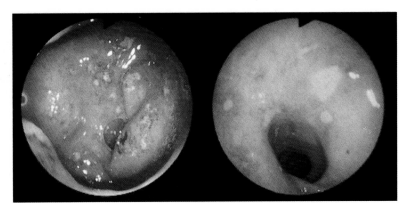

Figure 8.26 Erosive bulboduodenitis. Note the erythematous ring surrounding the defects.

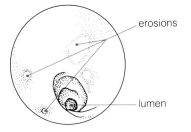

erosions

lumen

Epithelial destruction with discrete focal erosions is the predominant feature in more severe inflammation, and may be the source of upper GI bleeding (Fig. 8.25). Because of the adherent exudate, erosions usually appear as whitish areas, 1 to 3 mm in diameter or larger, often surrounded by a rim of striking erythema (Fig. 8.26). Patients with pronounced erosive bulboduodenitis often have gastric hypersecretion. Endoscopic signs are copious amounts of acid

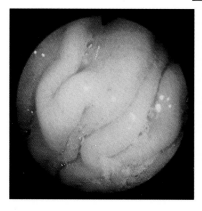 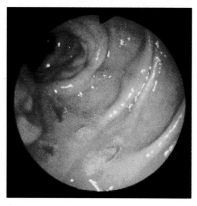 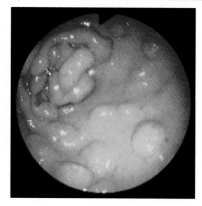 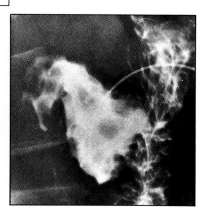

Figure 8.27 In patients with erosive bulboduodenitis, there is often evidence of gastric hypersecretion. Pronounced areae gastricae and copious amounts of acid fluid are apparent in this view of the stomach.

Figure 8.28 Erosive defects in the descending duodenum, with evidence of mild bleeding.

Figure 8.29 *Left,* Nodular deformity of bulb in a patient on renal dialysis. No alteration of the mucosal ap-

pearance can be seen. *Right,* Corresponding X-ray of bulb shows obvious nodularity.

fluid in the stomach and an accentuated pattern of areae gastricae in the corpus-fundic area (Fig. 8.27). In hypersecretion, the erosive defects may expand into the duodenum and may be the source of upper GI bleeding (Fig. 8.28). This lesion may be pronounced in Zollinger-Ellison syndrome.

Mucosal nodular deformity or excrescences are found in a minority of patients with bulboduodenitis. Such nodules are usually concentrated in the bulb, and may be discrete and small (2 to 4 mm) or in the 5 to 10 mm range. If they continue into the descending duodenum, they may be accompanied by thickened Kerckring's folds. Such nodules may show apical erythema with or without tip erosions, although in some patients mucosal coloration is normal. Histologically, a variable degree of acute and chronic inflammation is usually present. Patients with nodular bulboduodenitis have a high incidence of peptic ulceration. Nodular duodenitis is especially common in end-stage renal disease or in patients on chronic dialysis (Fig. 8.29).

PEPTIC ULCERATION OF THE BULB AND DUODENUM

INCIDENCE AND ETIOLOGY
Peptic bulboduodenal ulceration is a necrotic process in which the lesion destroys muscularis mucosae and extends into the submucosa or into the deeper muscle layers. It is common in the United States; about 10% of the population will experience duodenal ulcers sometime in their lives, men more often than women. For unknown reasons, however, the incidence has been decreasing over the last 30 years.

The cause of peptic ulceration is not known. Although many people with duodenal ulcers show hypersecretion of gastric acid, the secretory values overlap to a large extent with those of the general population. This implies that acid secretion cannot be the only etiologic factor. Other sug-

gested factors include more rapid emptying of the stomach in ulcer patients, or the possibility of genetic predisposition. In some patients, the fasting level of gastrin is normal, but there is increased release of gastrin in response to a meal. This, coupled with an increased response of the parietal cell mass to the gastrin and an impaired control of gastrin release in response to acidification of the antrum, may contribute to ulcer development. Cigarette smoking has been associated with an increased incidence of duodenal ulcers and with impaired response to therapy. Occasionally, drugs such as acetylsalicylic acid, other nonsteroidal anti-inflammatory agents, or potassium chloride medications cause ulcers (Figs. 8.30 and 8.31), which heal rapidly after withdrawal of the offending medication.

SYMPTOMS
The symptoms of a duodenal ulcer vary. The classical pattern in many patients is burning epigastric pain 2 to 3 hours after eating. While the pain is often severe enough to awaken the patient at night, it is rarely present in the morning. The pain is usually relieved rapidly by antacids or food. Occasionally, ulcers may occur without pain; in these cases, patients may present initially with a complication such as bleeding.

Recurrence rates of 50% in 1 year have been reported after healing of a duodenal ulcer. If all patients are reexamined after healing regardless of the presence of symptoms, the incidence of recurrent ulcer is even higher.

LOCATION
About 50% of all duodenal ulcers are located on the anterior wall. Ulcers on the posterior wall are less common (Fig. 8.32). The surfaces of the superior and inferior walls account for roughly 20% of all duodenal ulcers. Apical ulcers are relatively uncommon and usually associated with prominent folds and scar deformity.

About 15% of the time, patients with a duodenal ulcer

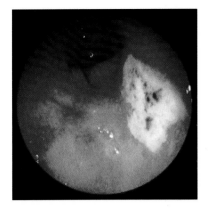

Figure 8.30 Combined drug-induced duodenal and gastric ulcer. The duodenal ulcer shows stigmata of recent bleeding.

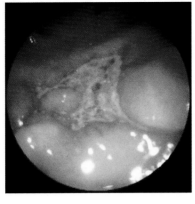

Figure 8.31 KCl-induced ulcer in the bulb. Note the irregular shape and absence of inflammatory changes in the surrounding mucosa.

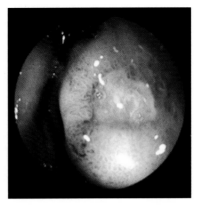

Figure 8.32 Duodenal ulcer of the posterior wall. Conspicuous erythema and swelling are apparent.

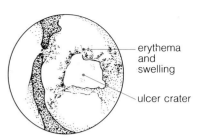

erythema and swelling

ulcer crater

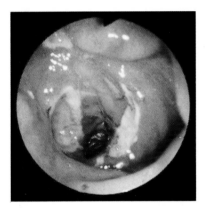

Figure 8.33 Kissing ulcers in the bulb are found on opposite walls at the same site.

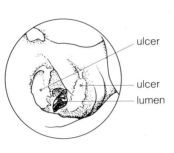

ulcer

ulcer

lumen

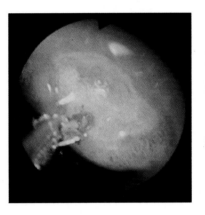

Figure 8.34 Open biopsy forceps as a measuring device. This ulcer recurred within 10 days after a 6-month course of maintenance therapy with ranitidine.

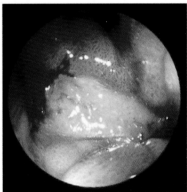

Figure 8.35 Large duodenal ulcer of the posterior wall with marked erythema and friability of the border.

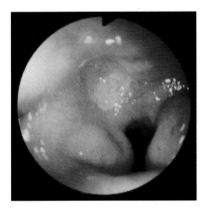

Figure 8.36 Round duodenal ulcer of the anterior wall with an erythem-

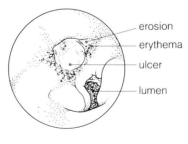

erosion

erythema

ulcer

lumen

atous rim. This ulcer is seen merging with an erosion.

SIZE AND SHAPE

The size of an ulcer may be estimated with reasonable accuracy by direct vision. Generally, error is on the side of underestimation. A more accurate estimation of ulcer size can be achieved using either the open-biopsy forceps method or a calibrated probe (Fig. 8.34).

Most duodenal ulcers are under 1 cm in greatest dimension, with roughly half having a diameter of between 5 and 9 mm. Twenty-five percent are large and have a diameter between 10 to 20 mm (Fig. 8.35). Giant duodenal ulcers have a diameter exceeding 20 to 25 mm. Most duodenal ulcers are 1 to 2 mm deep. Superficial ulcers may be difficult to distinguish from erosive defects, while deep ulcers have a depth of greater than 3 mm.

The single most striking feature of an ulcer of the bulboduodenum is the shape of the crater, which also has some bearing on its response to medical therapy, The round- or oval-shaped ulcer is the most common and responds most predictably to therapy (Fig. 8.36). The crater appears yellowish-gray; the margin is usually hyperemic and erythematous. Occasionally the ulcer crater may merge with an erosive patch. Histologically, the base shows a fibrinoid

have a second ulcer, often within a short distance of the main ulcer. Common sites of multiple ulcers are the pylorobulbar junction, the anterior and posterior wall of the midbulb, and the apex. Ulcers on opposite walls of the same site are called "kissing ulcers" (Fig. 8.33).

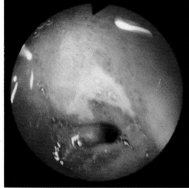
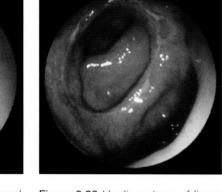
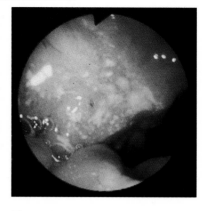
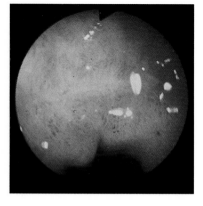

Figure 8.37 Irregular-type duodenal ulcer in a scarred bulb.

Figure 8.38 Healing stage of linear ulceration located along the ridge of the fold. Note the characteristic pseudodiverticular malformation.

Figure 8.39 Multifocal, patchy-type duodenal ulceration. Background mucosa shows erythema.

Figure 8.40 Complete healing stage. Edges surrounding the scar are erythematous.

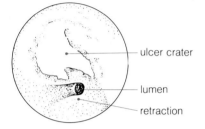

ulcer crater

lumen

retraction

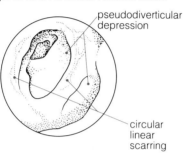

pseudodiverticular depression

circular linear scarring

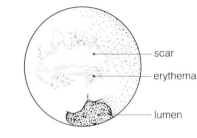

scar

erythema

lumen

necrosis, whereas the erythematous rim shows features of acute duodenitis.

Irregularly shaped ulcers account for about 10% of all ulcers, and are usually associated with scar deformity (Fig. 8.37). Presumably because of such scarring, these ulcers do not heal as readily in response to therapy.

About 10 to 20% of all ulcers are linear. These are also commonly associated with scar deformity and may be found along the ridges of one or more of the deforming folds (Fig. 8.38). Linear ulcers are the least predictable in response to treatment.

The multifocal, patchy, salami-type ulcer is distinctly less common. A discrete area of multiple, tiny ulcerations is seen on a background of intense erythema (Fig. 8.39). Such ulcers are generally less than 1 cm in diameter, are relatively slow to heal, and have a high recurrence rate.

In the rare mixed type, the ulcer pattern combines two or more of the above variations. Most often, the round or irregular shape is combined with the linear appearance. This mixed type is commonly associated with scar deformity.

HEALING AND SCAR FORMATION

Duodenal ulcers reepithelialize from the periphery. During the healing phase, the crater becomes progressively smaller and less deep at the average rate of 1 to 4 mm per week. Usually the healing phase is characterized endoscopically by marked erythema of the surrounding edges (Fig. 8.40). After healing, prominent folding in a hypermotile or hyperkinetic bulb may persist (Fig. 8.41).

Delayed healing may be seen in association with scar de-

formity, suggesting recurrent ulcer disease. Since duodenal ulcers tend to recur, there is often evidence of previous ulceration and scarring together with fresh crater formation (Fig. 8.42). Thus, ulcer scarring should always alert the endoscopist to search for the presence of an ulcer crater. Scarring is presumably the result of repeated injury at the same location, causing mucosal and submucosal fibrosis with some muscle hypertrophy around the site of ulceration. The combination of fibrosis and muscle hypertrophy tends to pull the adjacent layers toward the point of recurrent ulceration, producing the characteristic converging or projecting folds radiating from the ulcer toward the periphery.

Between these folds, one may appreciate pseudodiverticula. These are single or multiple outpouchings in the bulb within zones of scar deformity, possibly formed as a result of a pulsion effect on the lesser or uninvolved portion of the duodenal wall (Figs. 8.43 to 8.45). A pseudodiverticulum may simply be the result of a stretching effect of the uninvolved wall by material entering the bulb between fixed points of scarring. Pseudodiverticula usually occur at the fornices and middistal portion of the bulb (Fig. 8.46).

Midbulb or apical deformity alone or together may be sufficient to contract the bulb, shortening it to less than 3 cm (Fig. 8.47). In advanced stages of foreshortening, the bulbous structure may virtually disappear.

Breakthrough bulbar ulcers, observed during prolonged H_2 blockade therapy, have a peculiar appearance. Most often such ulcers are small and superficial without intense erythema and swelling of the surrounding mucosa (Figs. 8.48 and 8.49). Occasionally, they may be difficult to distinguish

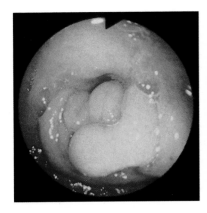

Figure 8.41 Heavy folds in a hyper-contractile bulb after duodenal ulcer healing.

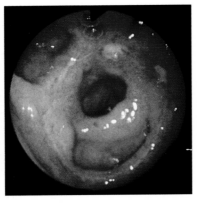

Figure 8.42 Recurrent duodenal ulcer. Fresh ulceration is seen together with scarring and deformity from previous ulcers.

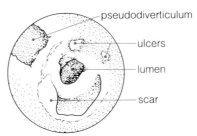

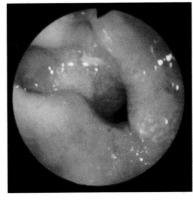

Figure 8.43 Partial healing with scarring and pseudodiverticular deformity. Pseudodiverticula commonly occur between the folds formed during scar formation.

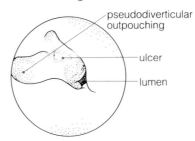

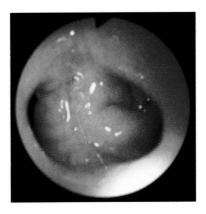

Figure 8.44 In this patient, excessive scarring and retraction caused pseudodiverticula formation, giving the appearance of a split pylorus.

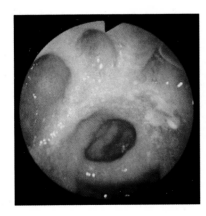

Figure 8.45 Marked pseudodiverticular deformity. Confluent erosive defects may also be observed along the folds formed by ulcer scarring.

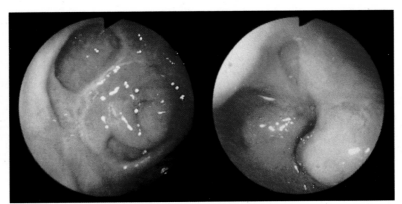

Figure 8.46 Examples of scar deformity with pseudodiverticula.

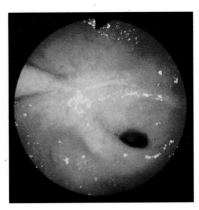

Figure 8.47 Extensive scarring and retraction caused foreshortening of the bulb in this patient.

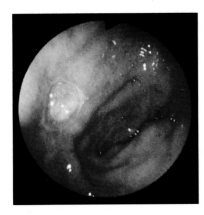

Figure 8.48 Breakthrough ulcer observed during H₂ blockade maintenance therapy. This ulcer is small

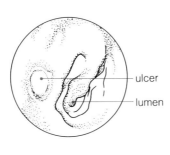

and superficial without prominent inflammatory changes in the surrounding mucosa.

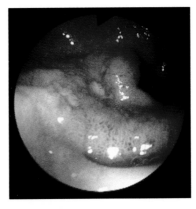

Figure 8.49 Breakthrough ulcers with more conspicuous inflammatory changes.

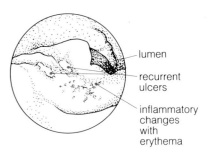

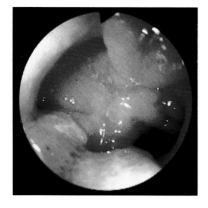
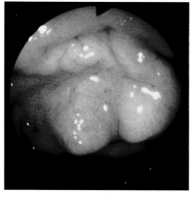
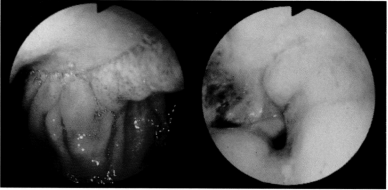

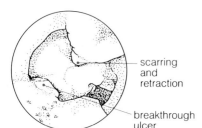

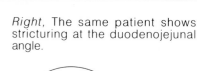

Figure 8.50 Breakthrough ulcer. In this patient, the bulb shows evidence of scarring and retraction, indicating a tendency for breakthrough ulcers.

Figure 8.51 Lush gastric mucosa with a prominent areae gastricae pattern is occasionally seen in patients with ordinary duodenal ulcer disease. This appearance is compatible with acid hypersecretion.

Figure 8.52 *Left,* Giant postbulbar ulceration in the horizontal part of the duodenum is due to gastrinoma.

Right, The same patient shows stricturing at the duodenojejunal angle.

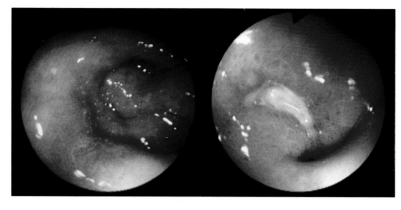
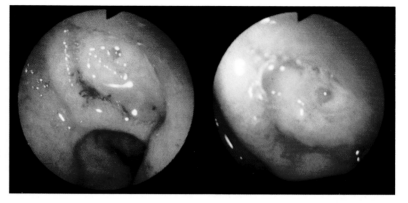

Figure 8.53 *Left,* In this view, a duodenal ulcer is hidden between swollen folds and is not immediately identified. *Right,* Upon close inspection, an oval-shaped ulcer is readily seen.

Figure 8.54 A side branch of the gastroduodenal artery is visible in this posterior wall duodenal ulcer. Bleeding is evident at the margin of the ulcer.

from a large erosion. Patients with marked scarring and deformity are especially prone to breakthrough ulceration (Fig. 8.50).

GASTRIC ULCERS
In patients with ordinary duodenal ulceration, the gastric mucosa usually looks normal. Occasionally, upon careful inspection one sees lush gastric mucosa with somewhat thickened folds and a prominent areae gastricae pattern, especially in the corpus and fundic area (Fig. 8.51). However, peptic ulcers of the bulb may be associated with gastric ulcers. Characteristically, such ulcers are in the prepyloric antrum, adjacent to or within 2 cm of the pyloric channel (see Fig. 8.4). Another common location for a secondary gastric

ulcer is the angle adjacent to the lesser curve. The presence of prepyloric ulcers indicates the need for a detailed examination of the bulb. Such ulcers are notoriously difficult to heal and have a high recurrence rate.

GASTRINOMA-RELATED ULCERS
Multiple extensive ulcers of the bulb and descending duodenum may be associated with gastrinoma and acid hypersecretion (Fig. 8.52; see also Fig. 8.28). Superficial, erosive/ulcerative destruction of the duodenum usually appears on the uppermost portion of the prominent, somewhat enlarged Kerckring's folds. The presence of postbulbar, superficial or large, and extensive ulceration of the descending and horizontal parts of the duodenum should

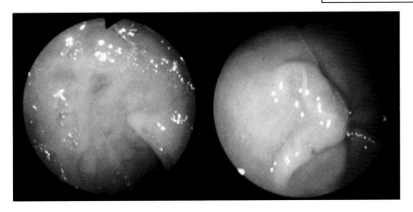

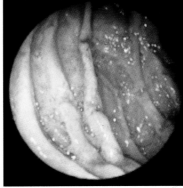

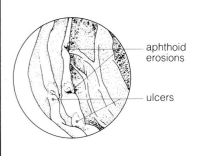

Figure 8.55 Parasitic duodenitis due to Strongyloides. *Left,* Small focal erythematous areas are clearly visible. *Right,* Strongyloides worms visible as tiny whitish threads.

Figure 8.56 Duodenal Crohn's disease. Note the discrete aphthoid erosions and small ulcers at the crests of Kerckring's folds.

always suggest the possibility of gastrinoma or Zollinger-Ellison syndrome. In such cases, inspection of the stomach usually reveals enlargement of the fold pattern with accentuation of the areae gastricae.

ENDOSCOPIC GUIDELINES

A small-caliber endoscope or a side-viewing instrument should be used when there is strong suspicion of an ulcer, especially along the proximal portion of the superior wall. In general, most ulcers are located within 1 to 2 cm of the pylorobulbar junction. Occasionally, an ulcer may be hidden between swollen folds (Fig. 8.53). Careful, gentle inspection and, if necessary, intravenous injection of antispasmodics such as glucagon usually allow identification of the ulcer.

Because of the risk of rupturing a deep penetrating ulcer, it may be wise to forego or limit the number of attempts to pass the endoscope for examination of the bulb in patients with severe symptomatic disease. This is especially true if antispasmodic medication does not sufficiently relax the bulb to allow easy passage of a small-caliber endoscope.

COMPLICATIONS

Major complications of severe ulcer disease include intractable pain (less common now because of antisecretory therapy), scarring, gastric outlet obstruction, penetration, perforation, and bleeding. The presence of a complication may be preceded by a change in symptoms. For example, obstruction must be suspected when pain is no longer relieved by food ingestion, and is accompanied by nausea and vomiting.

Bleeding from a posterior wall ulcer is dangerous because of the proximity of major arteries involving the stem or side branches of the gastroduodenal artery. Occasionally a vessel may be visible in the base of such an ulcer (Fig. 8.54). Especially in severe bleeding, the overlying blood, clot, or both may obscure the crater itself. Jet irrigation may clear the blood sufficiently to allow visualization of the crater and of

the bleeding spot. However, it can be difficult if not impossible in a contracted bulb to obtain full view of the bleeding site, which is a prerequisite for treatment with laser photocoagulation, electrocoagulation, heater probe application, or local injection therapy.

NONPEPTIC DISORDERS OF THE DUODENUM

The duodenum may undergo degenerative or inflammatory changes due to infection by viruses, bacteria, fungi, or parasites. In addition, the bulboduodenal mucosa may be involved in various diseases such as Crohn's disease and diseases which cause malabsorption, such as celiac sprue. Several other disorders can cause characteristic changes in the bulb or duodenum.

PARASITIC INFECTIONS

Parasitic duodenitis caused by hookworm, Strongyloides, Giardia, or Ascaris appears as a pronounced focal erythema with edema and partial or complete disappearance of the Kerckring's folds (Fig. 8.55). Occasionally there is some nodular deformity. The lesions usually start in the postbulbar area and are diffusely spread. Duodenal aspiration should be performed for diagnosis in patients with unexplained duodenal inflammatory changes that spare the bulb, especially if the patient has recently traveled in tropical areas.

CROHN'S DISEASE

Of all patients with gastrointestinal Crohn's disease, 0.5 to 4% will have manifestations in the duodenum. Whether isolated duodenal involvement in Crohn's disease exists is uncertain. Generally the bulb is involved in conjunction with the descending duodenum or prepyloric antrum. Discrete aphthoid erosions and shallow ulcerations are seen in the prepyloric antrum, bulb, and proximal or entire duodenum (Fig. 8.56). Surrounding the aphthoid erosions is a halo

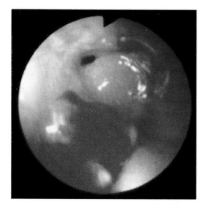 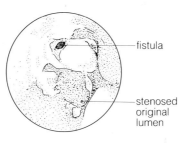

Figure 8.57 Crohn's disease of the postbulbar area can cause stricturing. In this case, stenosis of the lumen is seen along with a fistula leading to the intramural sinus.

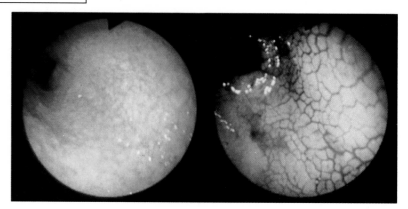

Figure 8.58 Celiac sprue. *Left,* Close examination of the mucosa shows complete villous atrophy. *Right,* Corresponding picture after methylene-blue dye-spraying shows the characteristic mosaic pattern of the flat mucosa.

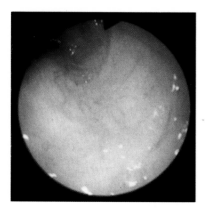 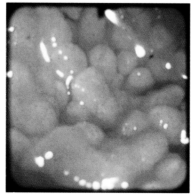

Figure 8.59 Hypogammaglobinemia. Total villous atrophy is seen along with giardiasis.

Figure 8.60 Hypogammaglobulinemia is associated with nodular lymphoid hyperplasia in this presentation.

of erythema; between the lesions the mucosa may appear normal. Occasionally nodular deformity may develop, creating a cobblestonelike appearance. There may be long or deep serpiginous ulceration within areas displaying a cobblestone pattern. In rare cases, discrete ulcers are present around a fistulous tract (Fig. 8.57). Other patients show only a nonspecific duodenal inflammation with erythema, exudate, and minor nodular deformity of the contour.

Stricturing with some obstruction of the proximal small intestine is not uncommon in Crohn's duodenitis (see Fig. 8.57). The apex itself may be ulcerated and stenotic. In addition, the lesions usually extend into the proximal midportion of the descending duodenum, giving the mucosa a nodular and ulcerated appearance. In approximately 50%

of the biopsies, epithelioid cell granulomas may be identified. These lesions in the proximal GI tract may be related to Crohn's disease or may be drug-induced.

CELIAC SPRUE

In most patients with celiac sprue, the mucosa appears superficially normal; there are no petechiae and the mucosa does not traumatize easily. However, on closer examination, villous atrophy can be seen (Fig. 8.58). In some patients, the duodenal mucosa may appear pale and atrophic with a pronounced vascular pattern. In other cases, the mucosa is conspicuously erythematous. Sometimes a mottled appearance of pallor and erythema may be noted.

The most common mucosal feature is the loss of the normal microgranularity. Instead, the mucosa appears smooth and shiny due to loss of villous excrescences, especially in the duodenal bulb. Sometimes a mosaic pattern or a finely convoluted appearance may be appreciated. Occasionally the openings of the crypts may be visible; such areas should be biopsied. Within the descending duodenum, the Kerckring's folds may be either normal, slightly prominent and erythematous, or—rarely—flattened.

A more detailed study of the mucosal surface morphology may be obtained using either indigo-carmine or methylene-blue dye-scattering techniques. Most characteristic is a flat mosaic appearance as the insufflated air forces the dye into the clefts between the islands of slightly elevated mucosa (see Fig. 8.58). Occasionally the dye enters the mouth of the slightly dilated crypts of Lieberkühn.

OTHER NONPEPTIC DISORDERS

Patients with hypogammaglobulinemia or common variable immunoglobulin deficiency syndrome may have a flat, avillous mucosa, nodular lymphoid hyperplasia, or both (Figs. 8.59 and 8.60). Raised 2 to 5 mm nodules may cover a portion of the mucosa. Usually they are a somewhat brighter color than the surrounding mucosa. The Kerckring's folds may be normal, or they may be pinkish because

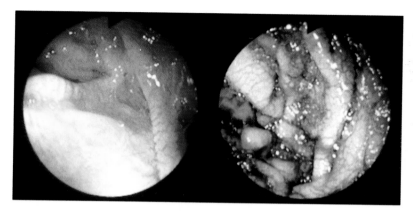

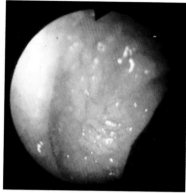

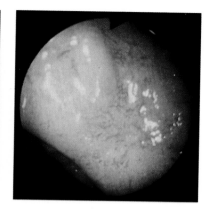

Figure 8.61 Bruton's agammaglobulinemia. Complete villous atrophy *(left)* is confirmed by the mosaic pattern *(right)* after methylene-blue dye-scattering.

Figure 8.62 Whipple's disease. Coarsening of villous pattern and patchy, whitish discoloration of the mucosa are characteristic.

Figure 8.63 Pseudo-Whipple's disease in an AIDS patient, caused by *Mycobacterium avium intracellulare.*

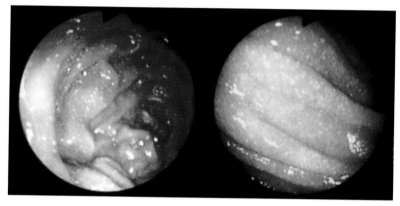

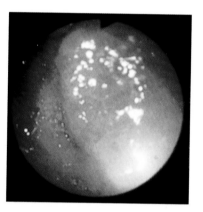

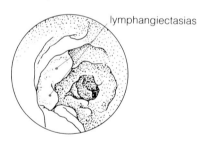

Figure 8.64 *Left,* Idiopathic small intestinal lymphangiectasia. Shiny white spots are characteristic of the ectatic lymph vessels. *Right,* Primary lymphangiectasia with severe protein loss.

Figure 8.65 Brown discoloration of the mucosa is due to duodenal melanosis.

of the abundance of superimposed nodules. In Bruton's agammaglobulinemia there usually is complete villous atrophy without nodular lymphoid hyperplasia (Fig. 8.61).

Whipple's disease has a characteristic endoscopic appearance with patchy, whitish discoloration, alteration of the villous pattern, and occasionally a markedly irregular mosaic pattern (Fig. 8.62). A related condition called pseudo-Whipple's disease, caused by *Mycobacterium avium intracellulare,* is occasionally observed in patients with acquired immune deficiency syndrome (AIDS). Analogous endoscopic abnormalities are seen with irregular coarsening of the villous pattern and conspicuous whitish discoloration

due to stagnant lipid in the lamina propria (Fig. 8.63).

Lymphangiectasia or chylangiectasia is usually characterized endoscopically by shiny, whitish spots in an otherwise normal-looking mucosa. These white spots are due to light reflection from the ectatic lymph vessels filled with chylomicrons (Fig. 8.64). In other patients, somewhat larger lymph or chyle cysts may be readily apparent. Yellow-white milky fluid may escape upon puncture of the cysts.

Duodenal melanosis is an unusual condition in which pigment is deposited in the mucosa (Fig. 8.65). Biopsies may show focal deposits of brownish-black pigment in the stroma of the villi.

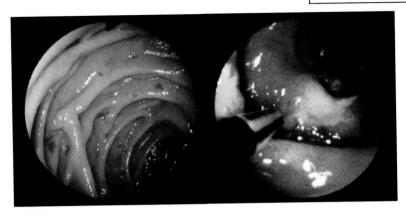
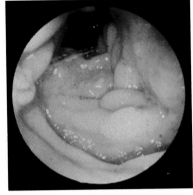
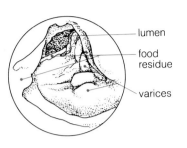

Figure 8.66 Rendu-Osler-Weber syndrome. *Left,* Hemorrhagic telangiectasia of the duodenum may be seen in this hereditary disorder. *Right,* Coagulation can be accomplished with bipolar electrodes.

Figure 8.67 Varices of the duodenum are discernible here as large tortuous protuberances.

VASCULAR ABNORMALITIES OF THE DUODENUM

Telangiectasis may be seen in Rendu-Osler-Weber syndrome. These irregular cherry-red spots range in size between 2 and 4 mm (Fig. 8.66).

The duodenum is occasionally the site of varices due to extrahepatic portal hypertension or extensive malignancy of the pancreatic bed. Large, serpiginous, undulating, tortuous protuberances are seen running between the Kerckring's folds, particularly on the posterior wall of the apex (Fig. 8.67). Sometimes they have a gray-blue or faint bluish discoloration; in other cases the color is that of the surrounding mucosa. The protruding nodular folds are soft and easily compressed when touched with a closed biopsy forceps, which is a useful clue to their identity.

Rarely, ischemic damage occurs in the duodenum. The overall endoscopic appearance is nonspecific, with loss of the fold pattern, patchy focal erythema, and mild friability. In more severe cases, a diffuse erosive or ulcerative defect may be seen, covered with a dirty exudate.

TUMORS OF THE BULB AND DUODENUM

Tumors of the proximal small bowel are uncommon. The etiology varies from benign conditions to invading malignancies.

BENIGN POLYPOID LESIONS
Polypoid lesions of the bulb and duodenum usually present as multiple small mucosal nodules. When there is no flat mucosa between the elevated surfaces, the term nodularity or mamillation may be preferred; otherwise, the term polypoid excrescence is appropriate. There is virtually no effective visual feature for distinguishing polypoid lesions of epithelial origin from those of submucosal origin.

Multiple Polypoid Lesions. Multiple small polypoid excrescences can be hyperplastic, inflammatory, or they may be due to heterotopic gastric mucosa, Brunner's gland hyperplasia, or lymphoid hyperplasia.

Hyperplastic-inflammatory polyps presumably correspond to the healing stage of nodular bulbitis. The mucosa can be histologically normal or it can show nonspecific duodenitis. At endoscopy the polyps appear as discrete, 2 to 4 mm elevations covered with normal-appearing mucosa (see Fig. 8.29). They may be found in the bulb alone or also in the descending duodenum. Larger polyps may become erythematous and even superficially eroded.

Polypoid lesions may also be composed entirely of heterotopic gastric mucosa. Heterotopic gastric epithelium is a common finding in bulboduodenal biopsies. Usually, several small sessile excrescences 1 to 3 mm in size are tightly grouped to form a granular, slightly elevated plaque. These excrescences are usually conical or round, and have a frosted-glass appearance with a pale pink or slightly reddened coloration (Figs. 8.68 to 8.70). In other cases a slightly raised, irregular, ill-defined patch of mucosa is seen, which has a fine cobblestonelike appearance. Heterotopic gastric mucosa is located preferentially in the proximal part of the bulb. Sometimes a single whitish polyp about 5 mm in size is seen in the second portion of the duodenum. Histologically, the lesion consists of full-thickness corpus-type gastric mucosa with both parietal and chief cells.

In Brunner's gland hyperplasia, multiple nodular elevations about 5 mm in size are spread throughout the descending duodenum. In most cases the bulb is not involved. The nodular elevation is mainly due to accumulation of somewhat enlarged Brunner's glands (Fig. 8.71). Nodular lymphoid hyperplasia is seen endoscopically as multiple small sessile nodules covered with shiny mucosa that is otherwise unremarkable.

Single Polypoid Lesions. Many conditions in the bulboduodenum typically cause a single polypoid lesion. Single hyperplastic-inflammatory polyps amidst normal mucosa are common. Their size (3 to 6 mm) and eroded appearance may cause the endoscopist to suspect an adenoma. Single submucosal polyps are either leiomyoma, lipoma, carcinoid, Brunner's gland adenoma, hamartoma, or adenoma. Other benign small bowel tumors such as fibromas, angiomas, lymphangiomas, and myomas are rarely encountered.

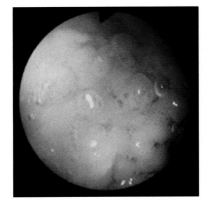

Figure 8.68 Heterotopic gastric mucosa in the bulb. A cluster of slightly elevated, pinkish, opalescent polyps, 5 mm in size, is obvious. Note the central red spot in several of the polyps.

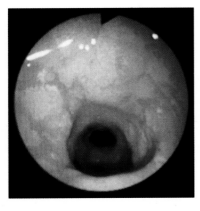

Figure 8.69 Heterotopic gastric mucosa, giving a flat appearance.

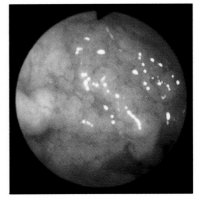

Figure 8.70 In this case, heterotopic gastric mucosa in the bulb presents a diffusely nodular appearance.

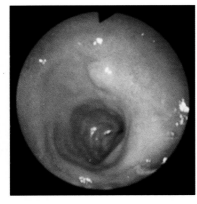

Figure 8.71 Brunner's gland hyperplasia with a single nodular elevation occurring in the apex of the bulb.

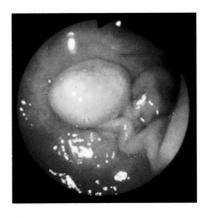

Figure 8.72 This submucosal polypoid lesion, consistent with a leiomyoma, is found at the apex of the bulb.

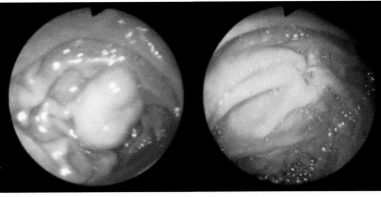
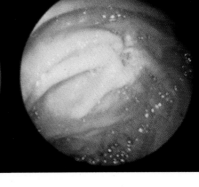

Figure 8.73 *Left,* Brunner's gland adenoma located in the proximal duodenum. *Right,* A small healing ulcer with converging folds remains after endoscopic removal with snare polypectomy.

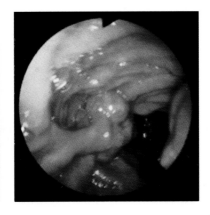

Figure 8.74 Hamartomatous polyp in the duodenum due to Peutz-Jeghers syndrome.

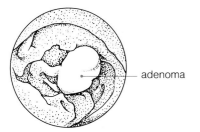

adenoma

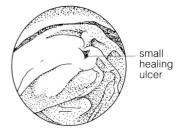

small healing ulcer

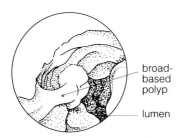

broad-based polyp

lumen

Leiomyomas are usually larger than 1 cm and are located at the junction of the apex of the bulb and the proximal descending duodenum (Fig. 8.72). Occasionally they may have a central ulceration or umbilication. Lipomas also occur preferentially at the bulboduodenal junction. These are slightly yellow and have a smooth surface. Unlike leiomyomas, they are usually not umbilicated or ulcerated. Most submucosal lipomas range from 1 to 6 cm and form intramucosal sessile growths which eventually become pedunculated. When pedunculated, the polyp is soft, freely movable on a stalk, and covered with normal shiny-looking duodenal mucosa.

A Brunner's gland adenoma may present as a sessile or pedunculated polypoid mass, 2 to 4 cm wide. These rare lesions are usually confined to the first part of the duodenum and are covered with normal-looking mucosa (Fig. 8.73).

Hamartomatous polyps in Peutz-Jeghers syndrome vary in size, are usually irregularly shaped, and have a somewhat dark-brownish color compared to surrounding mucosa (Fig. 8.74).

Adenomatous polyps in the duodenum are rare. Most are 1 cm or larger and may be singular or multiple, sessile or pedunculated. The surface mucosa is usually finely mamillated. Such polyps are seldom large enough to cause obstruction. Intussusception is also not a problem due to anatomical fixation of the duodenum. If a pedunculated polyp is endoscopically accessible, polypectomy should be considered. Occasionally, small adenomatous lesions are seen

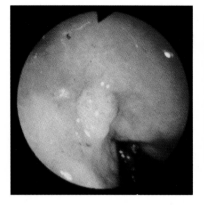

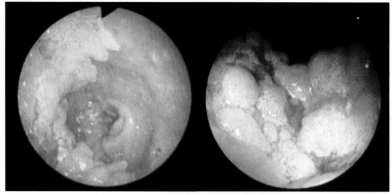

Figure 8.75 A small adenomatous polyp at the bulboduodenal junction is seen in this patient with familial polyposis coli and polyposis of the stomach.

Figure 8.76 Villous adenoma of the bulb. *Left,* Soft multilobular polyps are shown in this view. *Right,* Detail of the adenomatous tissue shows the cauliflowerlike appearance of this tumor.

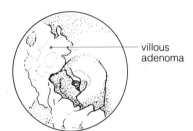

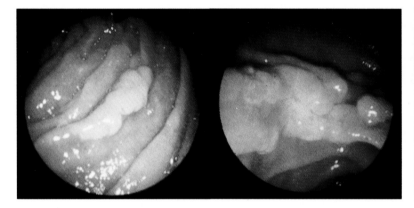

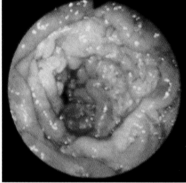

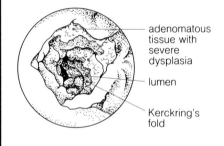

Figure 8.77 *Left,* A single, small adenomatous fold with severe dysplasia. *Right,* Villous adenoma involving a single fold in the descending duodenum. Note the shaggy, irregular surface and the difference in mucosal color.

Figure 8.78 Diffuse adenomatosis and dysplasia of the whole proximal small intestine. Note the color difference between adenomatous tissue and uninvolved Kerckring's folds. This rare presentation may be found in patients with familial polyposis coli.

in the duodenum in patients with familial polyposis coli (Fig. 8.75).

An association between familial polyposis coli or Gardner's syndrome and adenoma of the papilla has recently been observed. These lesions may be the precursor of adenocarcinoma of the papilla. When the association is clarified, we may have to screen patients with side-viewing duodenoscopy to rule out adenoma or carcinoma of the papilla. If there is a question concerning the papilla during endoscopy, biopsy and cytology are indicated.

Villous adenoma, a rare lesion of the duodenum, appears similar to villous lesions found in the colon. They are often sessile, irregular on the surface, and moderately large, often wider than 1 or 2 cm. Classically, a large, multilobular, soft, sessile polyp covered with a shaggy surface is seen at endoscopy (Fig. 8.76). Occasionally the villous adenoma appears limited to one large Kerckring's fold (Fig. 8.77). In exceptional cases there is diffuse adenomatosis of the whole proximal small intestine in conjunction with familial polyposis coli (Fig. 8.78). Endoscopic resection should not be attempted unless the tumor is small and pedunculated because of the danger of transmural damage. Biopsies may miss a deep-seated carcinoma.

DUODENAL MALIGNANCIES

Primary duodenal cancer is rare. The tumor usually appears as a nodular, ulcerated, exophytic, polypoid mass confined to the medial wall in the second portion of the duodenum (Fig. 8.79). This cancer may be limited or involve an entire segment of the duodenal wall.

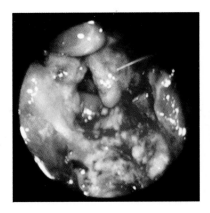

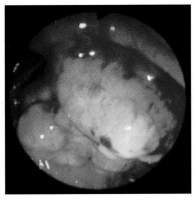

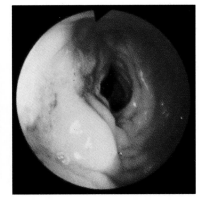

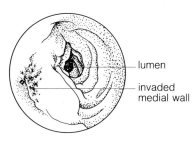

Figure 8.79 Primary cancer of the apical region of the bulb. An exophytic ulcerating mass is clearly discernible.

Figure 8.80 Cancer of the ampulla of Vater. A large, multilobulated, friable mass is seen.

Figure 8.81 Invasion of the medial wall of the duodenum by pancreatic cancer. Note asymmetry of the duodenal lumen.

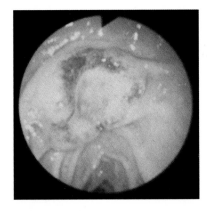

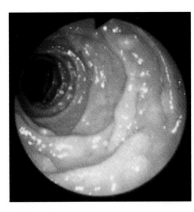

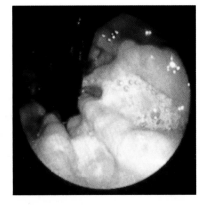

Figure 8.82 Centrally ulcerated mass due to primary lymphoma of the duodenum.

Figure 8.83 Generalized lymphosarcoma of the duodenum is seen as patchy, discrete, white lesions.

Figure 8.84 Generalized lymphosarcomatous involvement of the stomach in the patient in Figure 8.83. Note irregularity and broadening of folds.

Carcinoma more commonly arises directly from the duodenal papilla (Fig. 8.80). The papilla is enlarged two or three times its normal size, appearing as a cylindrically shaped mass. Usually a bulky raised tumor mass projects out from the hooded fold. In the typical case, the cancer infiltrates circumferentially, lifting the peripheral portion of the orifice in relation to a central depressed area, creating an excavated appearance. Tumor nodules and ulcerations may be seen within the excavated area.

Biopsies are obtained preferentially from the nodular periphery and from the excavated portion. When the papillary malignancy is largely covered with normal-looking mucosa, the diagnostic yield of direct biopsy may be enhanced by performing a limited-type papillotomy with a standard papillotome, a precut papillotome, or a papillotomy knife to expose the deep layers.

Direct extension of pancreatic cancer is the most common cancer of the duodenum. A widespread, ill-defined nodular mass of the medial wall is seen, usually involving the papilla and in some cases replacing the entire medial wall (Fig. 8.81). The mass often consists of 2 to 3 cm nodules.

Metastasis to the duodenum from a distant primary cancer is rare and is usually from a malignant melanoma; in this case, lesions may be small and pigmented or large with an ulcerated central portion and pigmented periphery. Other tumors which can metastasize to the duodenum include bronchus, breast, kidney, and uterine cervix. The typical metastatic implant appears as a 1 to 2 cm ulcerated mass set apart from the papilla.

Malignant lymphoma of the duodenum occurs most often in association with gastric lymphoma, which may extend through the pylorus. Multiple polypoid masses or large ulcerations may replace extensive portions of the bulb or duodenum, or the mucosa may have a diffusely infiltrated appearance with minor nodularity. Primary duodenal lymphoma may appear as nodular, sessile, ulcerated masses (Fig. 8.82). In generalized lymphosarcoma, the characteristic multiple, tiny, whitish, slightly elevated lesions in the duodenum may be easily overlooked (Fig. 8.83). Usually the stomach is also involved (Fig. 8.84).

Several other malignancies may present in the bulb or duodenum. Duodenal infiltration due to leukemia may present as plaquelike thickening of folds or as diffuse elevated nodular lesions and polypoid masses. Kaposi's sar-

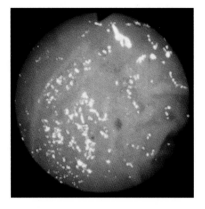

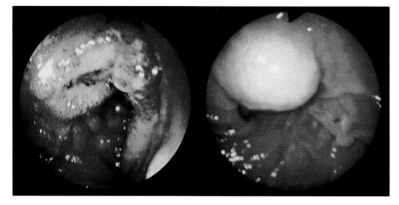

Figure 8.85 A reddish-brown lesion, characteristic of Kaposi's sarcoma of the duodenum.

Figure 8.86 *Left,* Destruction of the duodenal wall due to leiomyosarcoma. *Right,* Leiomyosarcomatous mass causing impression of the antrum.

Lesions of Terminal Ileum

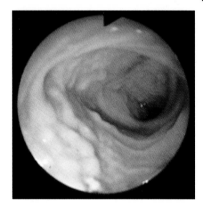

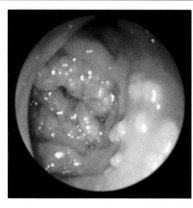

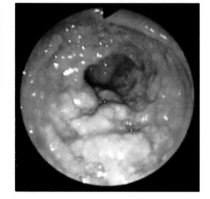

Figure 8.87 Lymphoid follicles in the terminal ileum.

Figure 8.88 Cobblestonelike appearance of coalescing lymphoid follicles in the terminal ileum.

Figure 8.89 Peyer's patches in the terminal ileum, with a slightly erythematous surface.

coma presents as variably sized, reddish-brown lesions, often associated with gastric lesions (Fig. 8.85). Duodenal involvement by leiomyosarcoma usually presents as a nodular, centrally ulcerated lesion with massive destruction of the duodenal wall. Concomitant lesions may be observed in surrounding structures such as the stomach (Fig. 8.86).

POLYPOID LESIONS OF THE TERMINAL ILEUM

The terminal ileum has a relatively small-caliber lumen. In teenage patients and young adults, the mucosa may appear somewhat uneven due to irregularly distributed, small nodular elevations corresponding to the presence of prominent lymphoid follicles (Fig. 8.87). Sometimes the mucosa is carpeted with tiny 1 to 2 mm lymphoid nodules, giving the mucosa a granular appearance. This abundance of visible lymphoid tissue may produce mucosal surfaces ranging from flat to granular to a cobblestonelike appearance (Fig. 8.88). Some endoscopists grade the appearance of the terminal ileum in four classes, 0 to 3:

Grade 0—absence of lymph follicles or only a few minute follicles distributed sporadically.
Grade 1—diffusely but sparsely distributed tiny follicles.
Grade 2—diffusely and densely distributed follicles, usually without conglomerations between follicles.
Grade 3—diffuse and densely distributed follicles. Individual follicles generally large; interfollicular conglomerations or fusions evident. Covering epithelium sometimes hyperemic or pale. Large conglomerations are referred to as Peyer's patches (Fig. 8.89).

9

Endoscopic Retrograde Cholangiopancreatography and Sphincterotomy

The field of biliary and pancreatic endoscopic treatment is one of the most exciting in clinical medicine today. Initial advances were in diagnosis. With endoscopic retrograde cholangiopancreatography (ERCP) it became possible to inspect the papilla of Vater and inject X-ray contrast material into the biliary and pancreatic ductal systems for precise diagnosis. Treatment of diseases of the biliary and pancreatic ducts then became feasible using endoscopic retrograde sphincterotomy (ERS). Today bile duct stones can be removed endoscopically, and drains and stents can be placed for benign and malignant biliary ductal obstruction. New developments in the use of ultrasound and mechanical crushers further expand the possibilities of stone removal. The future will likely hold many new applications.

In this chapter we will review ERCP and ERS. Normal and abnormal appearances of the papillae will be shown, followed by examples of successful ERS procedures. This chapter is not intended to be an instruction manual for ERCP and ERS. Therefore, X-ray interpretation of endoscopic cholangiography and pancreatography is not discussed, nor are the indications for these procedures.

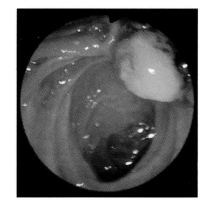

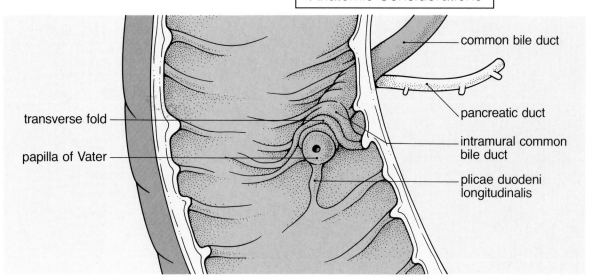

transverse fold

papilla of Vater

common bile duct

pancreatic duct

intramural common bile duct

plicae duodeni longitudinalis

Figure 9.1 The anatomy of the descending duodenum, with the intramural segment of the distal common bile duct cephalad to the papilla of Vater. Folds of the plicae duodeni longitudinalis run cephalad and end at the papilla.

ANATOMIC CONSIDERATIONS

Interest in the anatomy of the descending duodenum and the papillae began with the advent of ERCP as a diagnostic procedure in the early 1970s. There are two papillae. The major one, the papilla of Vater, derives from the ventral bud of the duodenum, developing into the ventral portion of the pancreas and the biliary ducts. The papilla of Vater is the structure which is cannulated routinely. The minor or accessory papilla, the papilla of Santorini, is the embryologic remnant of the dorsal bud of the duodenum which develops into the main body of the pancreas. In normal embryologic development, the two pancreatic ducts fuse so that the papilla of Vater drains the biliary system and ducts from both the ventral and dorsal pancreas. The accessory system often remains patent and serves as a second, minor drainage system for the main pancreatic duct.

The papilla of Vater is located 3 to 4 cm distal to the apex of the duodenal bulb on the medial wall of the descending duodenum. The papilla of Santorini is located on the same wall, usually 1 or 2 cm proximal to the papilla of Vater. The characteristic appearance of the major papilla is a red, reticulated surface and variable diameter (up to 1 to 2 cm). It is nearly always much larger than the minor papilla. The minor papilla is often smaller than the 2-mm cannula and appears fleshy and pale. Recognition of the characteristic appearance of the major papilla is critical because, when searching for the papilla, only a brief glimpse may be possible. Once the structure is recognized, time can then be spent getting the papilla directly in view and preparing to cannulate.

The anatomy of the papilla of Vater is especially important when considering ERS. Characteristically, the vertical fold or folds run cephalad and end at the papilla. Indeed, the papilla is often covered and may even be hidden by a fold. Cephalad to the papilla may be a bulge into the duo-

denum which is the intramural portion of the common bile duct as it runs in the duodenal wall (Fig. 9.1).

The papilla of Santorini is of less importance to the endoscopist. Recently, there has been interest in pancreas divisum, a condition in which the two pancreatic ducts do not fuse. The ventral pancreas drains at the papilla of Vater and the body and tail of the pancreas drain at the papilla of Santorini. This anatomy may predispose to development of pancreatitis in some patients.

Diagnosis of abnormalities of the accessory papilla requires cannulation of this papilla. This can be accomplished in some patients and is facilitated by using a tapered cannula; in other patients the papilla is too small to cannulate. Some groups have performed ERS of the accessory papilla to treat stenoses of this papilla in pancreas divisum with pancreatitis, but this procedure is not yet an established method of treatment.

Located above the intramural segment of the common bile duct is a branch of the gastroduodenal artery called the retroduodenal artery. This artery runs outside the duodenal wall and crosses over the common bile duct. It is located more than 3 cm above the papilla of Vater in approximately 85% of patients; however, it is as close as 1 cm in approximately 15% of patients. Massive, potentially life-threatening bleeding can result if this artery is cut as part of an ERS incision. Bleeding from this artery or other vascular structures occurs in moderate to severe degree in 1 to 3% of patients undergoing ERS. In the future it may be possible to identify this low-lying artery with an endoscopic Doppler probe and thereby reduce the risk of massive hemorrhage.

SIDE-VIEWING ENDOSCOPY

ERCP and ERS are the only clinical endoscopic procedures that use a side-viewing endoscope routinely. The viewing

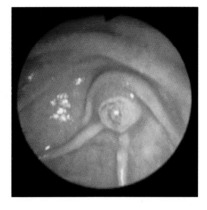
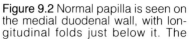
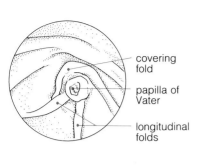

Figure 9.2 Normal papilla is seen on the medial duodenal wall, with longitudinal folds just below it. The configuration is papillary or protruding.

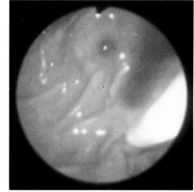

Figure 9.3 This normal papilla is relatively flat. A cannula for ERCP is being positioned.

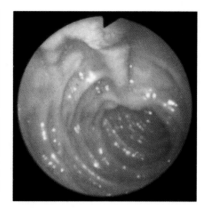

Figure 9.4 Here, the papilla is high in the duodenum and just distal to the duodenal bulb. The longitudinal fold is just below the papilla.

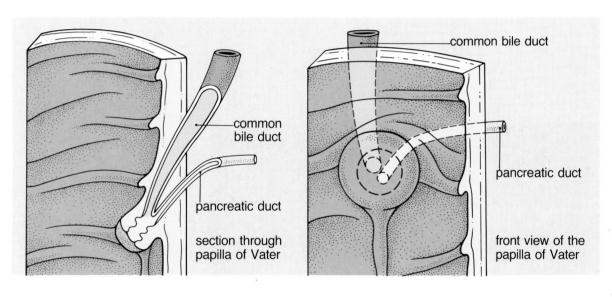

Figure 9.5 The orifice of the common bile duct on the papilla is located to the left and cephalad. The pancreatic duct is in the center of the papilla.

angle is at 90° to the long axis of the endoscope. In newer scopes, the viewing angle is actually more than 90° in a cephalad direction to facilitate visualization and cannulation of the papilla of Vater. Learning to use these endoscopes requires special instruction and patience. With experience, the endoscope can be passed without difficulty into the antrum of the stomach, through the pylorus, and into the descending duodenum. The papilla can be located, using the anatomic considerations noted above, and cannulation accomplished. The distal tip of the channel has an elevator which allows moderate control of the tip of the cannula during ERCP and ERS.

ERCP

One of the great advantages of ERCP over other imaging techniques is its ability to allow visualization of the papilla of Vater (hereafter, simply referred to as "the papilla"). The percutaneous transhepatic technique allows visualization of the biliary tree following injection of contrast but does not permit imaging of the pancreatic duct or inspection of the papilla.

THE NORMAL PAPILLA

The normal papilla may appear papillary (Fig. 9.2) or relatively flat (Fig. 9.3). Vertical folds may run cephalad and converge on the papilla. The papilla may be located proximally in the duodenum, just distal to the bulb, but even in this situation the longitudinal fold can be appreciated (Fig. 9.4).

The pancreatic duct is usually in the center or slightly to the right of the papilla, although this can be variable. The common bile duct is often in the left upper segment of the papilla as viewed endoscopically (Fig. 9.5). The direction

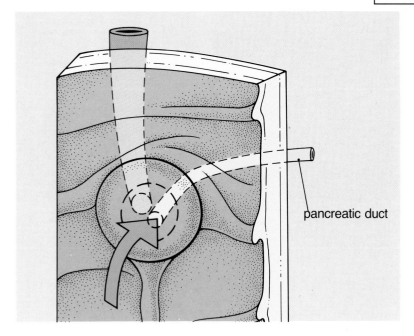

Figure 9.6 The most successful direction of approach to the pancreatic duct is to the right and horizontal.

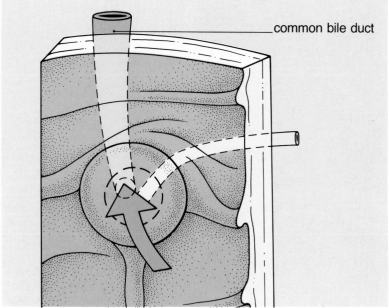

Figure 9.7 The direction for cannulation of the common bile duct is up and to the left of the papilla. Bowing of the cannula may permit a cephalad orientation.

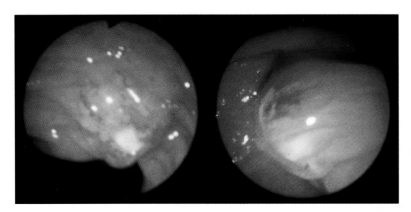

Figure 9.8 The white necrotic area on the tip of the papilla resulted from an impacted stone in the common bile duct.

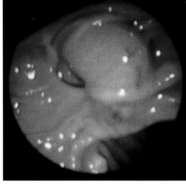

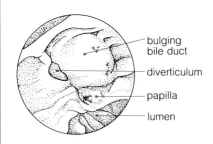

Figure 9.9 An impacted stone in the common bile duct causes the intramural portion of the duct to bulge. The papillary opening is at the tip of the bulge. A small perivaterian diverticulum is also seen.

of approach to the pancreatic duct is toward the right and horizontal (Fig. 9.6); the direction of approach to the common bile duct is cephalad and toward the left upper margin of the papilla (Fig. 9.7).

THE ABNORMAL PAPILLA

Once one is familiar with the characteristics of the normal papilla, it is possible to appreciate abnormalities. If findings are ambiguous, biopsy and cytology may be helpful to exclude a neoplasm (carcinoma or adenoma). If the biopsy and cytology are normal, it is prudent to reexamine the patient in a few weeks or months. If the papilla appears definitely abnormal, further workup for a periampullary carcinoma should proceed, even if biopsies and cytologies are negative.

PAPILLA WITH IMPACTED STONE

A bile duct stone impacted in the papilla may cause inflammation, with erythema of the overlying mucosa. A necrotic area may subsequently develop in the mucosa (Fig. 9.8). The papilla may bulge prominently and protrude into the lumen of the duodenum (Fig. 9.9). This bulge represents the intramural common bile duct, greatly distended from obstruction. The opening of the papilla is found at the caudad margin of this bulge. Often a small amount of exudate is present on or exudes from the papillary opening.

Acute infection of the biliary system (cholangitis) is an urgent indication for ERCP and treatment with ERS. In

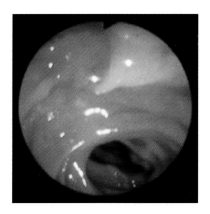

Figure 9.10 In this case of severe cholangitis caused by an obstructing stone, pus can be seen exuding from the papilla.

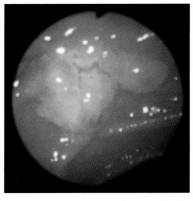

Figure 9.11 This abnormal papilla shows the characteristic "lava flow" appearance of an adenoma associated with FPC. The mucosa over the papilla appears pale and seems to spill over the papilla and adjacent tissue.

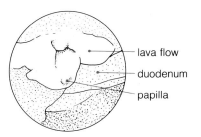

lava flow
duodenum
papilla

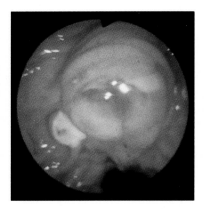

Figure 9.12 Mucus is seen covering an enlarged papilla in this patient with mucus-secreting pancreatic carcinoma. Since mucus is not normally seen over the surface of the papilla, this should suggest disease. The abnormal white area immediately adjacent to the papilla should be biopsied and brushed for cytology.

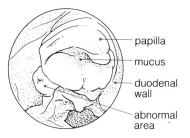

papilla
mucus
duodenal wall
abnormal area

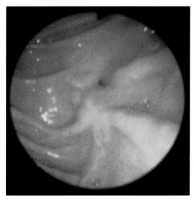

Figure 9.13 A suprapapillary choledoduodenal fistula is seen just cephalad to the papilla. Bile exits from the fistula.

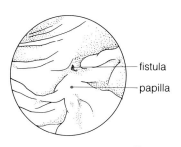

fistula
papilla

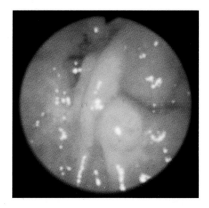

Figure 9.14 A silk suture from a previous choledochoduodenostomy is seen. The orifice of the anastomosis is not well seen.

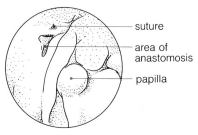

suture
area of anastomosis
papilla

most patients, stones pass spontaneously after incisions of the papilla, resulting in immediate relief of obstruction and infection. In severe cholangitis, pus may drip from the papilla (Fig. 9.10).

ADENOMA OF THE PAPILLA
Genetic predisposition to intestinal neoplasia is an increasingly important issue in gastroenterology. The clinical implications of the inherited polyposis syndromes are just now becoming apparent. An example is the association of duo-denal and periampullary adenoma and carcinoma with familial polyposis coli (FPC). A characteristic "lava flow" appearance has been described for the abnormal papilla in FPC. This appearance often indicates adenomatous change of the papilla, a possible forerunner of carcinoma (Fig. 9.11). The association of papillary problems and FPC may be sufficiently strong to warrant periodic screening of the duodenum and papilla with a side-viewing endoscope.

PAPILLA AFFECTED BY MUCUS-SECRETING PANCREATIC TUMOR
In such patients the papilla may be covered with mucus originating from a mucus-secreting tumor of the pancreas (Fig. 9.12).

SUPRAPAPILLARY FISTULA
A fistulous opening may be noted between the common bile duct and the duodenum. This may result from complications of common bile duct stones or as a result of an injury occurring during biliary surgery (Fig. 9.13).

PAPILLA FOLLOWING SURGERY
Postoperative changes may occasionally be seen. In Figure 9.14, a suture is apparent cephalad to the papilla, the remnant of a surgical choledochoduodenostomy performed several years earlier.

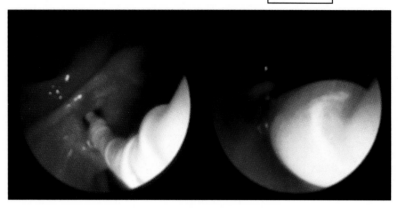 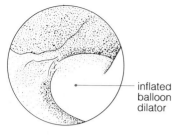

Figure 9.15 Stricture of the papilla after surgical sphincterotomy. *Left,* A saucer-shaped balloon catheter is introduced into the papilla. *Right,* On direct vision, the balloon is inflated to dilate the stricture.

BALLOON DILATION OF THE PAPILLA

A saucer-shaped balloon catheter can be passed into a strictured papilla to dilate the orifice. This technique may be used for stenosis after biliary surgical sphincterotomy (Fig. 9.15).

ERS

Precise, specific diagnoses of diseases of the hepatobiliary or pancreatic ducts are possible using ERCP. Another important aspect of this new technology is the ability to treat the patient endoscopically at the time of ERCP. This procedure is referred to as endoscopic retrograde sphincterotomy (ERS).

ERS has made possible endoscopic biliary surgery. Impacted bile duct stones can be pulled out using a balloon catheter or grasped with a basket. Researchers are examining the use of ultrasonic probes in the duct to shatter the stone, and wire baskets to mechanically crush stones. A temporary nasobiliary drain can be passed to relieve benign or malignant strictures, or permanent biliary stents can be placed. This new field of endoscopic biliary surgery will likely have a significant impact on clinical management of patients with diseases of the biliary tree.

TECHNIQUE OF ERS

ERS relies on both endoscopic and radiographic techniques. Fluoroscopy is essential to evaluate the state of the ducts, to ascertain the extent of disease, and to monitor the position of the catheters during ERS and for placement of drains and stents. Endoscopy is essential to locate and cannulate the papilla of Vater, to perform ERS, and to direct the insertion of the various catheters and drains.

The first step in ERS is to locate the papilla of Vater. The endoscope must be positioned to visualize the papilla en face. Next, the papilla is cannulated as in a routine ERCP. Contrast is injected and the diagnosis established.

Once ERS has been selected as the appropriate therapeutic procedure, the diagnostic catheter is replaced with a papillotome. A papillotome is a catheter with a wire exposed at the tip. Under fluoroscopic control, the papillotome must be deeply inserted into the papilla and up the common bile duct. If this is not possible, an initial small incision of the papilla may be necessary to allow passage of the papillotome. This is called a precut procedure (Fig. 9.16). The precut is just long enough to permit the papillotome to be passed into position for the full ERS. Some endoscopists separate the precut from the definitive ERS by days, while others perform the ERS immediately after the precut.

An alternative to a precut is to use a papillotomy knife. The instrument may be used in a manner similar to the precut papillotome to incise the papilla so that a regular papillotome can be passed (Fig. 9.17).

The technique of ERS is demonstrated sequentially in Figure 9.18. After locating the papilla and cannulating it, a papillotome is passed into the common duct. When fluoroscopy confirms the position of the papillotome in the bile duct, the wire is pulled taut and the tip bowed. The location of the wire relative to the papilla is critical. Endoscopically, the wire appears in the 9 o'clock to 12 o'clock position, corresponding to the location of the intramural portion of the common bile duct. In any other position the wire may cut laterally, away from the roof of the papilla, causing a perforation or injuring the pancreas. Only the intramural portion of the distal common bile duct can be safely incised during ERS. A diathermic current is then passed down the papillotome. A ground plate in broad contact with the patient completes the electrical circuit. A cutting current, occasionally mixed with coagulation current, is used to make the incision of the sphincteric fibers surrounding the distal bile duct. Under endoscopic guidance, a partial cut is made followed in a stepwise fashion by a complete cut 1 to 1.5 cm long. A balloon catheter can now be passed up the duct,

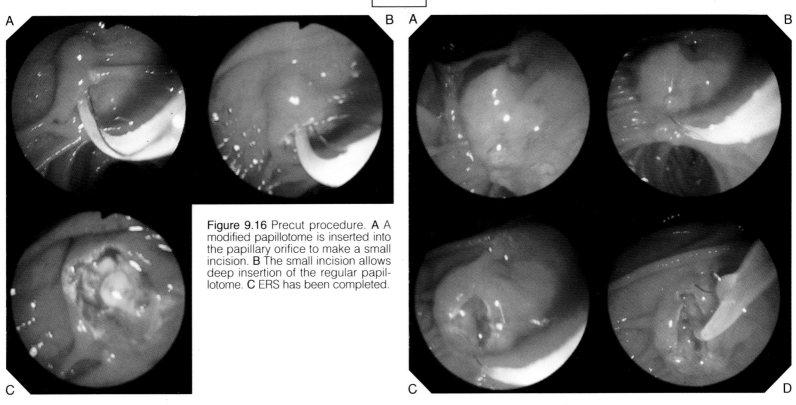

Figure 9.16 Precut procedure. **A** A modified papillotome is inserted into the papillary orifice to make a small incision. **B** The small incision allows deep insertion of the regular papillotome. **C** ERS has been completed.

Figure 9.17 Papillotomy knife sequence. **A** It was not possible to insert the papillotome into the papilla of Vater. **B** A papillotomy knife is used to incise the papilla **C** A small incision is made. **D** The regular papillotome was then inserted and full papillotomy incision completed. The wire can be seen at the cephalad border of the incision.

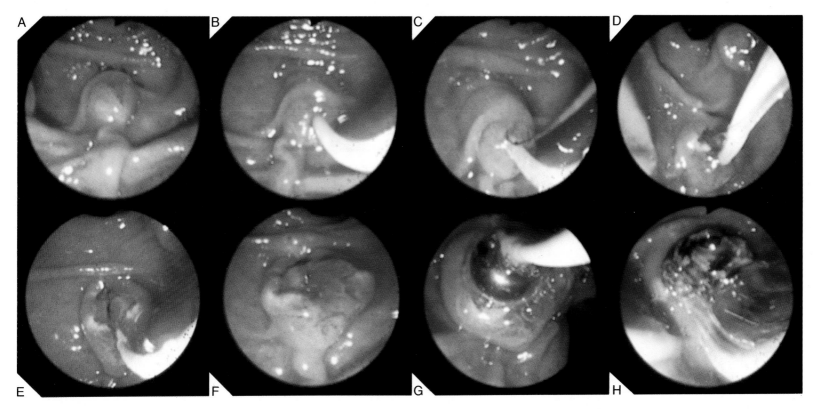

Figure 9.18 Technique of ERS. **A** The papilla is located in the descending duodenum. Note the longitudinal fold below the papilla. **B** The papilla is cannulated for diagnosis. **C** The cannula is replaced with a papillotome. After the position in the common bile duct is confirmed, the papillotome is bowed in preparation for ERS. **D** A cutting current is passed through the wire and a partial incision is made. **E** The incision is extended. **F** ERS is completed. **G** A balloon with a 1-cm diameter is passed, inflated, and withdrawn to calibrate the papillotomy orifice.

H The balloon has been passed above the retained stone, inflated, and pulled down to bring out the stone. The stone can be seen exiting the papilla.

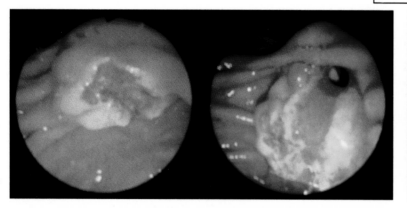

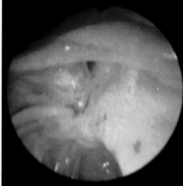

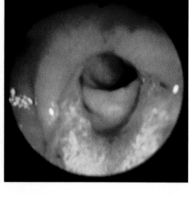

Figure 9.19 *Left,* Immediately following ERS, the incised tissue is edematous. *Right,* With a slightly different position of endoscope it is possible to see into the distal common duct and observe a retained stone.

Figure 9.20 The papilla 1 week after ERS, with less edema and whitening of the mucosa. Instead, a lacy erythematous appearance is noted. The common bile duct opening is also visible.

Figure 9.21 Six months after ERS, the papilla is still open and one can see into the common bile duct. There is no evidence of·stenosis and no residual evidence of inflammation.

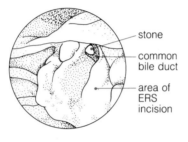

stone

common
bile duct

area of
ERS
incision

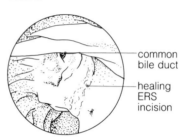

common
bile duct

healing
ERS
incision

inflated, and withdrawn to calibrate the size of the papillotomy. If a common bile duct stone does not pass spontaneously into the duodenum, a balloon catheter can be passed above the stone, the balloon inflated, and the catheter withdrawn, pulling the stone out of the papilla.

The endoscopic appearance of the papilla after ERS varies with time. Acutely, there is whitening of the mucosa surrounding the incision, edema (Fig. 9.19), and occasionally a small amount of bleeding. After 1 week, the periampullary tissue is less edematous, and the white coagulated appearance is replaced by a lacy, erythematous-appearing mucosa (Fig. 9.20). The opening of the common bile duct may be seen, which is unusual under normal circumstances. At 6 months, the papilla is usually less inflamed and is permanently open. It may be possible to look directly into the distal common bile duct (Fig. 9.21).

APPLICATION OF STENTS AND DRAINS

An exciting aspect of ERS is the ability to drain obstructions of the biliary ducts. In the past patients with unresectable tumors had surgery simply for palliation. With the use of ERS, a palliative bypass can be accomplished without invasive surgery.

First, a diagnostic ERCP is performed to determine the radiographic diagnosis, the location of the blockage, and the degree of stenosis. Observations must be made about invasion of the duodenal wall. Frank tumor masses are biopsied or brushed for cytology.

If a stent is to be passed, this can be accomplished with or without ERS. ERS facilitates passage of stents and drains but is not necessary in all cases. ERCP and ERS may be performed with a standard side-viewing endoscope. After papillotomy, the smaller endoscope is removed and a side-viewing scope with a large channel is passed into the duodenum. A Teflon catheter, usually containing a guidewire, is then passed into the papilla and up the bile duct. If the catheter will not pass the obstruction, the spring-tipped guidewire is advanced from the catheter to see if it will pass. If the guidewire passes, the catheter is then advanced over the wire above the narrowed area. The advancement of the catheter and wire is monitored fluoroscopically.

A pusher tube then pushes the stent down the endoscope channel over the catheter. The stent is advanced into the bile duct and positioned with fluoroscopic guidance until the proximal tip is above the stricture. The catheter and wire are then removed followed by the pusher tube, leaving the distal end of the stent free in the duodenum, protruding 1 or 2 cm from the papillary orifice. If the catheter and wire cannot be passed through the stricture, dilating catheters or balloon-tipped catheters may be used to dilate the stricture so that the catheter and wire can be passed above the stricture to guide the stent.

If a nasobiliary drain is selected to temporarily drain the

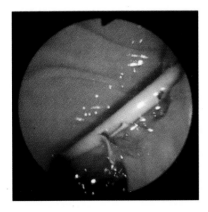

Figure 9.22 A biliary prosthesis from the common bile duct into the duodenum. The side flaps reduce the chance of migration.

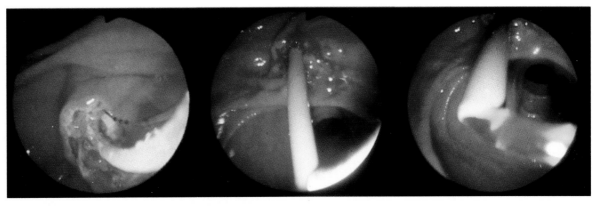

Figure 9.23 *Left,* ERS in a patient with malignant jaundice caused by an unresectable lesion in the bile duct. *Center,* A biliary prosthesis and pusher tube are inserted over a guidewire which cannot be seen here. *Right,* After removal of the guidewire, bile exits from the drain.

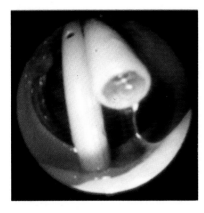

Figure 9.24 In this case two drains are seen exiting from the papilla. Multiple drains are used if the obstruction cannot be bypassed with a single drain, for example, if a tumor obstructs both the left and right main intrahepatic ducts.

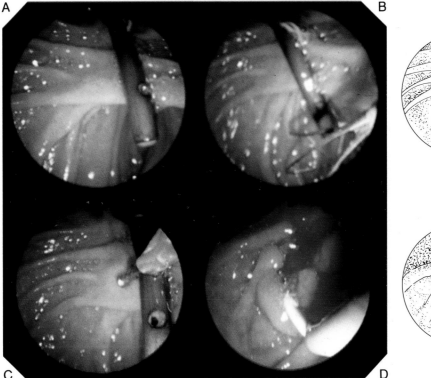

Figure 9.25 Clearing a clogged stent. **A** A biliary stent exiting from the papilla. The stent is clogged and has ceased to function. **B** A basket catheter has been passed and opened to grasp the end of the stent. **C** The basket has been tightened on the stent. The drainage hole in the stent is clogged with debris. **D** After removing the clogged stent, a guidewire and catheter are placed into the common bile duct and a new stent is about to be positioned into the duct.

duct, the tip of the drain is placed above the narrowed area. The proximal end of the drain is brought out through the mouth and then repositioned to exit from the nose.

Drains and stents are kept in place by either having a pigtail curvature on the end or a series by small spurlike protuberances on either end. These shapes reduce the chance of stent migration (Fig. 9.22). Figure 9.23 demonstrates ERS for a malignant obstruction, with the passage of a prosthesis or stent for drainage. In complicated cases, often involving malignant duct obstruction, multiple stents and drains may be necessary (Fig. 9.24).

Occasionally, drains become plugged with debris. Figure 9.25 shows a clogged biliary stent, its endoscopic removal, and the endoscopic passage of a new stent. The limiting

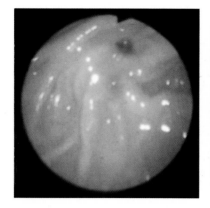

Figure 9.26 A normal papilla of Vater, with a diverticulum adjacent to it.

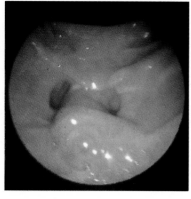

Figure 9.27 A papilla with diverticula on either side.

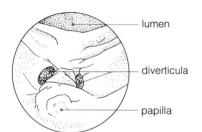

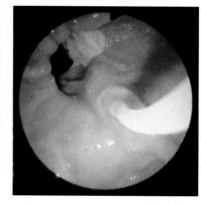

Figure 9.28 The papilla is located on the rim of this perivaterian diverticulum. Note the debris in the diverticulum. The papilla is easily cannulated.

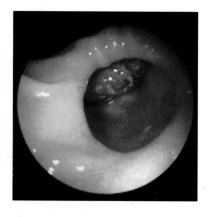

Figure 9.29 The papilla inside of a duodenal diverticulum.

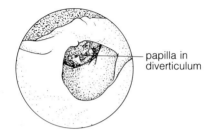

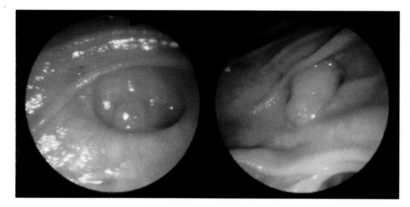

Figure 9.30 *Left,* Here, the papilla is located inside a diverticulum. *Right,* With manipulation and with suction via the endoscope channel, the papilla is everted out of the diverticulum.

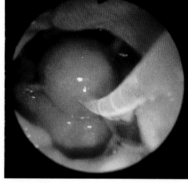

Figure 9.31 The papilla is being cannulated inside a duodenal diverticulum.

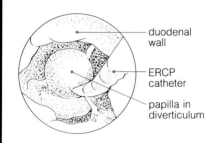

factor in the diameter of the stent or drain placed endoscopically is the diameter of the biopsy channel of the endoscope. Endoscopes with larger channels of 3.8 and 4.2 mm are available.

ERCP AND ERS IN PERIVATERIAN DIVERTICULA

Of patients undergoing ERCP, 10 to 15% have diverticula of the duodenum in the periampullary region. The diverticulum is most often seen as an opening adjacent to the papilla (Fig. 9.26), though sometimes there may be a diverticulum on both sides of the papilla (Fig. 9.27). The papilla is characteristically located on the rim of the diverticulum, often in the 4 o'clock position. The papilla in this position normally cannulates easily (Fig. 9.28). If the papilla is located inside the diverticulum (Fig. 9.29), it may be impossible to cannulate; however, in some instances the papilla can be everted out of the diverticulum with gentle suction (Fig. 9.30) or gentle manipulation with a catheter and then cannulated. In some instances the papilla can be cannulated in the diverticulum (Fig. 9.31).

Initially endoscopists were reluctant to perform ERS on patients with perivaterian diverticula because of the risk of perforating the diverticulum or the duodenal wall. However, it is now well accepted that ERS can be performed

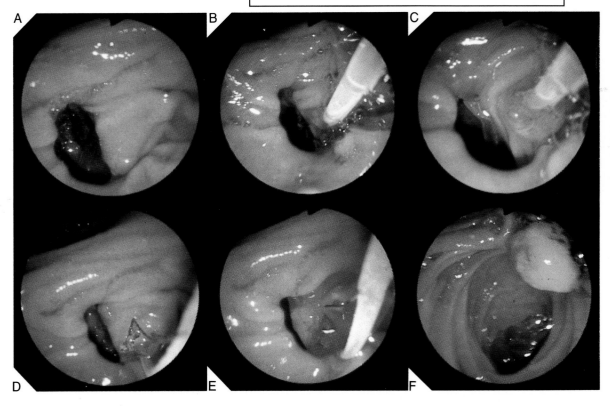

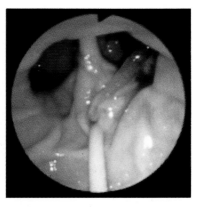

Figure 9.33 A nasobiliary drain has been placed into the papilla for drainage above a biliary obstruction. Diverticula are seen on either side of the papilla.

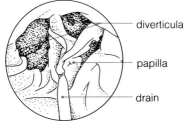

Figure 9.32 ERS in perivaterian diverticula. **A** A perivaterian diverticulum in the descending duodenum. The papilla is inside the diverticulum and cannot be seen. **B** With gentle manipulation with an ERCP catheter, the papilla is everted out of the diverticulum. **C** The papilla is then cannulated. **D** and **E** ERS is performed. **F** The stone freed by ERS is seen in the duodenum.

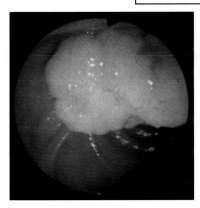

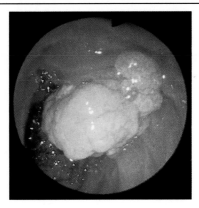

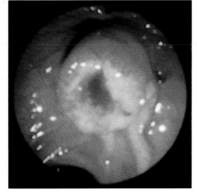

Figure 9.34 Periampullary carcinoma, seen as a large, pale mass in the area of the papilla. The surface is multilobed, slightly yellow, and irregular.

Figure 9.35 Multilobed periampullary carcinoma. Tumor appears to extend above and to the right of the papilla.

Figure 9.36 Periampullary cancer involving the papilla. The center is hemorrhagic and friable.

on these patients (Fig. 9.32). It is also possible to place drainage tubes to bypass bile duct obstruction in patients with diverticula (Fig. 9.33).

Anatomically, the common bile duct and pancreatic ducts pass through the duodenal wall at the level of the papilla of Vater, referred to as the duodenal window. This window may create a weak spot through which the duodenal mucosa can bulge and form a diverticulum. The same explanation may account for the association of colonic diverticula and penetrating blood vessels.

ERCP AND ERS IN PERIAMPULLARY CARCINOMA

Periampullary carcinoma usually has an appearance distinct from that of a normal papilla. The papilla may appear enlarged, irregular, multilobed, discolored (i.e., not a fine, erythematous, lacy color but rather white or yellowish), friable, and in some cases necrotic (Figs. 9.34 to 9.36). Periampullary carcinoid tumors may be seen as masses, occa-

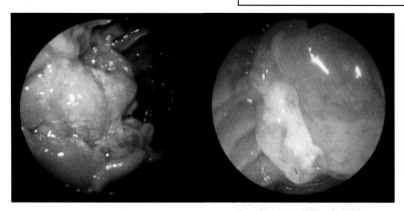

Figure 9.37 Periampullary carcinoid tumors present as masses, sometimes with ulcerations (*right*).

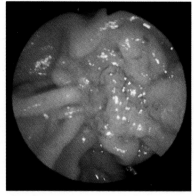

Figure 9.38 A pancreatic carcinoma has invaded the duodenal wall just above the papilla. The folds are irregular and nodular.

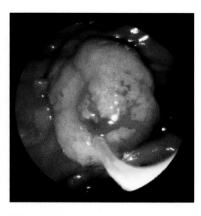

Figure 9.39 Periampullary carcinoma with an area of minimal bleeding in the center, cannulated for ERCP.

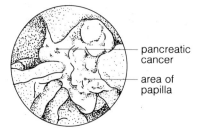

pancreatic cancer

area of papilla

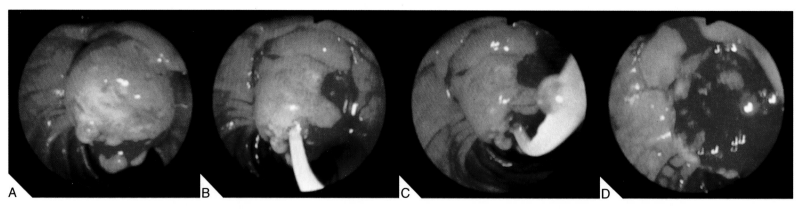

A   B   C   D

Figure 9.40 ERS in periampullary carcinoma. **A** The carcinoma presents as a friable, bleeding mass. **B** A cannula is inserted. **C** After ERCP, a papillotome is passed for ERS. The taut wire can be seen making an incision. **D** After ERS, a small amount of bleeding occurs. The open papilla allows for biopsy of the mass and/or placement of stents or drains to relieve obstruction.

sionally with an ulcer at the tip (Fig. 9.37). A pancreatic carcinoma may be seen invading the duodenal mucosa and the papilla (Fig. 9.38).

If a periampullary carcinoma is encountered, the endoscopist should obtain a sheathed brush cytology specimen and several directed biopsies. A decision has to be made concerning further diagnosis undertaken during that session. In many instances it is appropriate to cannulate the carcinomatous papilla to make a diagnosis and determine the extent of the obstruction by the tumor (Fig. 9.39). Endoscopic ultrasound may be useful to delineate the depth of infiltration and the presence of enlarged lymph nodes.

ERS can be performed in periampullary carcinoma for two reasons: first, to obtain a specimen of the deeper tissue of the papilla for histologic diagnosis, and second, to pass drainage tubes and stents for temporary (if surgery is planned) or permanent (if the problem is considered inoperable) relief of obstruction (Fig. 9.40).

CHOLEDOCHOSCOPY

In rare circumstances, a small-caliber end-viewing endoscope may be passed into the common bile duct, usually via a choledochoduodenal anastomosis. One may then visualize the common bile duct, common hepatic duct, and even the bifurcation of the major right and left intrahepatic ducts (Fig. 9.41). Although this technique may occasionally allow visualization of ductal stones and other pathology, it is only applicable in patients who have widely patent anastomoses.

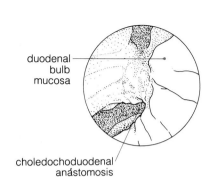

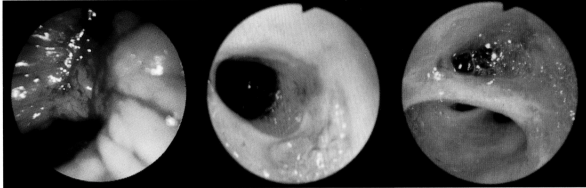

Figure 9.41 Choledochoscopy. *Left,* A choledochoduodenal anastomosis is seen in the duodenal bulb. *Center,* The common bile duct. *Right,* Bifurcation of the common hepatic duct.

duodenal bulb mucosa

choledochoduodenal anástomosis

HEMOBILIA

ERCP is also of importance in the detection of hemobilia. During the acute bleeding phase, blood may be seen exuding from the papillary orifice. After bleeding has stopped, clots may occasionally be seen escaping from the papilla. Upon retrograde choledochography, clots which have a characteristic appearance may be noted in the biliary system.

CONCLUSION

Overall, ERCP, ERS, and related therapeutic endoscopic procedures such as drain placement are among the most important advances in endoscopic diagnosis and treatment. These techniques are likely the forerunners of other types of endoscopic therapy that will significantly improve management of difficult medical problems.

10

Colon I: Polyps and Tumors

In this chapter we will briefly present general techniques for intubation of the colon. With colonoscopy it is possible to diagnose premalignant adenomatous polyps, remove the polyps, and detect colorectal cancers. Each of these entities will be presented in detail later in the chapter.

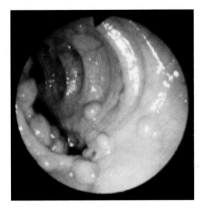

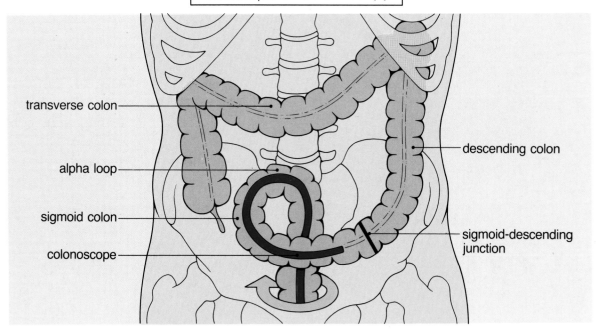

Figure 10.1 The alpha maneuver.

TECHNIQUE OF COLONOSCOPY

In experienced hands, 80 to 90% of patients can be colonoscoped to the cecum in 20 to 30 minutes without use of fluoroscopy. Failure to intubate the entire colon is mainly due to anatomical variations such as a long redundant sigmoid colon or transverse colon, fixation of the bowel from prior surgery, or other intra-abdominal problems such as diverticulitis. Fluoroscopy is only necessary in difficult cases requiring special maneuvers (the alpha maneuver, discussed later) or if external overtubes are used to stiffen the colonoscope to reduce formation of loops in the sigmoid colon. Fluoroscopy can also be used to identify the location of the tip of the colonoscope in the cecum, but other indicators are usually adequate to determine that the cecum has been intubated.

Before colonoscopy, most patients are given a narcotic (meperidine) and/or a sedative (diazepam). An IV access line may be used to administer these medications, and in the event of a vasovagal episode, to administer an anticholinergic or other medication.

Patients are examined lying in the left lateral recumbent position with the knees and thighs flexed. The patient may be rotated supine, prone, or onto the right side to assist in passing a difficult bend. In certain circumstances it is valuable to have an assistant press on the patient's abdomen so loops do not reform in the sigmoid colon. This also assists in passage of areas such as the proximal transverse colon.

Initially and throughout the procedure a generous amount of lubricating jelly is used at the anus to facilitate advancement of the endoscope by reducing friction at the anal verge, which will also prevent trauma to the anal canal. This is especially important if the anal sphincter tone is high or if large hemorrhoids are present.

Once in the rectum, the instrument is advanced by gently distending the colonic lumen with air and advancing under direct vision. Most experienced colonoscopists can intubate the entire colon with this technique. Occasionally, blind intubation—called the "slide-by" technique—is necessary although less desirable. This technique uses gentle pushing pressure while the mucosa slides past the visual field. The pushing pressure should be discontinued immediately if the tip stops moving and if the color of the mucosa changes, suggesting excessive pressure. Slide-by may be performed for short distances, providing the mucosa does not appear excessively whitened due to stretching. In general, advancing with the lumen in view is preferable to "slide-by."

Other general principles are to be gentle and not to advance with excessive force. One must try to follow the lumen and be careful not to traumatize a false lumen such as a diverticular orifice. It is also best to keep the amount of air insufflated to a minimum, and the instrument as straight as possible. The more experienced endoscopist will move the endoscope in and out or "jiggle" it to reduce the number of bends as the tip is advanced. Unnecessary loops tend to enlarge when the colonoscope is advanced, interfering with advancement. The colon is accordioned over the colonoscope, keeping the instrument as straight as possible. The straight position keeps the tip control optimal and allows the colonoscopist to approach flexures, especially at the sigmoid-descending colon junction, at a favorable angle for introduction of the tip of the instrument into the descending colon.

If intubation is difficult, lengths of the colonoscope may have to be withdrawn, allowing the colon to straighten, reducing bends, and thus permitting further intubation. It may be useful to remove as much gas as possible to reduce

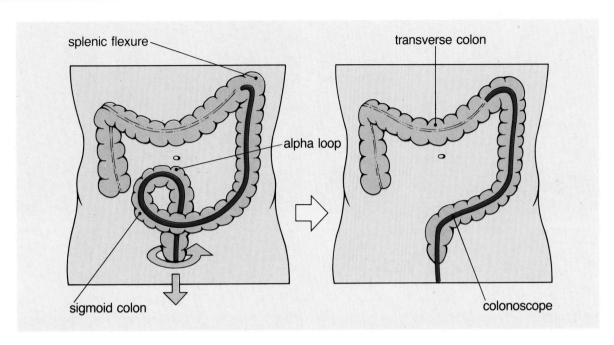

Figure 10.2 Derotating the alpha loop.

distension and the chance of loop formation. First, remove some of the colonoscope to see if the colon can be straightened. Next, gentle pressure over the area where the loop is forming can prevent further expansion of the loop. Repositioning the patient may facilitate passage into the transverse colon from the descending colon, or into the ascending colon from the transverse colon. This may require having the patient lie on his or her right side. Clockwise torque may assist passage in several difficult positions by reducing the tendency of the sigmoid colon to form loops.

Special maneuvers such as the alpha maneuver can be used to straighten acute angles and permit passage of the colonoscope. In this technique, usually performed with fluoroscopy, a loop which on X-ray resembles the letter alpha is created in the sigmoid colon (Fig. 10.1). This is accomplished by counterclockwise rotation of the colonoscope. In the alpha configuration it is possible to pass the tip of the colonoscope past the angle at the sigmoid-descending colon junction into the descending colon. When the tip has been advanced to the level of the splenic flexure or the left transverse colon, the alpha loop in the sigmoid colon is reduced by withdrawing the colonoscope, under fluoroscopy, with a simultaneous clockwise rotation (Fig. 10.2).

If a loop reforms in the sigmoid colon and prevents further advancement, it may then be necessary to use an external stiffener. This device is passed when the colonoscope tip is in the descending or transverse colon and the colonoscope is straight without any loops. The stiffener prevents recurrent formation of the sigmoid loop. This technique requires special instruction, carries a slightly increased risk to the patient, and must be performed with fluoroscopic guidance. Improvements in the flexibility of colonoscopes have reduced the need for this technique. The newest models have a flexible tip with a less flexible shaft closer to the controls which reduces the chance of forming loops when the tip of the colonoscope is up in the colon, for example, at the splenic flexure.

Other techniques which assist intubation of the ascending colon include removing a length of colonoscope to lift a bow in the transverse colon and to reduce the angulation of the instrument as it approaches the hepatic flexure. Clockwise rotation, aspirating air, and having the patient take a breath will also facilitate passage into the ascending colon.

The cecum has its own distinctive fold pattern, characterized by the appearance of three compartments as the tenial bands converge. The orifice of the appendix may be seen at the point of convergence. Light from the endoscope tip can be seen through the abdominal wall in the right lower quadrant. Other indicators of the cecum include identification of the cecal sling, a circular fold approximately 7 cm proximal to the cecal bottom, representing the frenula valvulae coli, and identification of the ileocecal valve next to the cecal sling. Fluoroscopy can also be used to confirm the position of the tip of the colonoscope.

After documenting depth of penetration of the colonoscope, the instrument is slowly withdrawn. Examination during withdrawal is a critical part of colonoscopy. Each examiner has an individual system for surveying various segments of the colon. Mucosal surfaces should be inspected meticulously. Careful inspection and reinspection of areas behind haustra and around flexures and bends may be required. The instrument may have to be advanced and withdrawn intermittently over varying distances to ensure that abnormalities have not been overlooked. The examiner should establish a set of survey arcs at a few cm intervals, scanning the circumference of the lumen while maintaining the tip at the center, thus describing the configuration of a helix as the tip is withdrawn to optimize inspection of the colonic mucosal surface.

10.3

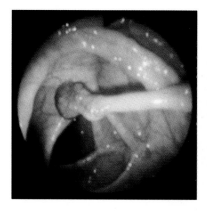

Figure 10.3 Small tubular adenoma on a long stalk. Note the erythematous mucosa at the polyp tip.

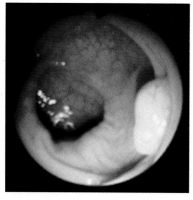

Figure 10.4 Small, sessile, tubular adenoma in a patient previously operated on for colonic cancer. Mucosa of this polyp appears normal.

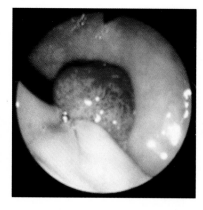

Figure 10.5 Moderate-size tubular adenoma on a short stalk shows conspicuous erythema.

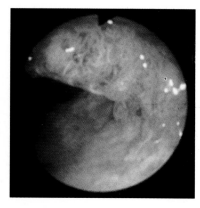

Figure 10.6 Villous projections of an adenoma in the distal rectum show hyperemia.

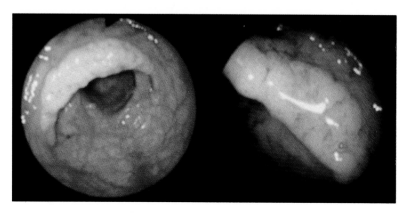

Figure 10.7 *Left,* This view shows a flat, sessile, villous polyp which developed around a valve of Houston. The yellow-white color of the multiple tiny nodules is typical of villous adenoma. *Right,* Closeup view.

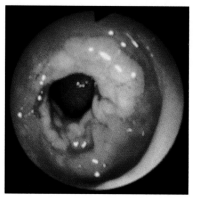

Figure 10.8 Small, circumferential, villous adenoma. The surface of the lesion consists of multiple tiny nodules.

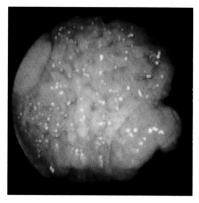

Figure 10.9 Extensive villous polyp covers the bowel wall circumferentially in a tapestry-like fashion.

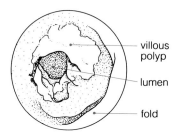

villous polyp

lumen

fold

POLYPOID LESIONS

Colonic polypoid lesions are the most common pathology found during colonoscopy. They may be single or multiple, and of epithelial or nonepithelial origin. Within the epithelial polyps, adenomatous, hyperplastic, juvenile, and inflammatory polyps are distinguished. Neoplastic and non-neoplastic polyposis syndromes are also discussed.

EPITHELIAL POLYPS

ADENOMATOUS POLYPS

The characteristic appearance of colonic adenomas varies. It is uncertain why this variation occurs but it possibly relates to the size of the polyp and perhaps to the rapidity of growth. What has been learned recently is that it is impossible to tell endoscopically whether a polyp is an adenoma or a hyperplastic polyp. When dealing with small polyps this distinction is important because we have learned that the presence of an adenoma (even a small one) is associated with synchronous and metachronous polyps and cancer.

The smallest or diminutive polyp is typically less than 5 mm, covered with normal-appearing mucosa and rarely large enough to have a stalk. Occasionally, even these small adenomas are red in appearance. Histologically, these adenomas are composed predominantly of branching tubules packed closely together surrounded by lamina propria.

As the size of the adenoma increases they may be sessile or pedunculated (Figs. 10.3 and 10.4). As with smaller pol-

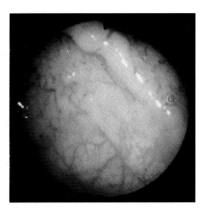

Figure 10.10 Early villous transformation is characterized by blurring and irregularity of vascular pattern.

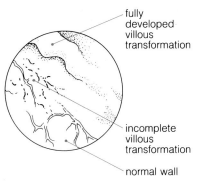

Figure 10.11 Moderate-size, sessile, tubulovillous adenoma. Several lobules are evident.

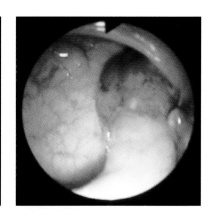

Figure 10.12 Large tubulovillous polyp in the sigmoid colon. Note the wide pedicle and erythematous, nodular polyp head.

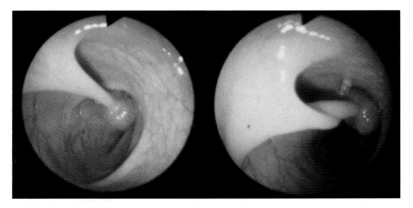

Figure 10.13 Pedunculated adenomatous polyp (left) can spontaneously twist on its stalk (right). Prolonged or repetitive twisting may cause ischemic damage and lead to autoamputation.

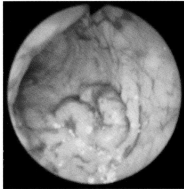

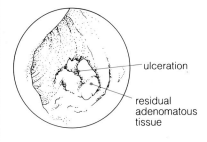

Figure 10.14 Autoamputation of a pedunculated polyp caused sudden massive hematochezia. This view shows the residual adenomatous tissue surrounding the central ulcerative defect.

yps, the covering mucosa may appear normal or slightly erythematous. When the polyp is larger than 1.0 cm, the contour of the surface may vary. The smaller polyps tend to be smooth; as they grow, a lobulated appearance may be noted (Fig. 10.5). These larger polyps have usually been present longer than the smaller polyps, and they are often pedunculated, occasionally with a long stalk.

Adenomas usually remain pedunculated as they grow and therefore are removable with snare techniques. Most endoscopists are concerned about the potential for immediate or delayed hemorrhage resulting from removal of larger lesions (over 2 cm). Therefore removal as an inpatient, with blood for transfusion available and with appropriate caution to watch for delayed hemorrhage, is appropriate. In several series, hemorrhage associated with polypectomy may be delayed by as long as 7 to 12 days.

There are two predominant histologic forms of adenoma: villous and tubular. In general there is more concern about the villous than the tubular form because the villous are generally larger, sessile, and more likely contain a carcinoma. It is not unusual to find lesions over 3 cm in diameter. The

polyp is frequently sessile, and the surface is often irregular or covered with small nodules several millimeters in height (Figs. 10.6 and 10.7). These polyps are often pale-yellow, rather than the typical erythema of tubular adenoma.

There are other common patterns of growth of villous lesions including a villous lesion growing in a diffuse pattern along the circumference of a segment of colon (Figs. 10.8 and 10.9). The mucosa at the edge of this type of lesion may have an indistinct vascular pattern referred to as incomplete villous transformation (Fig. 10.10).

Intermediate between these two forms is the tubulovillous adenoma. These lesions are often moderate in size and pedunculated with a thicker stalk than a typical tubular adenoma. The surface is often nodular, especially over the area containing villi (Figs. 10.11 and 10.12).

Polyps may disappear spontaneously. Twisting of the stalk of a long polyp or excessive aboral traction due to hypermotility may cause ischemia and autoamputation, characterized clinically by a brief episode of brisk rectal bleeding (Figs. 10.13 and 10.14). Endoscopically, a small mucosal defect surrounded by some inflammatory changes may be

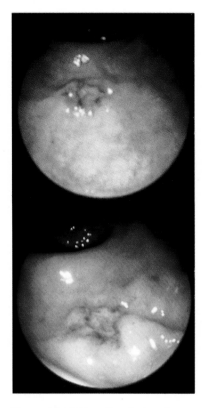

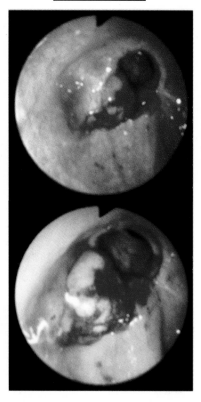

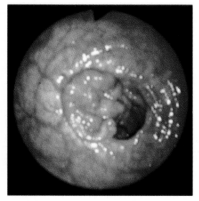

Figure 10.17 Superficial central ulceration in this rectal villous polyp is suggestive of malignancy.

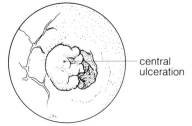

central ulceration

Figure 10.15 *Top*, Small ulcer in colon surrounded by slight inflammatory changes was caused by autoamputation of a polyp. *Bottom*, Detail view of the ulcerative defect.

Figure 10.16 *Top*, This malignant rectal polyp shows a discrete central ulceration and friable surface. After polypectomy, cancer was present in the transection line. *Bottom*, Detail view of the malignant polyp.

seen (Fig. 10.15). If the endoscopic examination is delayed, it may be difficult to recognize the site of the lesion. Because autoamputation may occur in adenomatous polyps bearing a focus of malignancy, biopsy of the postamputation ulcer or of the site is essential.

Adenomatous polyps are neoplastic and may undergo cancerous degeneration. Some polypoid structures are composed largely of cancerous tissue with little or no remaining adenomatous elements. These are often sessile or have a short stalk. Characteristic endoscopic features of malignant polyps include subtle changes such as deformity, deep ulceration of the head of the polyp, an excessively granular or friable surface, or bleeding (Figs. 10.16 and 10.17). Sharp, angular edges or a waxy, hard consistency, especially upon biopsy, are also suggestive of malignancy. If the polyp moves easily away from the colonic wall when touched with a catheter or biopsy forceps, invasion of the deeper layers of the wall is unlikely. If the polyp is fixed to the wall such that the polyp and colonic wall move together, invasion into and beyond the muscularis propria is likely. Discoloration of the head of the polyp may indicate foci of invasive cancer. Broad-based pedicles or pseudopedicles produced by peristaltic action may also suggest malignant invasion, especially when the pedicle has an ill-defined base.

HYPERPLASTIC POLYPS

Hyperplastic polyps are small sessile excrescences, usually less than 5 mm in diameter, most commonly found in the rectum. The tiny mucosal excrescences or slightly larger mamillations are pale or, more commonly, the same color as the surrounding mucosa (Figs. 10.18 and 10.19). In a rare case, hundreds of tiny hyperplastic polyps are visible, especially in the left colon. Giant hyperplastic polyps are an exceedingly rare presentation and may simulate carcinoma. They usually are single, but up to 10% of patients may have as many as 5 to 10 or more in a single segment of bowel.

While small hyperplastic polyps are invariably sessile, larger lesions may be pedunculated and therefore visually indistinguishable from small adenomatous polyps. If it is not known whether the patient forms adenomatous or hyperplastic polyps, such small polyps should be removed with a diathermy forceps (hot biopsy forceps), especially if the polyps are 4 to 5 mm and the patient is elderly. This technique destroys the potentially premalignant (adenomatous) tissue and, at the same time, obtains a biopsy for histologic interpretation. This is useful for future planning, as the treatment of the patient who forms hyperplastic polyps is different from that of the patient who forms adenomas.

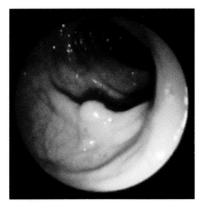

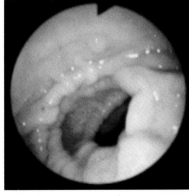

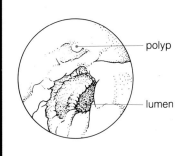

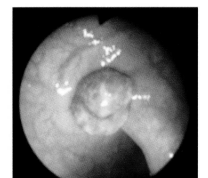

Figure 10.18 Small hyperplastic (metaplastic) polyp on top of a mucosal fold.

Figure 10.19 Tiny hyperplastic (metaplastic) polyp in the sigmoid

colon is the same color as the surrounding mucosa.

Figure 10.20 Juvenile polyp. The surface is eroded and erythematous.

JUVENILE POLYPS

Juvenile polyps, a type of hamartoma, are prevalent in children and adolescents. The typical endoscopic finding is that of a 1.5 to 3 cm sessile lesion with an intensely erythematous, friable, eroded, ulcerated surface (Fig. 10.20). Sometimes the surface is nodular but not ulcerated, making such polyps indistinguishable from a tubular adenoma. When examined histologically, the surface is usually ulcerated. The center of the polyp is composed of cysts with a large mucin component. There is an expansion of the lamina propria and increased inflammatory cells.

INFLAMMATORY POLYPS

Inflammatory polyps or pseudopolyps occur in the setting of inflammatory changes in the colon. They are nonspecific and indicate prior ulcerative epithelial destruction. They are made up of markedly inflamed, focally ulcerated epithelial bumps or granulation tissue. (See Chapter 11 for a detailed presentation of inflammatory bowel disease.)

NONEPITHELIAL POLYPS AND POLYPLIKE STRUCTURES

Submucosal tumors are much less common in the colon than in the upper GI tract. Lipoma is the most frequently encountered lesion of this type. These are important lesions to recognize endoscopically because they should not be removed with a snare cautery. When one attempts to snare and sever the polyp with radiofrequency current, it is difficult to coagulate the fat in the center of the lipoma, and bleeding or deep injury may result. These lesions appear yellow and translucent. They are usually sessile, often over 2 cm in diameter. Although they occur throughout the colon, they are most often found in the right colon. Endoscopically one suspects a lipoma by the color, the smooth surface, and by determining whether the lesion is soft and

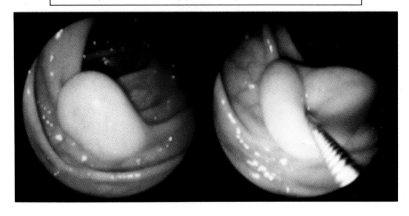

Figure 10.21 Left, Lipoma of the transverse colon is a soft, round, sessile lesion with yellow coloration.

Right, Easy indentation of the lipoma with a biopsy forceps is termed the "cushion effect" or "pillow sign."

indents when pressed by an accessory such as a closed biopsy forceps. This indentation is called the "pillow sign" (Fig. 10.21). If there is doubt concerning the type of lesion, a biopsy may be performed. Fatty tissue may exude from the biopsy site. A biopsy may be necessary when the surface of the lipoma is eroded or irregular in contrast to a smooth surface. The ileocecal valve may have a large amount of fat, referred to as lipomatous change, and may resemble a lipoma. The endoscopist should be careful to make this distinction and not attempt removal of the lipomatous valve.

Leiomyomas are rare submucosal tumors in the colon, ranging in size from 2 mm to 4 cm. At colonoscopy they appear smooth and sessile, and may be covered with a reddish, stretched mucosa.

Carcinoid tumors may be found in the rectum but are rare in the colon. Usually a carcinoid appears as a smooth,

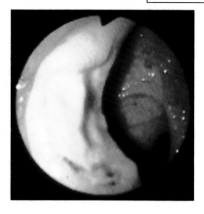
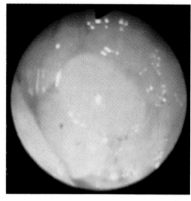
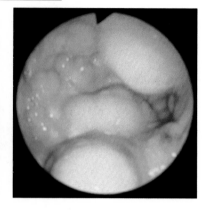

Figure 10.22 Rectal carcinoid. Note the peculiar yellowish discoloration. The superficial defect is due to prior biopsy.

Figure 10.23 Lymph cyst of the colon. Characteristic transparency and pale yellow color are evident.

Figure 10.24 Pneumatosis cystoides intestinalis is characterized by gas-filled cysts within the colonic wall.

sessile lesion with a glistening surface mucosa, which has a pale-yellow color (Fig. 10.22). Generally such tumors are nonulcerating and range in size between 1 and 2 cm. They often have a firm consistency when touched with the biopsy forceps.

Lymphangiomas are pale, smooth, round polypoid masses which are usually soft and easily compressible. Overlying mucosa may have a pale yellow coloration (Fig. 10.23). These cystic lesions in the submucosa are rarely reached by colonic biopsy because of their depth.

An endometrial implant via the serosal layer of the rectum or sigmoid occasionally presents as a submucosal polypoid mass. In addition to the mass there may be central erythematous discoloration, especially during episodes of intestinal bleeding at the time of menstruation.

Pneumatosis cystoides intestinalis is characterized by the presence of gas-filled cysts within the wall of the colon (Fig. 10.24). Cysts may be localized to one segment of the colon or occur throughout, with a predilection for the left side. They appear as submucosal polypoid masses ranging from 2 to 3 mm to well over 2 cm. These structures are soft and easily compressible. The overlying mucosa shows nonspecific erythema, especially at the top. Sometimes these masses obliterate the lumen and are mistaken for adenomas or even carcinoma. A biopsy will differentiate a cyst from a carcinoma or adenoma. A small biopsy will not usually penetrate into the cyst but a larger biopsy may. Because the cysts largely contain nitrogen, high-flow or hyperbaric oxygen therapy has been used to stimulate resorption of nitrogen from the cysts. When the cysts disappear, a focal area of brownish discoloration of the mucosa remains.

Other polyp-simulating structures include polyplike mucosal folds, which are occasionally seen in diverticular disease, especially of the sigmoid. (See Chapter 12 for a detailed presentation of diverticular disease.) Polypoid structures consisting entirely of granulation tissue occasionally develop, especially in the rectosigmoid area. These are due to breakthrough of inflammatory lesions originating from the pelvic organs, especially chronic salpingitis.

POLYPOSIS SYNDROMES

NEOPLASTIC POLYPOSIS SYNDROME
Familial polyposis coli (FPC) is a dominantly inherited disease in which the colon is studded with numerous adenomatous polyps prone to malignant degeneration. Three distinct patterns of FPC may be identified. The most common is the carpet of minute, 1 to 3 mm polyps (Fig. 10.25). These polyps are smooth and regular with normal-appearing mucosal coloration; no larger polyps are found (Fig. 10.26). In a less common variant, somewhat larger polyps (4 to 8 mm) are distributed throughout the rectum and colon with intervening areas of normal mucosa (Fig. 10.27). A third pattern consists of both large and minute polyps (Fig. 10.28).

Patients with adenomatous polyposis are always at risk for malignant transformation. Therefore, a prophylactic proctocolectomy or colectomy with rectal mucosal stripping, along with pelvic pouch and ileoanal anastomosis is the best treatment. If colectomy with ileorectal anastomosis is carried out, meticulous follow-up of the rectal stump is necessary to prevent cancer by removing all small adenomas and to detect early malignancy (Fig. 10.29).

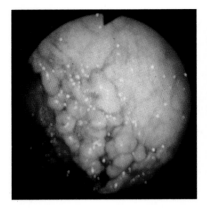

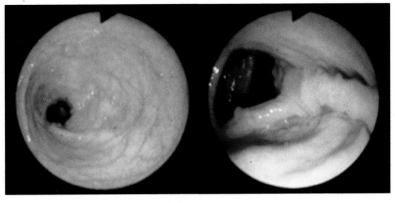

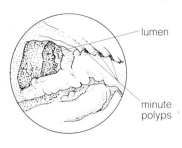

Figure 10.25 Conglomerate of innumerable small polyps covers the colon wall like a carpet. This is the most common presentation of FPC.

Figure 10.26 FPC. *Left,* Minute polyps scattered over the colon wall.

Right, Tenia of the transverse colon studded with minute polyps.

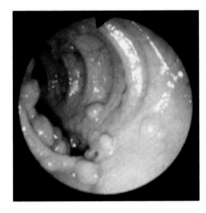

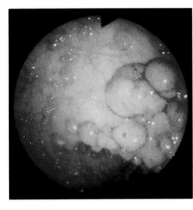

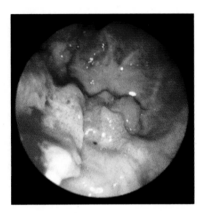

Figure 10.27 Small and larger polyps in FPC. The lesions are scattered, with normal-looking mucosa intervening.

Figure 10.28 Larger polyps appear with smaller ones in the combined pattern of FPC.

Figure 10.29 Rectal cancer developed after ileorectal anastomosis for FPC.

Differentiating FPC from inflammatory, parasitic, or lymphomatous polyposis may occasionally be difficult. Although inflammatory pseudopolyps of ulcerative colitis resemble those of FPC, the intervening mucosa in the latter is normal and the vascular pattern is preserved. In the case of ulcerative colitis, the intervening mucosa is abnormal and a distorted or absent vascular pattern is expected. Although inflammatory pseudopolyps may be numerous, they rarely carpet the mucosa to the extent of obliterating it. These pseudopolyps tend to vary considerably in size and shape, unlike the monotonous appearance of adenomatous polyposis. In addition, inflammatory polyps often exhibit exudate on their luminal surface.

NONNEOPLASTIC POLYPOSIS SYNDROMES
Several syndromes involving the intestinal tract are associated with polypoid lesions that are not true neoplasms.

These include juvenile polyps, Peutz-Jeghers syndrome, and lymphoid hyperplasia.

The multiple lesions of juvenile polyposis resemble those of single juvenile polyps. These lesions can occur throughout the GI tract or be confined to the colon. They may be associated with adenomatous polyps.

Peutz-Jeghers syndrome is a problem in gastroenterology in terms of management. These patients present with polyps throughout the GI tract, but especially the small intestine, which may be large and cause significant symptoms of obstruction, GI bleeding, or intussusception. They are hamartomas with a characteristic histologic appearance of an excessive and redundant muscularis mucosae covered by a nonneoplastic epithelium and lamina propria. Areas of the polyp may show evidence of infarction. The polyps vary in size but may be several centimeters in diameter. They are pedunculated or sessile and may have an irregular or lob-

10.9

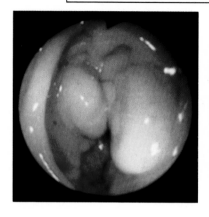

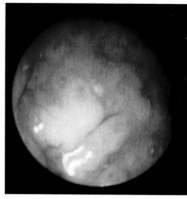

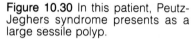

Figure 10.30 In this patient, Peutz-Jeghers syndrome presents as a large sessile polyp.

Figure 10.31 Lymphoid hyperplasia due to follicle enlargement.

ulated surface (Fig. 10.30). Because these polyps tend to recur, endoscopy during surgery may allow the endoscopist to enter the small bowel with guidance of the surgeon, find the polyps, and remove them without opening the bowel wall. This reduces the chance of further adhesion formation which can be a real problem in these patients.

Colonic lymphoid hyperplasia consists of lymphoid aggregations seen as slightly raised areas of multiple, 1 to 2 mm, closely spaced, yellowish-white polyps, similar in appearance to nodular lymphoid hyperplasia of the small bowel (Fig. 10.31). Colonic lymphoid hyperplasia may be noted in children and adolescents. Slightly raised, minute, polypoid structures due to lymphoid follicle enlargement may occasionally be seen in adults after severe intestinal infection or other colonic disease. The lesions have a central necrotic or slightly hemorrhagic patch. The significance of this finding is unknown.

TECHNIQUE OF ENDOSCOPIC POLYPECTOMY

Polypectomy is routinely used to remove polypoid lesions in the rectocolon. The technique is safe and effective for most colonic polyps, but selection of lesions appropriate for this procedure and performing polypectomy takes considerable training and experience. The colon must be carefully prepared so that endoscopic visualization is excellent, and to reduce the concentration of potentially explosive gases. Hospitalization may be recommended for patients with respiratory or cardiovascular disease or other significant medical problems, for debilitated patients whose colons are difficult to prepare thoroughly, and for patients with numerous polyps or large sessile polyps.

When an adenomatous polyp is known to be present anywhere in the colon or rectum, a total colonoscopic examination is important because of the increased incidence of synchronous polyps or cancer found at colonoscopy. Many of these lesions are undetectable radiologically. If a total colonoscopy cannot be done at the initial examination, it should be completed within 6 to 12 months.

The entire polyp and its base or pedicle must be inspected before a decision is made on endoscopic removal. Occasionally the lesion must be manipulated with a closed snare to facilitate evaluation. Polyps tend to locate in areas of acute angulation or flexures; patients may have to be repositioned to display the polyp to best advantage (Fig. 10.32).

Multiple polyps are usually removed at a single session unless they are scattered throughout the colon, in which case they are usually removed in separate right and left excision sessions. In this way problems can more easily be localized in a patient with numerous large polyps. In general, the most anatomically proximal polyp is removed first. After retrieval of the specimen, the colonoscope is inserted to the level of the next polyp and the procedure repeated until all polyps are removed. Several sessions may be required to remove all polyps. Occasionally India ink is injected into the submucosa to mark a polypectomy site in case of the need for further endoscopic or surgical therapy. Histologic examination of all fragments is essential for correct diagnosis.

REMOVAL OF PEDUNCULATED POLYPS

Virtually all pedunculated polyps can and should be removed endoscopically using snare electrosurgical techniques (Figs. 10.33 and 10.34). The plane of transection or coagulation of the stalk is best located near the head of the polyp rather than close to the normal bowel wall to minimize the risk of heat penetration and damage. The snare should not be tightened until it is precisely at the proposed plane of transection on the stalk. Grasping the stalk too snugly prior to application of current can cause premature mechanical transection with resulting hemorrhage and impaired vision. One must be certain that the tip of the colonoscope can be controlled so that the polyp does not move out of sight once it is snared, as a complication may occur if the polyp is excised blindly.

Once the wire loop is around the polyp, the tip of the snare sheath is advanced to the point of desired separation on the stalk. Once the snare has been tightened, it should not be loosened for repositioning, for the partially cut tissue may bleed and impair vision. Instead, that portion should be transected by diathermic current. The snare can then be repositioned to the proper place on the stalk and polypectomy completed. This method of partial or piecemeal polypectomy is often recommended for polyps in which the head is too large for safe, complete encirclement with the snare.

It is essential that the entire thickness of a polyp stalk be adequately coagulated. Ideally, coagulating current is applied as the wire loop is closed around the polyp stalk. Further tightening is done only after the effect of coagulation

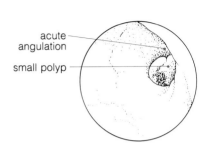

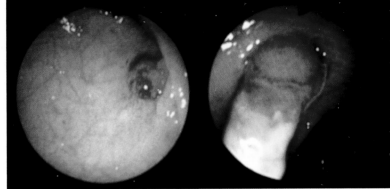

Figure 10.32 *Left*, Small polyp with minor bleeding is located in an area of acute angulation. *Right*, Larger polyp is found in an acute sigmoid bend.

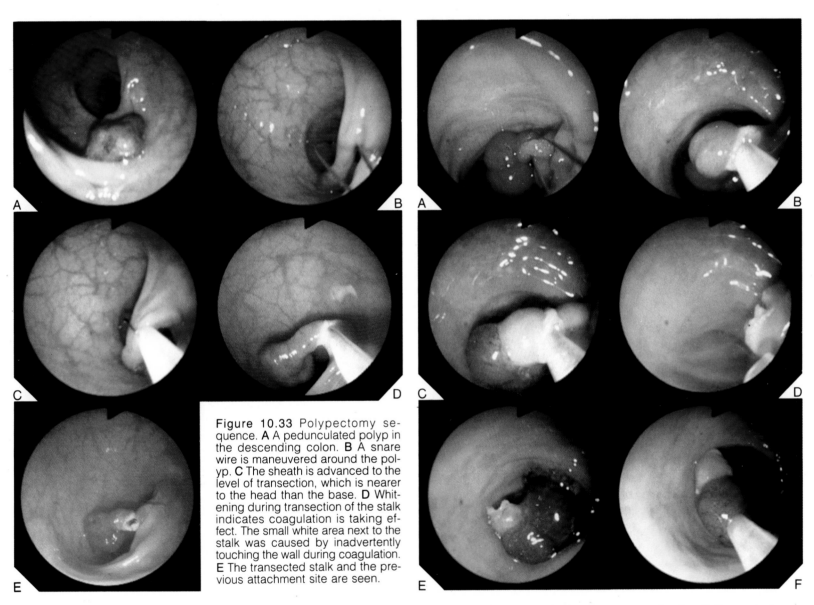

Figure 10.33 Polypectomy sequence. **A** A pedunculated polyp in the descending colon. **B** A snare wire is maneuvered around the polyp. **C** The sheath is advanced to the level of transection, which is nearer to the head than the base. **D** Whitening during transection of the stalk indicates coagulation is taking effect. The small white area next to the stalk was caused by inadvertently touching the wall during coagulation. **E** The transected stalk and the previous attachment site are seen.

Figure 10.34 Sequence of polypectomy of a multilobulated, peduncular polyp. **A** A snare wire is maneuvered around the pedicle. **B** During transection, white discoloration indicates coagulation is taking effect. **C** Edematous swelling is evident at the transection line. **D** Transected pedicle is seen; faint wisps of smoke generated by application of electrical current are evident. **E** Released polyp lies in the lumen. **F** A grasping device holds the polyp for retrieval as the colonoscope is withdrawn.

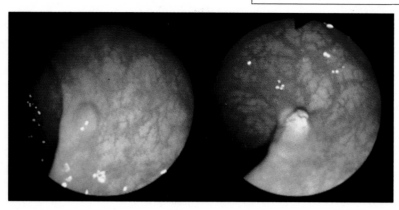

Figure 10.35 *Left*, Small sessile polypoid lesion before removal with hot biopsy forceps. *Right*, Appearance after removal.

is seen to spread a short distance along the pedicle. Higher current power or cutting current modes are used only if resistance to wire closure persists after sufficient coagulation is accomplished. If high power or cutting current is used before coagulation of the stalk, rapid transection may occur and result in hemorrhage. Smoke may be generated while applying current during polypectomy, but can be cleared via aspiration.

REMOVAL OF SESSILE POLYPS

The appearance of the sessile polyp is the most important criterion for determining whether it should be removed endoscopically. In general, soft, smooth, nonulcerated, sessile polyps less than 2 cm in size are benign and endoscopically excisable. Sessile lesions larger than 2 cm, especially those containing ulcerations or areas of firm consistency, are usually malignant and therefore not appropriate for endoscopic polypectomy. Transrectal sonographic examination will likely become an important means of differentiating benign and focally malignant, sessile villous lesions.

Sessile lesions are directly and broadly attached to the rectal or colonic wall. Electrosurgical snare excision is therefore always applied at the level of the bowel wall, making this a delicate and risky procedure. Selected larger lesions can be removed by an experienced endoscopist familiar with the segmental or piecemeal technique.

Small sessile polyps less than 0.5 cm are most easily eradicated using a hot biopsy forceps (Fig. 10.35). This allows a biopsy specimen to be obtained and, in addition, coagulates the entire base of the lesion. Routine use of this technique is not universally accepted because of the risk of delayed bleeding and perforation.

Sessile polyps in the 0.5 to 1.0 cm range can usually be removed by a single transection using the snare cautery technique (Fig. 10.36). One end of the wire snare is hooked on the edge of the polyp, while the other is eased over the widest diameter of the polyp. The wire should be placed at the base of the abnormal tissue to avoid grasping a margin of normal bowel mucosa. With the catheter sheath advanced to the point of transection at the base of the polyp, the snare is tightened gently. The polyp tissue is then pulled or tented slightly into the lumen. If correctly snared, it moves easily back and forth. If the normal mucosa around the polyp is caught in the snare, the polyp will be difficult to move. After proper placement of the snare, the lumen is distended slightly to prevent the grasped tissue from touching the adjacent or opposite wall. The diathermy current coagulates the residual abnormal tissue at the base of the polyp.

Sessile polyps larger than 2.5 cm with a small attachment site should be treated like pedunculated polyps. Those with wide-based attachment are usually removed by segmental transection in several sessions, usually separated by 3 to 6 weeks, with subsequent removal of fragments becoming easier with each attempt. In the segmental transection technique, one end of the wire is hooked at the junction of the polyp and the mucosal surface, and the other flipped over to engage a large portion of the polyp head. Diathermy current is then applied for a few seconds, followed by simultaneous application of current and closure of the wire snare. The transections are applied obliquely, so that only a portion of the base is cauterized each time.

Sometimes the cumulative cauterizations injure the bowel wall before the lesion is completely removed. After 4 to 6 weeks, the cautery effect resolves, allowing resumption of polypectomy and cauterization. Bleeding is rarely a problem in segmental transection since the large blood vessels supplying the polyp rapidly branch, with only small capillary-size vessels extending into the polyp.

After segmental transection polypectomy, the patient should be examined endoscopically at 3- or 6-month intervals until the polyp site completely heals. The exact site of a large sessile polyp may be difficult to ascertain after removal. Usually an area of whitish discoloration due to fibrosis or telangiectatic vessels may be seen at the reepithelialized polyp base, or a notch in the colonic wall remains at the site (Fig. 10.37).

If a sessile polyp is wrapped around a fold, the portion of polyp on the distal side of the fold should be removed first. Achieving total polypectomy on the proximal side may require considerable manipulation. Delaying until the coagulation ulcer has healed on the distal side may facilitate removal since retraction exposes the proximal side more favorably.

Ideally, the polyp should be shaved so that the base is flat; however, if this cannot be accomplished, it is wise to stop and have the patient return in 4 to 6 weeks. Upon reinspection, there may be complete healing or an ulcer may be present with minimal polypoid tissue around it. Sometimes the residual polyp may have reformed as several small polypoid excrescences at the site of the polypectomy. The residual polypoid tumor may be removed completely at this time or the piecemeal process may be continued. If tiny foci of adenomatous tissue are still present, a mono- or bipolar

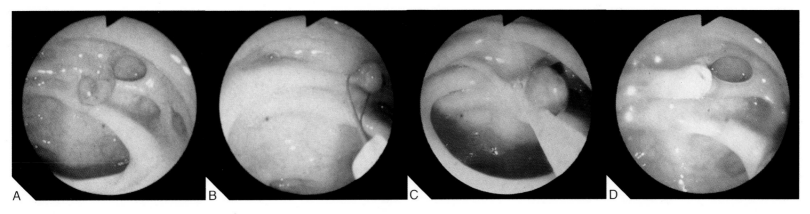

Figure 10.36 Polypectomy of a small sessile polyp at the edge of a diverticulum. **A** Appearance of polyp before removal. **B** Polypectomy snare wire is maneuvered around the polyp. **C** White discoloration occurs during transection. **D** This view shows the appearance of the coagulated insertion base.

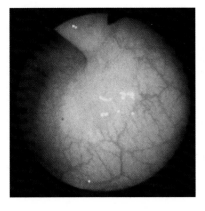

Figure 10.37 Appearance of the colon wall 3 months after destruction of a villous polyp with Nd-YAG laser. Note an area of whitish scarring and conspicuous telangiectatic vessels at the margin.

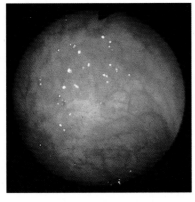

Figure 10.38 In this patient, nearly invisible adenomatous tissue remains after the polyp was removed.

electrocoagulation probe or laser photocoagulation may more easily destroy the remaining neoplastic tissue (Fig. 10.38).

Removal of large postage-stamp or tapestry-type sessile polyps which cover extensive areas of the circumference may be difficult. The recommended method at present combines debulking with the snare wire technique, followed by eradication of remaining polypoid tissue with Nd-YAG laser photocoagulation. Using this elegant technique it is usually possible to eradicate even extensive villous polyps. Destruction with laser requires several sessions to prevent circumferential necrosis and retraction, especially when the entire contour is covered with polypoid tissue.

An alternative technique is to use mono- or bipolar electrocoagulation devices. If these electrocoagulative devices are used, one must reduce the chances of a perforation by not pushing against the wall and by keeping the device's tip moving across the mucosa in a steady movement.

RETRIEVAL OF POLYPECTOMY SPECIMENS

Retrieval of all polypectomy tissue is extremely important to assure accurate histologic diagnosis. Single polyps or pol-

yp fragments in the 0.5 to 1.5 cm range can be retrieved by suctioning the fragment to the tip of the scope and maintaining the suction power as the scope is removed. However, larger polyps may fall loose while maneuvering the scope through the narrow and angulated sigmoid colon, especially in patients with diverticular disease. Therefore, for polyps larger than 1.5 cm, it may be easier to grasp the specimen by the stalk with the snare (Fig. 10.34F). By keeping the grasped specimen 3 to 4 cm from the tip of the scope, other polyps can be detected during withdrawal. In withdrawing a large, snared polyp through the anal canal, it is wise to bring the specimen flush to the tip of the scope just prior to bringing the specimen through the anal canal. Having the patient bear down may help passage, but this maneuver should be gentle as it may increase the chance of bleeding from the colonic wall at the site of the polyp resection.

If a polyp specimen is lost from sight and cannot be relocated, it can often be retrieved by using the endoscope to flush the area with 50 to 100 ml tap water or saline. This fluid can then be aspirated and the polyp can often be found and retrieved. An enema can also be used as a retrieval technique, but this is uncomfortable for the patient. Specimens retrieved 10 to 12 hours or more after polypectomy are often too autolysed for accurate histologic examination.

Several passes of the instrument may be necessary to remove all the fragments of a large sessile polyp. Retrieval of the resected portion closest to the base of the polyp is especially important for histologic examination to determine the depth of invasion if cancer is detected.

COMPLICATIONS OF ENDOSCOPIC POLYPECTOMY

Errors in identifying or labeling the site of a malignant polyp could lead to surgical resection of the wrong colonic segment. Exacting technique is especially critical in patients with a high risk of malignancy, such as patients from families in which one or more family members have colon or breast

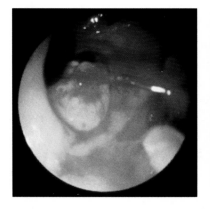

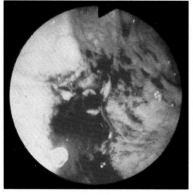

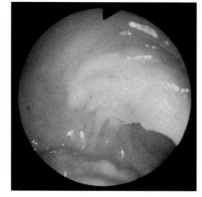

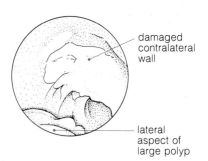

damaged contralateral wall

lateral aspect of large polyp

Figure 10.39 Spurting arterial hemorrhage after polypectomy.

Figure 10.40 Profuse bleeding results from premature mechanical transection with polypectomy snare.

Figure 10.41 Damage to the contralateral wall after endoscopic transection of a large polyp.

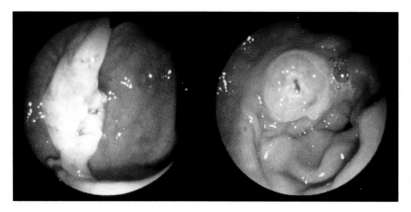

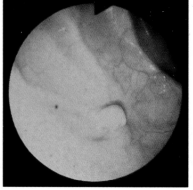

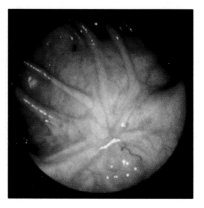

Figure 10.42 After polyp transection. *Left,* Whitish discoloration and swelling of insertion site. *Right,* Peculiar appearance with marked edema.

Figure 10.43 Granulation tissue developed at the site of a previous polypectomy.

Figure 10.44 Scarring and retraction 1 year after snare polypectomy with deep intramural burn.

cancer. This familial aggregation is referred to as the cancer family syndrome.

In several large series of colonoscopic polypectomy complications, the most common serious complication is that of hemorrhage (Fig. 10.39). Although this complication may occur with an endoscopist of any degree of experience, it is more common with inexperienced examiners. Bleeding after polypectomy may be immediate or delayed by up to 14 days. Immediate hemorrhage occurs when the stalk of a polyp is severed before sufficient coagulation has occurred to thrombose the arterial vessels in the stalk (Fig. 10.40). This may occur by mechanical transection or by the application of cutting R.F. current before adequate coagulation has been accomplished.

Serious postpolypectomy bleeding requires the immediate application of standard emergency measures, continuous monitoring of the patient, endoscopic attempts to control the bleeding, and angiographic treatment in selected cases. Surgical intervention is a last resort. If immediate bleeding occurs after the stalk is transected, it may be possible to place the snare over the stalk and gently close the snare to achieve hemostasis. If the snare is held closed for approximately 10 minutes, hemostasis may be achieved. To check the area for further bleeding, the snare is released just slightly. If there is any oozing or bleeding, additional coagulation may be cautiously attempted. Alternative methods

to control hemorrhage include local injection of epinephrine or a sclerosing agent to induce vasospasm and mechanically compress the bleeding vessel. Laser photocoagulation can also be applied to the bleeding spot.

If blood obscures the polypectomy site, the patient's position should be shifted to drain blood away from the area. Aspiration of blood and clots through a standard colonoscope is usually unsuccessful and nearly always plugs the suction channel. Ice water lavage or enema of the bleeding polypectomy site is probably not effective.

The colonic wall opposite the lesion may be damaged, especially during resection of large polyps in contact with the wall during application of diathermy current. Damage may be avoided or minimized by moving the polyp slightly during transection to prevent overheating of a narrow segment of colonic wall. Some damage is occasionally unavoidable (Fig. 10.41).

Transmural damage may lead to serosal irritation or outright perforation. Perforation is mainly encountered with resection of sessile polyps. Prolonged pain and signs of peritoneal irritation should lead to prompt investigation and, if necessary, surgical exploration.

The endoscopist should be aware of the endoscopic changes brought about by application of diathermy current or laser photocoagulation. The base of a recently coagulated polyp may rapidly take on a peculiar, edematous appearance

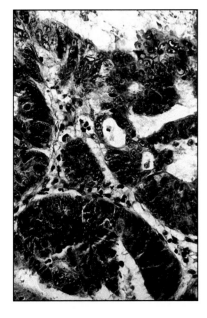

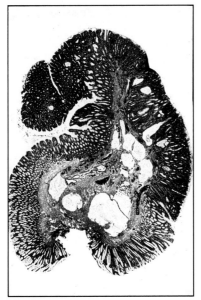

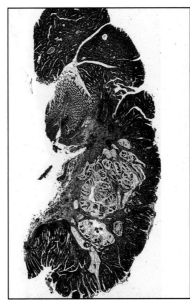

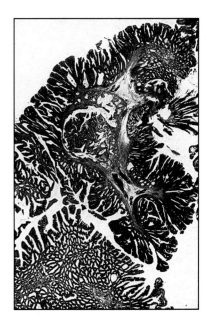

Figure 10.45 Detail of a focus of severe dysplasia located at top of adenomatous polyp. Note irregular, hyperchromatic nuclei, loss of polarity, and absent mucous secretion.

Figure 10.46 Pedunculated malignant polyp with deep infiltration of the stalk near the transection line. Note the precise orientation of the polyp, allowing histologic interpretation.

Figure 10.47 Sessile tubulovillous adenoma with mucoid carcinoma invading the submucosal layer close to the line of transection.

Figure 10.48 Fragment of a large villous polyp removed with piecemeal polypectomy technique. Because of poor orientation, it is impossible to analyze the depth of penetration of the malignant focus.

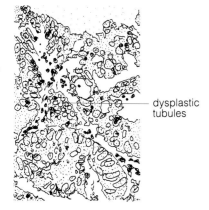

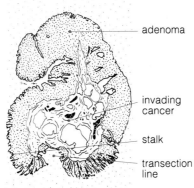

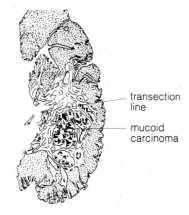

(Fig. 10.42). This is followed by sloughing of the necrotic tissue, and formation of an ulcerative defect which gradually forms granulation tissue (Fig. 10.43). After reepithelialization and healing, the area retains some whitish discoloration due to subepithelial scarring. In the early phases of healing, neocapillaries can be seen, especially at the rim between the coagulated base and surrounding mucosa. After extensive and deep coagulation, widespread scarring may cause convergence of folds and retraction (Fig. 10.44). Occasionally, excessive granulation occurs, and a granulation polyp forms. These small polyps are highly vascularized and easily traumatized.

ENDOSCOPIC REMOVAL OF MALIGNANT POLYPS

Correct orientation of the excised polyp is the most crucial aspect of endoscopic removal of malignant polyps. The pathologist must identify the coagulation site to evaluate the depth of invasion of the cancer. In this way it can be determined whether endoscopic excision is adequate therapy. Orientation may be aided by placing a small needle into

the coagulated polyp base before fixation of the tissue in formalin. Multiple tissue sections are examined.

Risk of malignant transformation increases with the size of the polyp, the villous character of the adenomatous proliferation, and the degree of dysplasia. The relationship of the malignant focus to the level of the muscularis mucosae is crucial. When malignancy crosses the muscularis mucosae, there is potential for lymphatic spread, and surgical resection may be required. A focus of malignant tissue at the top of a polypoid structure, well above the level of the muscularis mucosae, is best referred to as severe dysplasia rather than intramucosal cancer or carcinoma in situ (Fig. 10.45). Such very superficial lesions have negligible capacity for lymphatic spread.

When cancer cells invade into or through the muscularis mucosae of a polyp, the lesion must be regarded as a true cancer. For pedunculated polyps, the depth of penetration of malignancy into the stalk or insertion base of the polyp can usually be precisely delineated (Fig. 10.46). For large villous polyps (Fig. 10.47) removed by multiple transections this is more difficult, as it is virtually impossible to correctly orient all the tissue fragments (Fig. 10.48). The risk of a

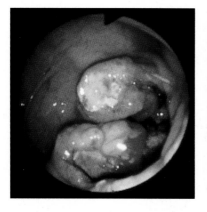
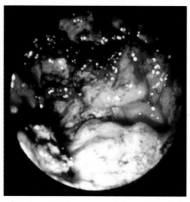
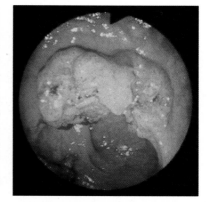

Figure 10.49 Adenocarcinoma of the cecum presenting as a centrally excavated mass with exophytic overhanging edges.

Figure 10.50 Adenocarcinoma presenting as a huge necrotic tumor cavity with a fecaloid exudate.

Figure 10.51 Polypoid mass without excavation developed around a valve of Houston.

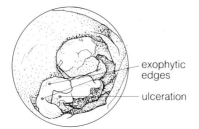
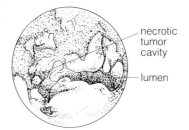

noncurative endoscopic excision of a sessile or pedunculated polyp appears to be greatest if the cancer is poorly differentiated, comes close to or within the margin of the transection, or if malignant cells are present in blood vessels or lymphatics of the polyp stroma.

There is a debate as to whether malignant polyps should be removed endoscopically or surgically. The decision depends in part on the age and health of the patient. Some physicians do not recommend surgical bowel resection in the area of a cancer if there is adequate clearance between the level of cancer invasion and the line of cautery, especially if the tumor does not invade the submucosa of the colonic wall at the site of attachment of the polyp. In these cases, the risk of lymph node metastasis is low, unless the malignancy is poorly differentiated or there is evidence of vasoinvasion. When the malignant growth is at or near the line of transection, surgical removal is recommended because of the risk of residual cancerous tissue at the polypectomy site, and of lymph node metastases.

For patients in whom surgical risk might approach or exceed the risk of cancer or metastases, the therapeutic approach is different. If cancer invades or approaches the line of transection, the next step usually is endoscopic removal of any remaining stalk. Multiple biopsies are then obtained from the base and edges of the coagulation ulcer. If positive, additional coagulation of the gut wall, preferably with laser, is carried out until there is no further histologic evidence of malignant tissue. Transmural endosonographic examination is useful to document the potential presence and depth of remaining malignant tissue.

COLONIC MALIGNANCY

Most adenocarcinomas of the rectocolon follow the adenoma-dysplasia-carcinoma sequence. De novo carcinomas are rare, as are nonepithelial malignancies such as lymphomas and metastatic tumors to the colon.

EPITHELIAL MALIGNANCIES

ADENOCARCINOMA

Adenocarcinoma, the second most common cancer in the United States, accounts for about 13% of cancer-associated deaths. The adenomatous polyp is a premalignant condition associated with colorectal adenocarcinoma. With early detection and removal of such polyps, the incidence of adenocarcinoma can hopefully be reduced. In addition, colonoscopy helps the physician diagnose and treat colorectal cancer at an early pathologic stage, before patients become symptomatic. Although it has not been definitively proved that screening and early detection reduce mortality from these cancers, there is agreement that patients with early-stage tumors have higher 5-year survival rates.

Adenocarcinomas may occur throughout the rectocolon but are most common within the distal 40 cm. An ulcerated mass is a commonly encountered configuration of adenocarcinoma (Fig. 10.49). The ulcer is irregular, deep, and gray or pink, with a necrotic appearance. Feces may be noted

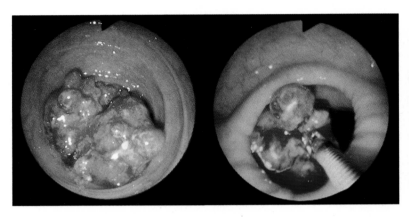 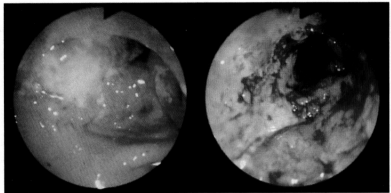

Figure 10.52 *Left,* This polypoid, nonulcerated, exophytic mass ob- structs the transverse colon. *Right,* Directed biopsy of the cancer.

Figure 10.53 *Left,* This annular, cir- cumferential, rectal mass in a young patient was missed for over 6 months in another institution. *Right,* This view shows details of circum- ferential infiltration and ulceration.

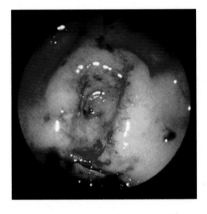 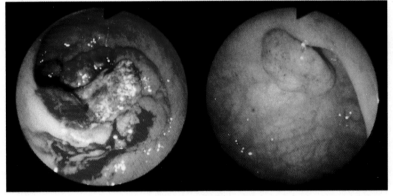

Figure 10.54 Stenosing type of ad- enocarcinoma with complete luminal cancerous obstruction.

Figure 10.55 *Left,* A large, excavat- ed, bleeding cancer in the midrec- tum was found in conjunction with a second, synchronous, smaller pol- ypoid malignancy *(right)* at the rec- tosigmoid junction.

in the base of the ulcer (Fig. 10.50). The surrounding mu- cosa is heaped up, red, and friable, accounting for the bleeding which occurs in the majority of these lesions. The lesion is hard when touched with the biopsy forceps. Sharp angles occur where the tumor tissue meets the adjacent co- lon wall.

About one-third of colorectal malignancies present as polypoid, nonexcavating masses of variable dimensions (Figs. 10.51 and 10.52). The raised, sessile mass typically has nodular surface distortion, with sharply angulated bor- ders showing focally eroded surface areas and, occasionally, striking friability. The mass is obviously fixed to the bowel wall.

An annular mass is a third presentation. This large ul- cerated mass spreads circumferentially, enveloping and penetrating the colonic wall. Generally, only the distal mar- gin of the mass can be seen, although a glimpse of the central ulcerated area is possible (Fig. 10.53).

A distinctly uncommon appearance is that of a plaque- like, slightly raised, flat, or discoid mass with a central depression or ulceration. Also uncommon is the stricturing type, seen as an abrupt termination of the lumen without an obvious mass. The growth pattern is infiltrative and linitis plastica-like; no tumor rim is apparent. The stricturing or stenotic appearance also occurs when the lumen has been narrowed by extension of the tumor into the pericolic fat, causing distal compression and obscuring the exophytic mass (Fig. 10.54).

Synchronous polyps and carcinoma also are common. Carcinomas occur in approximately 5% of patients, and pol- yps in up to 25%. Therefore, it is important to perform total colonoscopy to rule out a synchronous lesion prior to surgery because the findings may change the surgical ap- proach (Fig. 10.55). If the tumor is obstructing, the ex- amination of the total colon may be performed 1 to 2 months after surgery, but it is essential to examine the entire

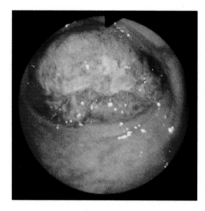 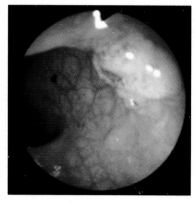 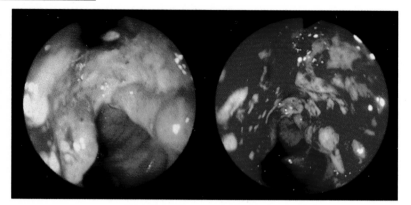

Figure 10.56 This recurrent carcinoma was found in a young patient after resection of rectal cancer.

Figure 10.57 Metachronous cancer at the rectosigmoid junction in a young patient with familial colon cancer syndrome. The patient had been treated for cecal cancer 2 years previously.

Figure 10.58 *Left,* Large, ulcerating epidermal carcinoma invading the distal rectum. *Right,* Diffuse bleeding after a single pass of the colonoscope.

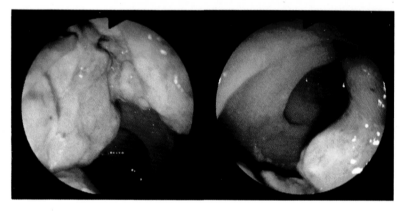

Figure 10.59 *Left,* Cloacogenic tumor invades the distal rectum. *Right,* This view shows the proximal extent of the cancer.

colon. The same is true for polyps—the entire colon must be surveyed for other polyps or carcinomas. A lifelong screening program is essential for these patients to detect metachronous lesions.

Several lesions may be confused with colon cancer. A sessile, adenomatous polyp of the sigmoid colon may be mistaken for carcinoma if the lesion is obscured by associated diverticular disease and luminal narrowing. Large villous adenomas may show enough surface irregularity and friability to suggest malignancy.

The distinction between a diverticular stricture and underlying malignancy can be difficult. In contrast to diverticular stricturing, carcinomatous narrowing is usually characterized by the distinctly irregular and heaped-up appearance of the folds, together with some discoloration or destruction of the mucosa at the level of the narrowing.

When the strictured area cannot be passed with a small-caliber colonoscope, the endoscopist should be reluctant to make a macroscopic diagnosis, even if the visible mucosa appears normal. If, on the other hand, the strictured area is passed with a small-caliber colonoscope and no macroscopically suspicious tissue is recognized upon slow withdrawal, the lesion most likely represents benign diverticular disease. Abnormal-appearing tissue should be biopsied to confirm the macroscopic suspicion.

The endoscopist should also be familiar with the appearance of recurrent cancer at a resection line, since this occurs in up to 10% of operated patients (Fig. 10.56). Most recurrences are found at sites outside the colon, such as lymph nodes or liver. In lymph node recurrences, the narrowed area usually shows marked nodularity, but is lined with normal-looking mucosa. Mucosal breakthrough is seen only in the case of suture-line recurrences.

After operation and anastomosis, examination with the colonoscope may be undertaken to rule out a suture line recurrence. The distinction may be difficult because of deformity caused by the suture line and the occurrence of nodules at the suture line resulting from suture granulomas. When a recurrent tumor is encountered, the mass is usually hard, friable, and may be ulcerated, presenting a different appearance from that of a granuloma. Echo imaging of this area may be important in the future to distinguish a small granuloma from a recurrent tumor with a large extracolonic mass.

Patients treated for colonic cancer should be seen at regular intervals to screen for metachronous polyps and cancer (Fig. 10.57). The timing of follow-up is not yet established; however, colonoscopic reexamination at 6 and 12 months is recommended. A schedule for lifelong screening must then be planned. This includes combinations of testing for carcinoembryonic antigen, occult blood testing, and full colonoscopy. The timing of colonoscopy is suggested to be yearly and then gradually advanced to every 2 or 3 years if no lesions are found on subsequent colonoscopic examination.

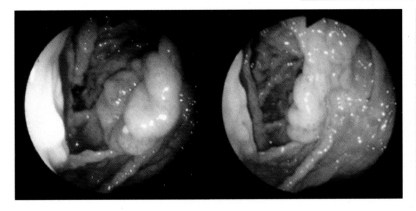

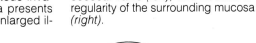

Figure 10.60 Lymphomatous invasion of the ileocecal area presents as mild erythema of the enlarged ileocecal valve *(left)*, and nodular irregularity of the surrounding mucosa *(right)*.

lymphomatous involvement

nodular transformation

small nodules

ileocecal valve

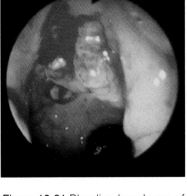

Figure 10.61 Bleeding lymphoma of the sigmoid colon in a patient diagnosed with AIDS.

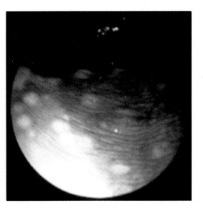

Figure 10.62 Monotonous lymphomatous invasion mimics FPC. The numerous, slightly raised, whitish structures are easily overlooked without dye-scattering.

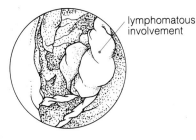

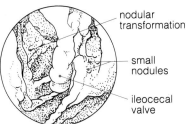

Figure 10.63 Numerous, minute, whitish lymphomatous foci are easily overlooked.

Figure 10.64 Solitary Kaposi's sarcoma lesion in the colon is visible as a slightly raised, purple-red macule.

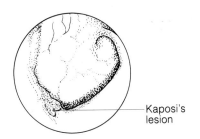

Kaposi's lesion

EPIDERMOID CANCER

Epidermoid or squamous-cell carcinoma originating from the anal verge may occasionally invade the distal rectum (Fig. 10.58). Also, a cloacogenic cancer originating from transitional epithelium may invade the distal rectum (Fig. 10.59).

NONEPITHELIAL MALIGNANCIES

LYMPHOMA

The colon may be involved with lymphoma in two ways: first, with a primary lymphoma and second, as part of a generalized lymphoma. With primary disease the cecal area is usually involved. On occasion, multiple areas are affected such as the cecum and transverse colon. Generalized lymphoma typically involves the left colon and rectum.

In the primary type of involvement, the lesion presents as polypoid masses of various sizes (Fig. 10.60). The masses may be multiple and large enough to obstruct the lumen (Fig. 10.61). These masses are firm, indurated, and may be friable. When the colon is involved as part of a generalized process, the findings are less specific and may present as a friable, indurated, erythematous mucosa. Rarely, an exophytic, malignant, annular stricture develops, indistinguishable from that seen in adenocarcinoma. The occurrence of multiple tiny, flat or slightly raised polypoid lesions is rare and easily overlooked unless dye-scattering techniques are used (Figs. 10.62 and 10.63).

KAPOSI'S SARCOMA

Kaposi's sarcoma, a tumor seen with increasing frequency mainly in the homosexual population with AIDS, may involve any segment of the intestine including the esophagus, stomach, small intestine, and colon. When Kaposi's involves the GI tract, the colon is involved in approximately one-half of the cases.

The most common appearance is an intensely red, raised macule (Fig. 10.64). The surface is often slightly irregular.

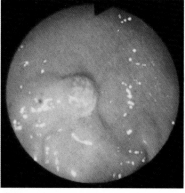

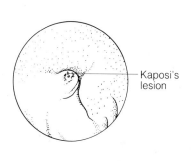

Kaposi's lesion

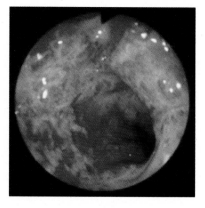

Figure 10.65 Early Kaposi's sarcoma lesion in the colon of a patient diagnosed with AIDS. The lesion mimics an inflammatory pseudopolyp.

Figure 10.66 Extensive Kaposi's sarcoma of the rectum in an AIDS patient. This is rarely seen.

Biopsy of Malignancies

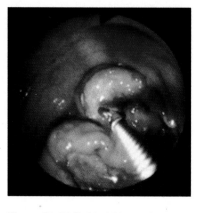

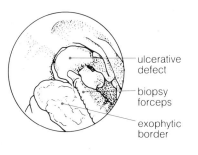

ulcerative defect

biopsy forceps

exophytic border

Figure 10.67 Guided biopsy from rim between overhanging border and excavated area.

Palliative Treatment

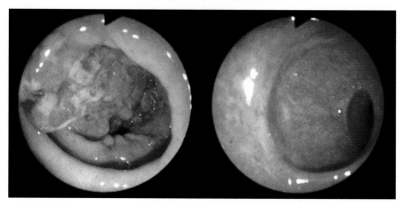

Figure 10.68 *Left,* A bulky, exophytic rectal cancer before laser treatment. *Right,* Full eradication of the cancerous mass is apparent after four Nd-YAG applications.

Two other appearances are less common. The lesions may be multiple and resemble small polyps of an inflammatory nature (Fig. 10.65). Or the lesions may present with a configuration of a dense cluster of polyps with destruction of long segments of the colonic wall (Fig. 10.66). Biopsies of these lesions show the typical elongated cells with increased blood vessel components.

METASTASES TO THE COLON

Involvement of the colon with carcinoma of other organs occurs in two forms: direct extension and distant metastases to the colonic wall. Both are rare.

When an organ adjacent to the colon invades the colon it may produce a submucosal mass or a narrowed segment. The tumor often spreads submucosally so the overlying mucosa is normal or minimally abnormal with slight erythema. This pattern may occur with cancer of the pelvic organs. In the future, echo endoscopy may help to define the presence of a mass and the extent of the involvement.

The second type of spread is that of metastases to the wall. These lesions may grow in the wall and then extend through the mucosa so that the appearance from inside the bowel lumen is that of an abnormal mucosa covering a small polyp up to 2 cm in diameter. These tumors can outgrow their blood supply and present with a depression or ulceration on the tip. The common tumors which metastasize in this manner include gastric, renal, pancreatic, breast, and melanoma. When the tumor is a melanoma, as in the upper GI tract, it may be pigmented with brown or black coloration or, if large, may be amelanotic.

BIOPSY OF COLONIC MALIGNANCIES

Any suspicious abnormality of the rectocolon should be extensively biopsied to establish a diagnosis and to direct therapy. In general, necrotic tumor tissue should not be biopsied. Biopsy of fresh, nonulcerated, malignant tissue or tissue from the edges between the exophytic, overhanging borders and the ulcerative defects increases the likelihood of obtaining a positive specimen (Fig. 10.67).

Simple forceps biopsy is a relatively high-yield procedure in most cases of exophytic growth pattern of cancer. Low yield, even for exophytic lesions, may be related to inability to position the instrument "en face" with the lesion. When the lesion is seen tangentially, it may not be possible to sample the surface of the cancer where it has broken through the mucosa. Moreover, biopsy forceps may fail to penetrate deeply enough to allow diagnosis of invasive cancer.

Sampling normal-looking mucosa at the edge of a malignant stricture is usually not productive. Even biopsies taken blindly from within the strictured area may not reveal malignancy. Brush cytology is most valuable in this situation, as brushing deep within the stenotic portion of a lesion may recover neoplastic cells.

PALLIATIVE TREATMENT

High-grade obstruction of the colon must be relieved with proximal diversion, resection, or endoscopic palliation. Ultimately, therapy depends on the cause of the obstruction. Palliative tumor destruction may be carried out with electrocoagulation, freezing, or with Nd-YAG laser energy. Laser photodestruction is especially indicated for chronically bleeding tumors or to open up obstructing colorectal malignancies (Fig. 10.68). This palliative approach is especially useful in elderly patients to avoid emergency colostomy in an unprepared colon. Usually one or two sessions are sufficient to reopen the bowel. Laser treatment may not be possible for tortuous lesions or lesions located at acute bends. Occasionally complete irradiation of bulky exophytic malignancies can be obtained with laser photocoagulation.

11

Colon II:
Inflammatory and Infectious Disorders

In this chapter we will discuss idiopathic inflammatory bowel disease including ulcerative colitis and Crohn's disease. We will also present a variety of other types of colitis including infectious, antibiotic-associated, ischemic, radiation-related, and assorted other types.

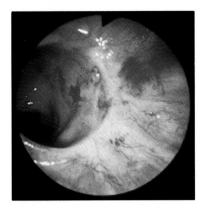

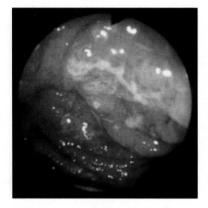

Figure 11.1 Abundant mucous discharge is an early sign of acute flare of ulcerative colitis.

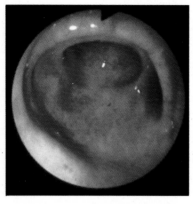

Figure 11.2 Vascular pattern is blurred in quiescent ulcerative colitis or early flare. Minimal erythema is present.

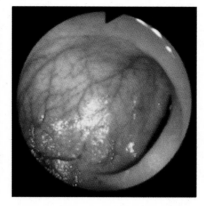

Figure 11.3 Ulcerative colitis in remission. Fine granular appearance is shown by multiple tiny dots of reflecting light. Note mild blurring of vascular pattern.

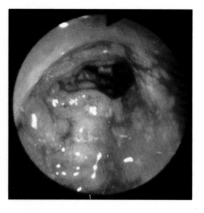

Figure 11.4 Active ulcerative colitis. Markedly friable mucosa which bled profusely after one pass with the colonoscope.

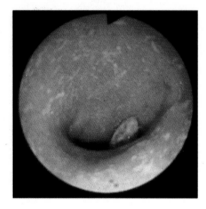

Figure 11.5 Scattered mucopurulent exudate with obvious erythema and blurring of vascular pattern in active ulcerative colitis.

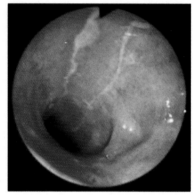

Figure 11.6 Linear, longitudinal ulceration in the descending colon of a patient with ulcerative colitis. Diffuse erythema, friability, and hemorrhage are also evident.

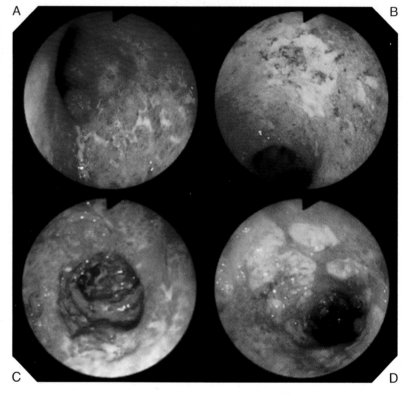

Figure 11.7 Examples of ulceration in active ulcerative colitis. Background mucosa shows marked erythema and friability.

IDIOPATHIC INFLAMMATORY BOWEL DISEASE

Ulcerative colitis and Crohn's disease are called idiopathic since neither their etiology nor pathogenesis is completely understood. The basic features indicating inflammation are swelling, erythema, mucoid or purulent exudation, mild or severe epithelial destruction (ranging from tiny, superficial erosive defects to serpiginous, linear, or deep ulcers), fine or coarse granular deformity of the contours, pseudopolyp formation, retraction, and stricturing.

Colonoscopy is an established procedure for evaluating patients with inflammatory disorders of the large bowel.

Direct inspection of the mucosa and the ability to obtain mucosal biopsies provide high diagnostic accuracy. Few endoscopic changes, when considered separately, are specific. In addition, the range of abnormalities produced by the mucosal lining in response to injury is limited.

Despite the lack of specificity, a presumptive diagnosis of idiopathic inflammatory bowel disease usually is possible by a compilation of the relevant findings. Idiopathic disease must be differentiated from the various forms of infectious colitis, antibiotic-associated colitis, and ischemic damage of the colon. In a vast majority of patients, colonoscopy may enable precise determination of the distribution of the abnormalities and the extent and severity of involvement.

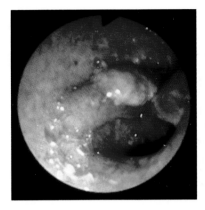

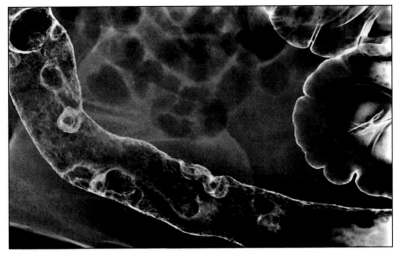

Figure 11.8 Large pseudopolyps in chronic ulcerative colitis *(left)* give a characteristic X-ray appearance *(right)*.

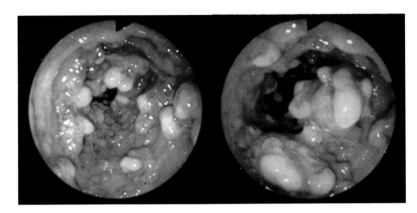

Figure 11.9 *Left,* Multiple pseudo-polyps in ulcerative colitis. Their surface is smooth and glistening. *Right,* Detail view of exudate creating the whitish caps.

Consideration of previous topical or systemic therapy is essential because this may obscure or interfere with the more characteristic elements of the inflammatory features.

ULCERATIVE COLITIS

Active ulcerative colitis inflames the mucosa in a continuous symmetrical fashion. The colitis may extend throughout the colon or may involve only part of it; characteristically, the rectal mucosa is affected. The diagnosis is usually made by history and proctosigmoidoscopy, but colonoscopy may provide a more exact evaluation. An accurate determination of extent depends upon total intubation to the cecum, which most often is relatively easy because of the foreshortening and tubularization of the colon.

ENDOSCOPIC APPEARANCE

There is no unique, macroscopic, mucosal abnormality pathognomonic for the endoscopic diagnosis of ulcerative colitis. Copious amounts of mucoid discharge seen as white creamy material covering the mucosa may be the most conspicuous sign of early disease or flare-up (Fig. 11.1).

With minimal inflammation, the mucosal vascular pattern may disappear or look blunted or blurred (Fig. 11.2). The obliteration is caused by edema and inflammation of the lamina propria. The vascular appearance is abnormal in that the branching pattern is markedly irregular and distorted in contrast to the normally smooth, gradual tapering and arcading of the vessels (Fig. 11.3). Abnormal vascular patterns are caused partially by the loss of mucosal transparency, which may be the only visible abnormality in the quiescent or healing stage of ulcerative colitis.

Erythema is caused by mucosal capillary dilation and is usually diffuse. The erythematous mucosa is friable and bleeds easily after trivial amounts of pressure (Fig. 11.4). Erythema indicates active mucosal involvement, especially when associated with granularity and a distorted or absent vascular pattern. The presence of loosely adherent yellow-brown mucopurulent exudate indicates even more active disease than does erythema (Fig. 11.5).

Granularity is a visual manifestation of fine or coarse surface irregularity. The normally homogeneous light reflex disappears, indicative of the granular changes in the normally smooth mucosa (see Fig. 11.3).

Superficial or deep epithelial necrosis or ulceration results from extensive epithelial destruction and crypt abscess formation. Single or multiple ulcerations varying from a few millimeters to several centimeters are an expected finding in active ulcerative colitis. They may be linear (Fig. 11.6), serpiginous, circinate, or ovoid. Whatever the ulcer form or shape, their most common characteristic feature is the erythematous and friable mucosa in which they are located (Fig. 11.7).

INFLAMMATORY PSEUDOPOLYPS

Inflammatory polypoid structures or pseudopolyps are thought to develop from epithelial buds which remain in areas of extensive ulceration or at margins of ulceration. As the ulcerations heal and the acute inflammation subsides, focally nodular areas of remaining mucosa protrude, resulting in the formation of inflammatory polyps or pseudopolyps. These are usually multiple, and range from little more than mucosal excrescences of a few millimeters up to 1 centimeter. Occasionally single lesions may exceed 1.5 cm (Fig. 11.8).

Inflammatory polyps may be broad-based, sessile, or pedunculated. They have a soft texture, and are easily compressible and friable. Often, they are covered with a whitish cap of exudate (Fig. 11.9). The larger pseudopolyps in par-

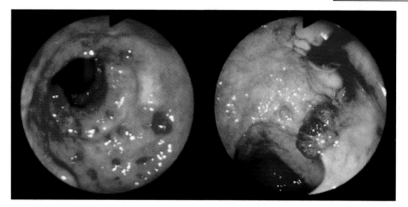

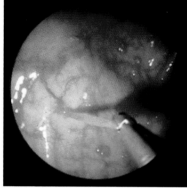

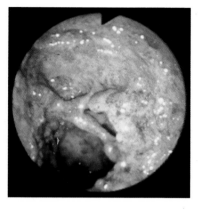

Figure 11.10 *Left,* Pseudopolyps in ulcerative colitis present here as cherry-red spheres. *Right,* Larger pseudopolyp shows striking erythe- ma, which contrasts with the paler mucosa. Ulcerative colitis is in the quiescent phase.

Figure 11.11 Filiform polyps. A bi- opsy forceps demonstrates their fi- lamentous nature.

Figure 11.12 Active ulcerative colitis with bridging mucosal folds.

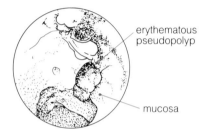

erythematous pseudopolyp

mucosa

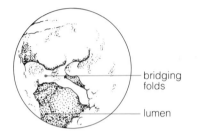

bridging folds

lumen

ticular may be eroded or ulcerated on the surface. Some-times the pseudopolypoid bulges show a striking erythema, contrasting with pale surrounding mucosa seen in the re-mission phase of the disease (Fig. 11.10).

A less common appearance is many clusters of flimsy, fingerlike, mucosal projections (Fig. 11.11). Such long fi-lamentous pseudopolyps, especially those arising in grape-like clusters, are characteristic of ulcerative colitis. Rarely, the pseudopolypoid structures are interconnected by bridg-ing mucosal folds (Fig. 11.12). These probably form as a consequence of undermining ulcers which leave a lattice-work-type appearance.

In cases of severe ulceration with intervening large in-flammatory pseudopolyps, coarse nodular deformity of the mucosal contour occurs. Typically, the mucosa surrounding the ulcerations is abnormal with pronounced erythema and friability (Fig. 11.13). This is in contrast to the cobble-stonelike appearance in Crohn's disease, where the mucosa is only slightly erythematous or even normal-looking with a preserved mucosal vascular pattern.

ANATOMIC VARIATIONS CAUSED BY ULCERATIVE COLITIS

Inflammatory changes within the mucosa may produce structural abnormalities. Many of the structural changes are primarily the result of edematous swelling, inflammatory infiltration, muscle contraction, and muscle hypertrophy. Loss of sharpness of the interhaustral folds or valvulae is an early structural change (Fig. 11.14). The thickened and blunted appearance is due to swelling and inflammation, and is most noticeable in the transverse colon where the expected sharp, thin, triangular folds become rounded and appear broader. Disappearance of the interhaustral fold pattern, which is generally thought to result from hyper-trophy and contraction of the teniae coli, suggests chronic disease (Fig. 11.15).

Ongoing muscle hypertrophy and retraction may sub-stantially decrease the width of the colonic lumen. Some-times the lumen contracts to less than 13 mm, barely ad-mitting a standard colonoscope. Loss of the haustral pattern and narrowing of the lumen create a tubular appearance (Fig. 11.16).

Strictures may form in ulcerative colitis, due mainly to focal muscle hypertrophy and retraction. They tend to be composed of thickened smooth muscle; by contrast, stric-tures in Crohn's disease are fibrotic. At the area of narrow-ing, one characteristically sees superficial or deep ulceration with markedly erythematous, friable, intervening mucosa (Fig. 11.17). The presence of intact, nodular, indurated mucosa without ulceration is atypical and suggests possible malignancy.

Strictures resulting from inflammation are relatively short; since they are distensible, they can be entered using a nar-row-caliber endoscope. Strictures longer than 5 cm should raise suspicion of malignancy. Benign strictures are easily distensible. However, all strictures must be biopsied since a smooth contour does not exclude dysplasia or underlying malignancy. Strictures too narrow for an endoscope are usually surgically removed since future surveillance will be impossible.

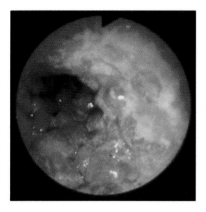

Figure 11.13 Coarsely nodular deformity of mucosal contour in ulcerative colitis. Mucosa is intensely erythematous and friable.

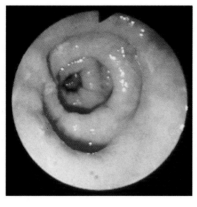

Figure 11.14 Thick and blunt interhaustral folds in the distal transverse colon are an early structural abnormality in ulcerative colitis.

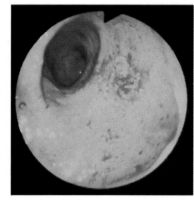

Figure 11.15 Loss of interhaustral fold pattern in chronic ulcerative colitis. Note the friability of the mucosa.

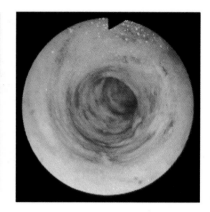

Figure 11.16 Tubularization of the colon occurs in long-standing ulcerative colitis. Plaques of exudate and punctiform petechial hemorrhages are also apparent.

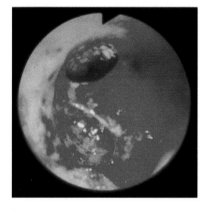

Figure 11.17 Ulcerative colitis with stricturing. Attempts to pass the stricture caused bleeding. Ulceration is present around the mouth of the stricture.

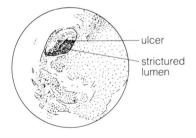

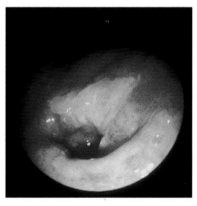

Figure 11.18 Severe, unhealed ulcerative colitis resulted in this ulcerated and incompetent ileocecal valve.

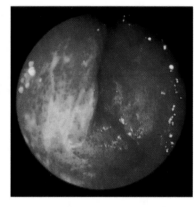

Figure 11.19 Severe inflammation and ulceration of the distal terminal ileum are due to backwash or reflux ileitis.

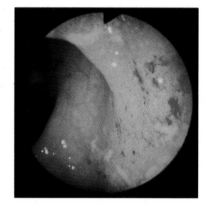

Figure 11.20 Sharp transition from normal to inflamed bowel is discernible at the rectosigmoid junction. Erythema and superficial ulceration of diseased mucosa contrasts with the normal vascular pattern.

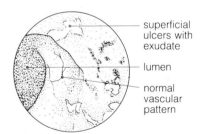

Chronic, long-standing, ulcerative colitis may lead to effacement of the ileocecal valve, usually associated with narrowing in caliber of the right colon (Fig. 11.18). The valve appears patulous with a diameter approximating that of the terminal ileum. Because the ileocecal valve is effaced and patulous, the terminal ileum can be easily entered with the colonoscope. Not uncommonly there is evidence of backwash ileitis: tubularization of the terminal ileum with disappearance of the mucosal fold pattern. This occurs in patients with total colonic involvement. The smooth mucosa may show evidence of inflammatory activity such as patchy or diffuse erythema and friability (Fig. 11.19). In rare cases, there is an inflammatory exudate. Mucosal ulceration is not part of this entity except in severe cases of backwash.

DISTRIBUTION OF LESIONS

Before treatment, a conspicuous gradient in disease activity is usually apparent, with more severe disease located toward the rectum. There is often a sharp transition from normal to diseased intestine (Fig. 11.20). In some instances, how-

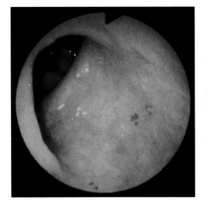

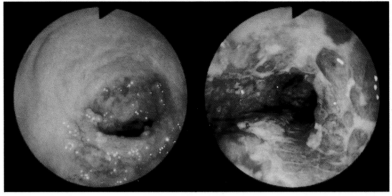

Figure 11.21 Distal transverse colon of an ulcerative colitis patient displays patchy distribution of erythema and blurring of vascular pattern at the proximal border.

Figure 11.22 Topical therapy causes obvious improvement of rectal disease with reappearance of a vascular pattern. Notice the transition to the markedly abnormal sigmoid *(left)*. Above this transition there is ongoing severe disease with marked ulceration in the sigmoid colon *(right)*.

ever, the abnormalities at the proximal extent of the disease may appear patchy (Fig. 11.21). In severe disease there may be rectal sparing or less pronounced rectal involvement, with deep ulceration starting at or beyond the rectosigmoid junction. A continuous symmetrical involvement from the rectum to the point of the highest extent of involvement is characteristic.

Distinct patterns of involvement may be recognized based on the extent of the disease. Total colitis is diagnosed when the entire colon is involved. Usually the activity is more severe distally, especially in the distal descending colon, sigmoid colon, and rectum. In subtotal involvement, the disease usually terminates at the hepatic flexure. In left-sided involvement, the disease stops at or just proximal to the splenic flexure, where a relatively sharp demarcation can usually be seen. An occasional patient may have predominantly right-sided involvement of the colon in a diffuse manner with ulceration and pseudopolyp formation, while the left side of the colon shows only minimal or discrete abnormalities.

In rectosigmoid colitis, the disease is confined to the rectum and sigmoid colon. When only the rectum is involved, this is termed proctitis. As a rule, there is a sharp inflammatory demarcation between the rectum and the sigmoid colon.

LEVELS OF ACTIVITY

In nonactive or quiescent ulcerative colitis, the colitic mucosa appears normal except for some alteration of the vascular pattern or the presence of fine granularity. There may also be slight friability and a few petechiae.

There is no universally accepted system for determining activity of ulcerative colitis. Stages of activity include:

1. Mildly active colitis: Unequivocal erythema, either diffuse or focal. The mucosal vascular pattern may be either distorted or absent.
2. Moderately active colitis: Single or scattered small ulcerations in a limited section of the colon. In addition, there is erythema, friability, granularity, and mucopurulent exudate.
3. Severe colitis: Deep, larger, more numerous ulcers, often with spontaneous bleeding, marked friability, and excessive amounts of mucopurulent exudate.

The severity of the colitis may be underestimated if only the rectum is evaluated and if topical therapy with corticosteroids or 5-aminosalicylic acid has already been given. The rectal mucosa may even look normal despite unequivocal edema, erythema, and friability in the more proximal colon (Fig. 11.22). Presumably also due to previous topical therapy, reappearance of inflammatory changes during flare may be more obvious in the more proximal colon than in the distal (previously topically treated) segment. Therefore, evaluation of the severity of a flare may be misleading if only the rectum is inspected.

The loss of the rectal indicator function after topical therapy is unfortunate because many clinicians use the macroscopic appearance of the rectum to titrate therapy. Increasingly, flexible sigmoidoscopy is used to visualize the sigmoid colon. This should more precisely mirror overall disease activity.

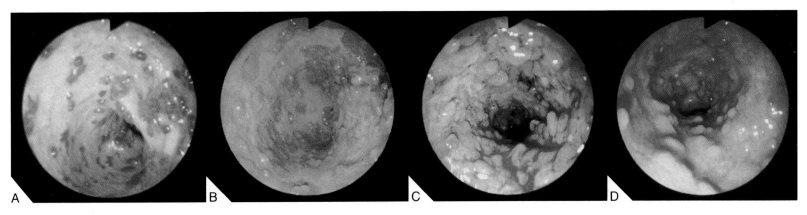

Figure 11.23 Sequential study of severe pancolitis. Massive ulceration of the colon was studied at intervals of 4 to 6 weeks after institution of medical therapy. A This view of the proximal sigmoid shows extensive ulceration prior to therapy. Some islands of remaining mucosa are visible. B Regression of inflammation and early reepithelialization are noted here. C In this view ulcers are regressing with pseudopolypoid elevation of nonulcerated mucosal islands. D Full reepithelialization and pseudopolypoid transformation characterize healing.

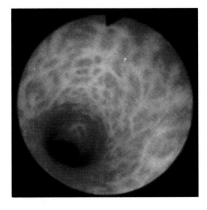

Figure 11.24 Healing stage after extensive ulceration of rectum. Interconnecting, lacelike whitish stripes correspond to areas of previous ulceration.

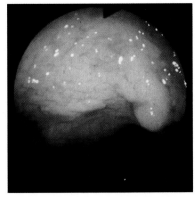

Figure 11.25 Irregular wartlike deformity of the mucosal lining due to severe dysplasia. Small nodular elevations are also present.

Frequent inspection of the inflamed mucosa using a small-caliber endoscope without bowel preparation may improve clinical evaluation during severe attacks and may be helpful in deciding whether medical therapy should be continued. Healing through reepithelialization may occur even after extensive ulceration, provided that medical therapy controls the inflammatory process (Fig. 11.23). Occasionally the appearance of the healing stage is bizarre (Fig. 11.24).

As the mucosa responds to medical therapy, the symmetrical diffuse pattern of involvement may be lost or may become less evident. Such inequality of involvement may occasionally lead to error in diagnosis. As a rule, the endoscopic aspect prior to therapy is always more informative with respect to the differential diagnosis than the appearance during or after medical therapy.

RISK OF DYSPLASIA OR MALIGNANCY

Patients with universal, subtotal, and perhaps even left-sided ulcerative colitis are considered to have an enhanced cancer risk after 10 years. The magnitude of the increased risk is not definitively established. Colonoscopy has been suggested as a means of identifying patients particularly at risk by looking for histologic evidence of severe dysplasia. Surveillance may be important in selected patients, but will have little impact on overall colon cancer mortality rates since only 1% of colorectal cancer is associated with a history of previous ulcerative colitis.

During screening colonoscopy, as much of the surface as possible should be inspected for a macroscopic appearance of colonic cancer or dysplasia-associated lesions or masses. Biopsies should be taken at approximately 10-cm intervals for histologic evidence of dysplasia. Additional biopsies should be obtained from areas showing surface irregularity and from large polypoid lesions. Areas that differ in appearance from the small, shiny, or wormlike benign inflammatory pseudopolyps frequently seen after a severe attack of colitis should also be sampled.

Dysplasia may be identified as an unequivocal neoplastic alteration of the colonic epithelium. Dysplastic mucosa is arbitrarily divided into low- and high-grade, the latter including carcinoma in situ. The presence of high-grade dysplasia, especially if present on more than one examination or in several locations, carries a high risk of a coexisting cancer or impending cancer formation. Because these cancers may still be intramural, they could easily escape endoscopic detection.

Flat dysplasia and macroscopic dysplasia may be studied by colonoscopy. There may be no macroscopic feature to suggest flat dysplasia. Rather, abnormal tissue is detected in routine, random biopsies. Occasionally, a flat, focal, villous-like or wartlike appearance can be recognized as different from the granular-type mucosal unevenness common to quiescent ulcerative colitis (Fig. 11.25).

Macroscopic dysplasia is associated with polypoid masses or other macroscopic appearances termed dysplasia-associated lesions or masses (DALM). The appearance of

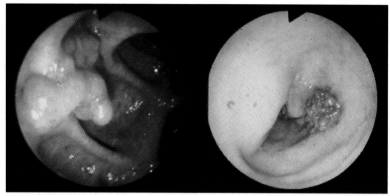

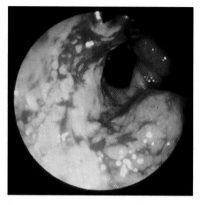

Figure 11.26 Examples of DALM in long-standing, inactive ulcerative colitis.

Figure 11.27 Advanced infiltrating ulcerated cancer in ulcerative colitis.

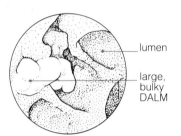

lumen

large, bulky DALM

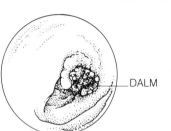

DALM

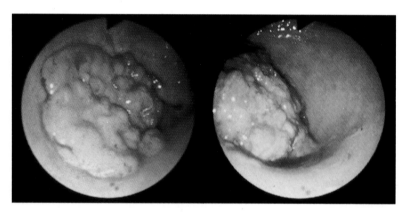

Figure 11.28 *Left,* A single, nonulcerative, sessile, cancerous mass presents in the sigmoid colon of a patient with long-standing, inactive ulcerative colitis. *Right,* In another patient, carcinoma presents as an indurated polypoid mass in the sigmoid.

DALM may be variable (Fig. 11.26). Occasionally, one may see a single, 2 to 4 cm, sessile, polypoid mass with a slightly irregular, nonulcerated surface. Sometimes multiple 5 to 15 mm polypoid bulges of firm consistency are clustered together; these usually present with ill-defined borders. DALM may also appear as slightly elevated nodular, plaque-like areas extending over a finite distance. Hence, any irregular or elevated area or polyp should be carefully inspected and biopsies taken of the apex and in particular any nodularity surrounding the lesion.

It may be impossible in chronic ulcerative colitis to distinguish an isolated adenoma from a polypoid area of dysplasia since both are composed of identical-looking neoplastic epithelium. There is an arbitrary tendency to regard such lesions as examples of dysplasia in younger patients, with the implication of an impending need for colectomy, whereas in older patients they are usually considered un-

related to the colitis and treated simply by polypectomy. It is best in all cases to seek further evidence of dysplasia in the mucosa immediately adjacent to the polyp or along its stalk because the polyp may prove to be part of a larger area of dysplasia. Polypectomy may not be curative if dysplasia is present in these other sites. When in doubt, any nonstalked adenoma, as reported by the pathologist, should be assumed to be a local area of precancerous dysplasia.

BIOPSY

During endoscopic examinations, biopsies should be taken from plaques; from nodular, thickened, or villous-appearing areas; from slightly elevated areas; from areas that appear velvety or show minor roughness; and from other unusual polypoid lesions and stenotic regions. Polypoid lesions should be especially biopsied when they show irregularities and friability of the mucosal surface, and when they are large and of firm consistency.

If no suspicious areas are visible, multiple random biopsies of otherwise flat or uninvolved mucosa should be taken from all regions of the colon at 10-cm intervals so that a total of eight or nine biopsy sites are covered. Ordinary-appearing inflammatory pseudopolyps and small areas of active inflammation are best avoided as histopathologic interpretation may be difficult and such areas are virtually never dysplastic. Because of the difficulties of histologic interpretation during the active phases of colitis, patients should be preferentially examined during a quiescent phase of their disease. Mucosal biopsies should be separately labeled to permit return to a specific area in the event of a suspicious or positive finding.

Although a high proportion of patients with dysplasia in colonoscopic biopsies also have dysplasia in rectosigmoidoscopic biopsies, most experts agree that multiple

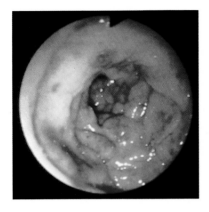

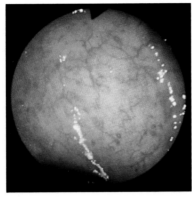

Figure 11.29 Focal erythema occurring in early flare of Crohn's disease.

Figure 11.30 Distortion of vascular pattern with spotty reddening is common in early Crohn's disease.

biopsies from various parts of the colon are desirable. The frequency of colonoscopy with biopsies is a matter of opinion, logistics, patient acceptance, and results of previous examinations. Most large centers are doing annual colonoscopy in patients with a 10-year or longer history of chronic ulcerative colitis involving the whole colon. The procedure may be performed more often in patients with suspicious findings on previous examination. Other patients with normal findings may have rectal biopsy done each year and colonoscopy with biopsies every 2 years. Whether patients with colitis confined to the left half of the colon should be submitted to a surveillance program is a matter of debate.

Biopsies yielding high-grade dysplasia justify serious consideration of colectomy in view of the high rate of synchronous occult carcinoma. This recommendation must be weighed against the immediate and long-term morbidity and mortality of the operation and sequelae. It is always wise to have an experienced pathologist confirm the diagnosis by demonstrating dysplasia in more than one biopsy specimen taken at the same colonoscopy, and in biopsies from the same area during repeat colonoscopy. A second pathologist should review the biopsy findings.

Because repeat colonoscopy is occasionally needed, the examination must be carried out with minimal discomfort to the patient. As the colon in extensive colitis is sometimes shortened and tubular, the endoscopic procedure is often relatively easy and may be done comfortably without sedation. If the colon is tortuous and difficult to examine, patients should be sedated to ensure compliance for repeat examinations.

CANCER IN ULCERATIVE COLITIS
The overall risk for cancer in patients with long-standing ulcerative colitis is increased, particularly for patients with universal involvement or onset during childhood. The risk is felt to be significantly increased with disease of more than 8 to 10 years and especially with disease in excess of 20 years. The exact risk, however, is uncertain, since most published reports are from special centers whose patient populations are often skewed toward the most severe cases.

Since 50% or more of early cancers in ulcerative colitis are located proximal to the splenic flexure area, screening colonoscopy is a means for detecting cancer while it is still curable.

The predominant growth pattern in colitic cancers is intramural and infiltrating, presenting a variety of endoscopic findings (Fig. 11.27). A local infiltrating malignancy may give rise to a flat or slightly elevated plaque-like mass with ill-defined edges. Colitic cancer may also present as an ulcerated, exophytic mass, indistinguishable from noncolitic cancer. In the case of infiltrating colitic cancer, biopsy may fail to show malignancy. However, biopsies usually reveal high-grade dysplasia.

A malignant stricture presents at endoscopy as an abrupt narrowing of the lumen. The mouth of the stricture appears nodular and friable but is usually nonulcerative. Biopsies from the mouth of the stricture give the impression of a firm surface. Occasionally, brush cytology may be a useful procedure for detecting malignancy in stricturing lesions.

Cancer may also present as a single, 2 to 4 cm, nonulcerated, sessile, polypoid mass (Fig. 11.28), with a smooth or slightly irregular mucosa. Only about one-third of the cancers in ulcerative colitis are of this protuberant variety and may appear similar to polypoid cancer. Less often, cancer may present as multiple, 1 to 2 cm, sessile, polypoid masses with a friable but nonulcerated surface lining. The absence of ulceration, along with the hard rubbery consistency appreciated on biopsy, distinguishes this lesion from clustering inflammatory pseudopolyps.

CROHN'S DISEASE

Crohn's disease is a chronic inflammatory disease, usually involving the terminal ileum and segments of the colon. Ileocecal or ileocolonic involvement is present in up to 50% of cases. Overall, some colonic involvement is expected in two-thirds of the patients. The focal, asymmetrical, patchy, discontinuous distribution of the lesions contrasts with the diffuse, symmetrical involvement in ulcerative colitis.

ENDOSCOPIC APPEARANCE
Occasionally, the only endoscopic abnormality in Crohn's disease is diffuse or patchy erythema and mild friability of the mucosa, more or less indistinguishable from that seen in ulcerative colitis (Fig. 11.29). Sometimes zones of redder color alternate with patches manifesting a peculiar, whitish opaqueness. Tiny erythematous spots may also occur during the early phase or early flare of Crohn's disease.

Spotty reddening with localized edema is a dominant abnormality during the preaphthoid phase of Crohn's disease. Such erythematous mucosal spots or plaques presumably consist of intramucosal hemorrhage, associated with focal crypt abscesses and destruction of crypt epithelium. This spotty erythema may distort the vascular pattern (Fig. 11.30).

Aphthoid erosions are generally regarded as an early, specific endoscopic finding in Crohn's disease. They are flat

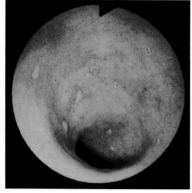

Figure 11.31 Characteristic superficial aphthoid erosions in Crohn's disease have erythematous rings.

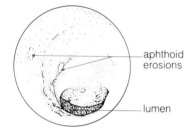

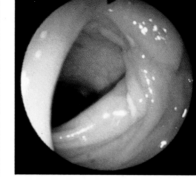

Figure 11.32 This view shows an example of skip lesions. The entire colon appears normal, except for a tiny patch of abnormality in the sigmoid colon.

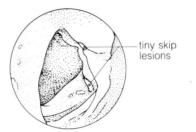

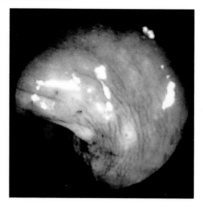

Figure 11.33 Microerosions are seen as tiny white spots amidst normal methylene-blue-stained mucosa. Failure to absorb dye is due to distorted architecture of the gland pits.

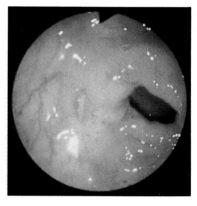

Figure 11.34 Small flat ulcer in Crohn's disease is surrounded by a zone of edema. Blurring of vascular pattern is also evident.

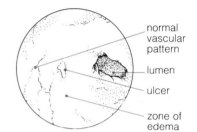

or just slightly depressed and usually less than 5 mm in diameter. They have a characteristic small rim of erythema in the absence of a raised margin, and usually a grayish or yellowish central crater (Fig. 11.31). Often occurring in groups, aphthoid erosions may develop from preaphthoid erythematous spots or plaques. They presumably result from partial or total destruction of crypts and surrounding surface epithelium in areas of previous focal inflammation.

Aphthoid erosions may be seen in otherwise normal-appearing mucosa at some distance from more severe lesions (Fig. 11.32). This discontinuity, often termed skip areas, is a key finding. Segments of normal bowel are interspersed between abnormal areas, or one wall will be normal with the opposite or adjacent wall abnormal.

Using dye-scattering techniques, very small aphthoid erosions (microerosions) have a worm-eaten appearance. Such lesions are probably due to distortion and destruction of the surface epithelium covering lymphoid aggregates, and are often rich in granulomas. The normal honeycomb pattern becomes distorted and the mucosa fails to take up the dye (Fig. 11.33). In some patients, larger lesions may be seen which resemble white spots. These are likely more advanced lesions than microerosions since they are larger and very slightly raised because of local edema.

From an endoscopic viewpoint, ulceration is a dominant abnormality in Crohn's disease. Between tiny aphthoid erosions and large deep longitudinal ulcers, there is a progression of intermediate forms, varying greatly in shape and depth (Figs. 11.34 to 11.38). Characteristically, such epithelial defects are sharply outlined and abruptly surrounded by normal or only slightly diseased mucosa.

The most common ulcers in Crohn's disease measure more than 5 mm in size. They vary from flat to deep, and often are irregular and tortuous in shape. There is a distinct margin to such ulcers because of their depth. Some ulcers look serpiginous, presumably due to coalescence of several smaller ulcers (Fig. 11.39). Deep serpiginous ulcers, greater than 1 cm in length, are most characteristic of Crohn's disease.

There is a peculiar tendency for linear ulcers to align longitudinally, creating a railroad-track appearance (Fig. 11.40). This appearance is more typical of Crohn's disease than of ulcerative colitis. Such linear ulcers are easily seen in smooth, even mucosa but are sometimes difficult to detect in coarsely nodular mucosa.

Severe hemorrhage may occur when a large ulcer penetrates and destroys blood vessels deep in the submucosa. In contrast, more diffuse bleeding is associated with acute exacerbations of Crohn's disease which are characterized by marked ulceration. The bleeding may be worsened by medicines that disturb platelet function given for arthritis or arthralgias (Fig. 11.41).

Cobblestoning—a rough, irregular, nodular, mucosal relief pattern with or without intersecting depressions or ulcerations—is characteristic though not pathognomonic for Crohn's disease. The cobblestone pattern is usually created by the interplay of parallel, longitudinal ulceration and transverse, fissuring-type ulceration. Thickened, slightly

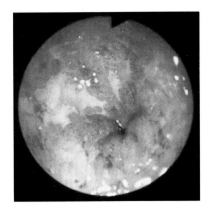

Figure 11.35 Irregular, superficial, serpiginous ulcer in Crohn's disease.

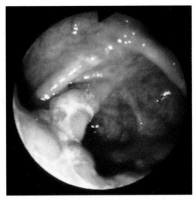

Figure 11.36 Linear ulcers dissect the mucosa in this presentation of Crohn's disease. Erythematous spots are also apparent.

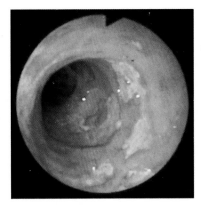

Figure 11.37 Multiple large, deep, excavated ulcers in severe ulcerating Crohn's disease show distinct margins. This patient has concomitant sclerosing cholangitis.

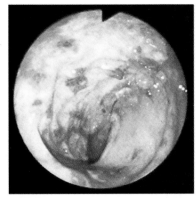

Figure 11.38 Extensive confluent ulceration in Crohn's disease involves half of the circumference of the bowel wall, while the other half appears normal.

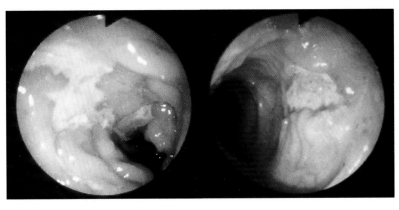

Figure 11.39 *Left,* Extensive, deep, confluent ulceration in Crohn's disease. *Right,* A deep excavated ulcer.

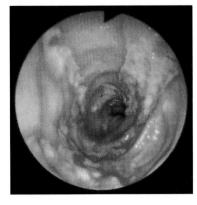

Figure 11.40 Longitudinal alignment of ulceration causes a railroad-track appearance in Crohn's disease.

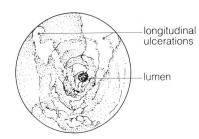

longitudinal ulcerations

lumen

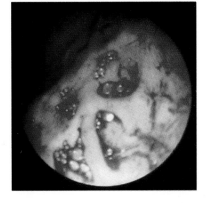

Figure 11.41 Severe flare-up of Crohn's disease with concomitant arthritis. Platelet dysfunction due to antiphlogistic medication is responsible for diffuse bleeding from ulcer margin.

edematous, mucosal bumps occur between intersecting ulcerations (Fig. 11.42). The mucosa of the cobblestone area between ulcerations may be pinker than the surrounding epithelium, but it is not typically friable. In contrast with pseudopolyps, the base of the cobblestones is usually wider than their height. Because focal involvement in Crohn's disease is common, the cobblestone appearance is often contained in segments of less than 5 cm. Cobblestoning is particularly prevalent at the mouth of inflammatory strictures.

INFLAMMATORY PSEUDOPOLYPS

Inflammatory pseudopolyps are found somewhat less frequently than in ulcerative colitis. They tend to be focal, localized to one distinct portion of the colon, although

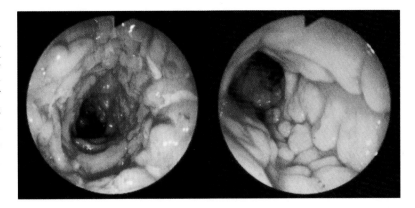

Figure 11.42 *Left,* Active phase of Crohn's disease shows cobblestoning, caused by interconnecting ulcerations. *Right,* Area of cobblestoning after therapy.

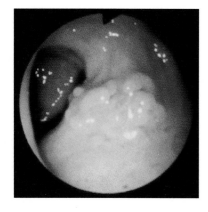

Figure 11.43 Cluster of small, smooth, shiny pseudopolyps with a transparent appearance is seen in quiescent Crohn's disease.

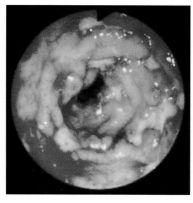

Figure 11.44 Coarse nodular deformity of luminal contour may occur in long-standing, severe Crohn's disease.

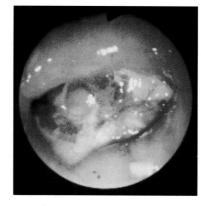

Figure 11.45 Moderately severe, irregular stricture in Crohn's disease. Interconnected ulcers are visible around the mouth of the stricture.

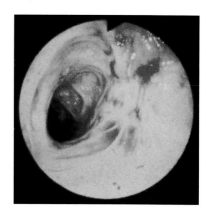

Figure 11.46 Severe longitudinal scarring and retraction leads to the formation of pseudodiverticular outpouchings.

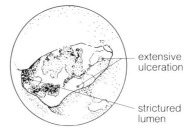

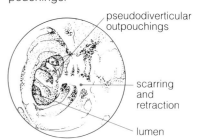

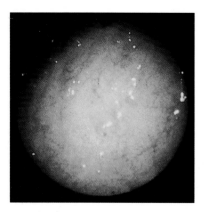

Figure 11.47 Broad, longitudinal scar is seen as a white band interrupting the vascular pattern.

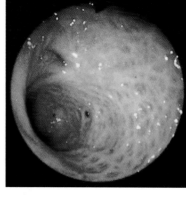

Figure 11.48 Extensive confluent scarring gives the bowel wall a bizarre appearance.

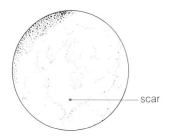

ANATOMIC VARIATIONS CAUSED BY CROHN'S DISEASE

Structural alterations often accompany changes in the mucosal lining as a consequence of fibrosis and scarring following deep ulceration and transmural fissuring. Thickening and blunting of the interhaustral folds may often be seen in segments in which there is ulceration, and occur as a consequence of submucosal edema and fibrosis. Occasionally, there is a striking predilection for ulcers to cluster in and around areas of convergence of the interhaustral folds. In severe cases, the haustral pattern may be completely lost due to major architectural derangements.

The thickened interhaustral folds and muscularis retraction may decrease the luminal diameter of the colon. Extensive underlying ulceration may result in the creation of mucosal bridges across the lumen once the acute phase has subsided and reepithelialization has occurred.

Fibrotic long (more than several centimeters) strictures are common in Crohn's disease and are a consequence of intense, deep ulceration and fissuring into the submucosa. The lumen is compromised to varying degrees; diameters after stricturing may range from 10 to 15 mm to less than 5 mm. Low-grade and moderately severe strictures can be examined with a small-caliber colonoscope but not with the standard 13-mm colonoscope. Strictures are often irregular, with evidence of inflammation and focal epithelial destruction (Fig. 11.45). Ulcerations are generally found within the strictured area, especially at the opening. Cobblestoning is common in the area leading to the stricture. Strictures caused by active inflammation are lined by edematous, erythematous, friable, and ulcerated mucosa. Smooth, inactive-

within any one area more than one may be noted. Generally, inflammatory pseudopolyps are less than 1.5 cm in greatest dimension (Fig. 11.43). Coarse, nodular deformity of the mucosal contours may occur in long-standing, severe disease through the combination of cobblestoning and pseudopolyp formation (Fig. 11.44).

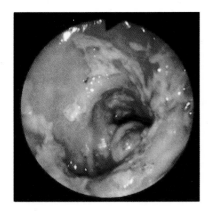

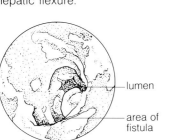

Figure 11.49 *Left,* Colocolonic fistula in Crohn's disease. Mucosa also shows evidence of ulceration. *Right,* Corresponding X-ray shows fistula at hepatic flexure.

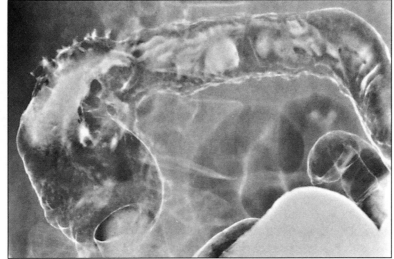

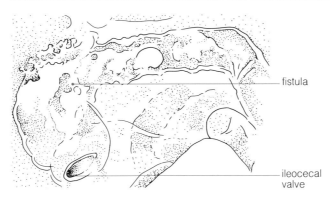

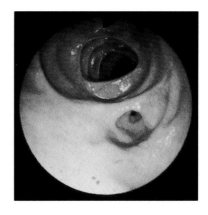

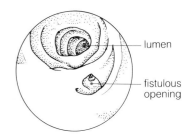

Figure 11.50 Healed fistulous communication between terminal ileum and transverse colon shows normal mucosa.

looking strictures are usually lined by fairly normal-appearing mucosa.

Healing of deep ulceration may result in thick bands of scar tissue in both the small and large bowel. Between these bands, diverticular outpouchings of the wall may occur (Fig. 11.46). Such extensive scarring, which dissects the mucosal lining, is always indicative of severe previous damage (Figs. 11.47 and 11.48).

Fistula formation is a well-known complication of Crohn's disease. A variety of fistulas may occur, such as colocutaneous, colocolonic, coloenteric, and colovesical. Usually a focal area of edema and erythema surrounds the fistulous opening, which itself may not be readily apparent. In other instances, the orifice of the fistula is a deep, rounded, ulcerlike cavity. The presence of epithelial defects adjacent to and at a distance from the fistulous opening is an indication that the fistula-bearing bowel segment is intrinsically involved in Crohn's disease (Fig. 11.49). When the inflammatory activity subsides and the epithelial lesions heal, the mucosal aspect of the fistulous opening may appear inactive (Fig. 11.50). When fistulas develop between the small bowel and colon, it is important to determine whether they are a manifestation of small bowel disease only or whether the large bowel is also involved. In the former case, there is only edematous swelling and some reddening around the fistulous opening. In the latter case, there usually is evidence of ulceration in the region of the fistulous opening.

Often a combination of mucosal and structural abnormalities are spread out over the colon (Fig. 11.51). The

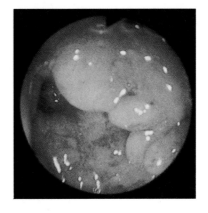

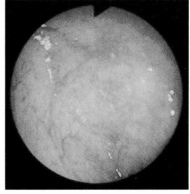

Figure 11.51 In this patient with Crohn's disease, cobblestoning and mild stricturing are combined.

Figure 11.52 Crohn's disease may take on a subtle appearance. This area of patchy aphthoid erosions in the cecum is barely visible.

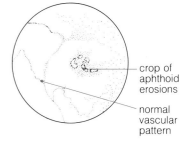

variability and severity of the defects are important elements in the differential diagnosis. Early lesions may be subtle, requiring careful inspection of the mucosal lining (Fig. 11.52). New lesions superimposed on older abnormalities

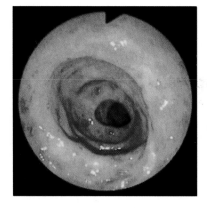
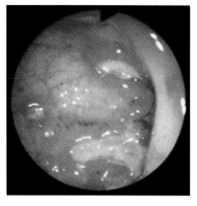
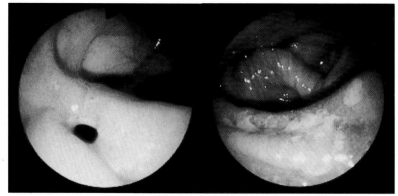

Figure 11.53 Spectrum of new lesions is superimposed on older abnormalities in Crohn's disease. Red spots and tiny aphthoid erosions appear on a whitish background due to scarring.

Figure 11.54 Characteristic focal lesions in Crohn's disease. The discontinuous abnormalities have intervening normal-appearing mucosa.

Figure 11.55 Involvement of the ileocecal valve in Crohn's disease can present as stenosis *(left)* or ulceration *(right).*

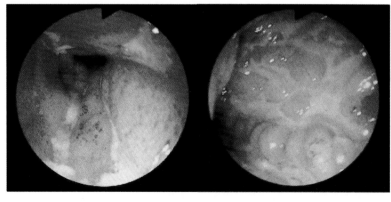
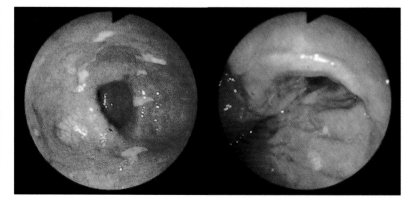

Figure 11.56 *Left,* Diffuse, concentric involvement of the distal terminal ileum in Crohn's disease presents as swelling, erythema, punctiform bleeding, and ulceration. *Right,* Circumferential involvement of the distal terminal ileum with longitudinal ulcers and cobblestoning.

Figure 11.57 In contrast to the distal portion, the more proximal segment of the terminal ileum shows smaller, patchy ulcerative lesions, with normal-appearing intervening mucosa.

occasionally produce bizarre appearances (Fig. 11.53). The characteristic finding is focal lesions with normal intervening mucosa (Fig. 11.54).

EXAMINATION OF THE TERMINAL ILEUM
Involvement of the ileocecal valve in Crohn's disease is often associated with stenosis resulting from ulceration and fibrosis. This inflammatory narrowing may prevent entry of the colonoscope tip into the terminal ileum (Fig. 11.55). Nevertheless, the terminal ileum should be inspected whenever possible. Since the terminal ileum and ileocecal valve are usually involved simultaneously, patchy inflammation or ulceration of the valve alone can be sufficient to make a correct diagnosis, even if the endoscope cannot be passed into the terminal ileum.

The same abnormalities described for the colon can also be seen in the terminal ileum. A characteristic finding is the presence of either aphthoid erosions or ulcers, ranging in size from small, superficial defects to large lesions measuring up to 1 cm. Some of the larger ulcers may be associated with stricture formation. Long, longitudinal parallel ulcers may result through coalescence of smaller lesions. Surrounding the ulcers, there may be evidence of inflammation

shown by the presence of erythematous spots or punctiform hemorrhage. Between ulcerations, there may be "skip" areas of normal-looking mucosa. In general, the inflammatory changes tend to involve the entire circumference in the distal terminal ileum (Fig. 11.56), but are patchy and focal in the more proximal involved ileal segment (Fig. 11.57).

Crohn's disease may affect younger patients, and nodular lymphoid hyperplasia of the terminal ileum is not uncommon in that age group. The typically nonfriable excrescences of lymphoid hyperplasia in the ileal mucosa should not be confused with cobblestoning of Crohn's disease.

Recrudescence of Crohn's disease after extirpation of diseased segments of the terminal ileum is common. In the majority of patients, tiny aphthoid or small superficial ulcers are left behind in the neoterminal ileum (Fig. 11.58). Progression of such lesions presumably leads to clinically manifest recurrent disease (Fig. 11.59). Recrudescent disease is nearly always within 20 cm of the anastomotic line, although not necessarily involving the anastomosis. When examining patients in the symptomatic stage after recurrence, one should carefully inspect the anastomosis itself before entering the neoterminal ileum (Figs. 11.60 and 11.61). It is

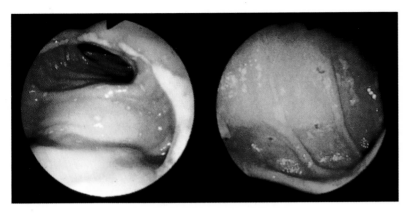

Figure 11.58 Recrudescent Crohn's disease. *Left,* Postsurgically, tiny aphthoid erosions are discernible scattered throughout the neoterminal ileum. In addition, the margin of a larger ulcer is seen. *Right,* In this case, a hemorrhagic spot is seen in the center of superficial ulcers.

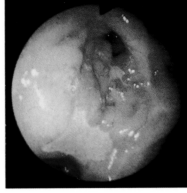
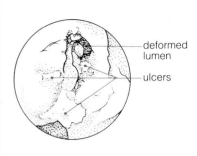

Figure 11.59 Recrudescent Crohn's disease in the neoterminal ileum with large ulcers. Note the luminal deformity.

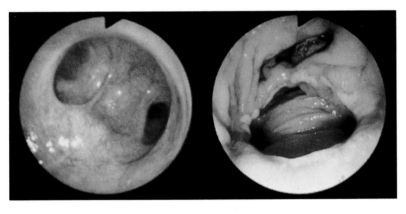
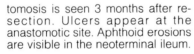

Figure 11.60 *Left,* The normal appearance of a side-to-end ileocolonic anastomosis after resection for Crohn's disease. *Right,* Early recrudescence at side-to-end anastomosis is seen 3 months after resection. Ulcers appear at the anastomotic site. Aphthoid erosions are visible in the neoterminal ileum.

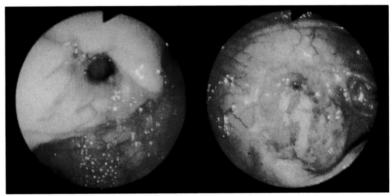
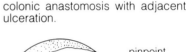

Figure 11.61 *Left,* The normal appearance of ileocolonic anastomosis. *Right,* Severely strictured ileocolonic anastomosis with adjacent ulceration.

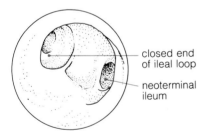
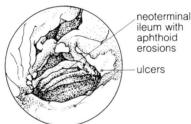
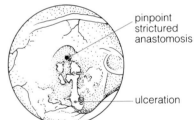

through the use of colonoscopy to examine the anastomotic line and inspect the neoterminal ileum that we have learned about the form that recurrent disease takes in this clinical circumstance.

Ulcerative defects are most often seen just at and proximal to the anastomosis (Fig. 11.62). When the terminal ileum is involved in recurrent disease, the ulcers initially tend to be circumferential and preferentially located on the ridge of the Kerckring's folds. They are apt to be superficial and may be accompanied by aphthoid erosions. Not uncommonly, normal mucosa may be present between areas of active disease. When the ulcerations are deep, the intervening mucosa may be edematous and appear thickened, accentuating the basic nodular character of the anastomotic line, which results from its construction with interrupted sutures (Fig. 11.63). Occasionally, deep ulcerations at the

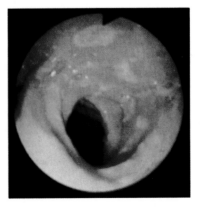

Figure 11.62 Small and large ulcers can be seen in the neoterminal ileum of this patient with recrudescent Crohn's disease.

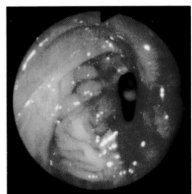

Figure 11.63 Moderately severe narrowing of an ileocolonic anastomosis can be barely bypassed with the colonoscope. The nodular configuration of the anastomosis follows the suture line.

11.15

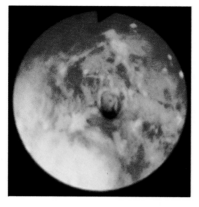
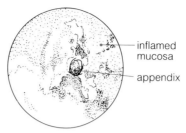

inflamed
mucosa

appendix

Figure 11.64 Crohn's disease with obvious involvement of appendix and cecum.

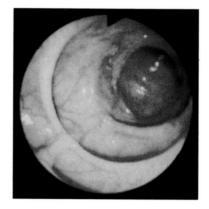

Figure 11.65 Distal colon has a normal appearance except for patchy anal involvement.

anastomosis seem to follow the lines of the previous sutures. With extensive ulceration, the intervening mucosa may disappear altogether, with the anastomotic line resembling one continuous area of ulceration. This type of ulceration ultimately leads to a high-grade strictured anastomosis. Adjacent to such areas of deep ulceration, the segment may show cobblestoning.

DISTRIBUTION OF LESIONS

One of the hallmarks of Crohn's disease is the focal, patchy, discontinuous distribution of the lesions. Although Crohn's disease is probably a panenteric disease, predilection for certain areas of the bowel occurs sufficiently often to allow some patterns to be distinguished.

1. Right-sided involvement: The ileocecal area is the most common site of involvement in up to 60% of all cases. In an additional 20 to 30%, the right colon is involved exclusively. Thus, in the majority of cases, the disease tends to be right-sided. Overall, nearly 70% of patients have largely, if not exclusively, right-sided involvement, including the ileocecal valve and terminal ileum.
2. Rectal-sparing: Often disease begins at the rectosigmoid junction. Deep ulceration and strictures are characteristic. In some cases the anus and 3 to 4 cm of the distal rectum are involved, but the rectum above this point is normal.
3. Segmental involvement: Skip lesions are the rule in the majority of the cases. Areas of normal bowel appear preserved between areas of obvious disease. Segmental involvement may be seen in any area of the gut, including the anal canal and the appendix (Figs. 11.64 and 11.65). In some cases ulcerations are seen on only one side of the colonic mucosal surface.

LEVELS OF ACTIVITY

Crohn's disease is called inactive when the vascular pattern is only slightly distorted and there is fine granularity without obvious friability or epithelial defects. There is no standardized system for staging the activity of Crohn's disease. The term mildly active is used when there is unequivocal erythema, either focal or confluent, and some friability

without epithelial necrosis. Arbitrarily, the stage is moderately active when a few aphthoid erosions or small ulcers are noted. Cases are described as severe when ulcers are larger and more numerous. Complications of Crohn's disease such as stricturing, fistula formation, and massive bleeding usually indicate severe disease.

RISK OF DYSPLASIA OR MALIGNANCY

There may be a slightly increased incidence of cancer in Crohn's disease patients, especially in cases of extensive colonic involvement with early onset, and after previous surgery and bypass. Tumors may occur in the excluded intestinal loop. The cancers occur in relatively young patients, tending to locate on the right side and in areas of fistula formation. Such cancers are often infiltrative in nature. However, a variety of gross morphologic appearances may be encountered such as polypoid masses which are often sessile and nodular. Flat or plaque-like cancers may also be encountered. In Crohn's disease, the appearance of such infiltrating cancer may be obscured by the endoscopic findings of Crohn's disease itself, including strictures, cobblestoning and ulceration.

DIFFERENTIAL DIAGNOSIS OF ULCERATIVE COLITIS, CROHN'S DISEASE, AND ACUTE SELF-LIMITED COLITIS

The main differential diagnosis with respect to idiopathic inflammatory bowel disease centers around ulcerative colitis and Crohn's disease. Colonoscopy is useful to help in the differential diagnosis and to assess the extent and severity of the disease. Despite increased experience, for 5 to 10% of patients the diagnosis remains difficult and changes back and forth over the years. Differential aspects of ulcerative colitis and Crohn's disease are summarized in Figure 11.66.

FACTORS FAVORING DIAGNOSIS OF ULCERATIVE COLITIS

Diffuse involvement of the rectum is almost a prerequisite for the diagnosis of ulcerative colitis. Most often, some evidence of rectal involvement is present initially. Conversely,

Differential Diagnosis of Ulcerative Colitis and Crohn's Disease

Characteristics	Ulcerative Colitis	Crohn's Disease
Distribution	Symmetrical	Asymmetrical
Continuous involvement	Always	Exceptional
Patchiness	Absent	Frequent
Rectal involvement	Almost always	Often absent
Vascular pattern	Blurred or lost	Often normal
Profuse bleeding	Common	Rare
Granularity (fine/coarse)	Common	Less common
Cobblestoning	Absent	Characteristic
Erythema	Characteristic	Less pronounced
Edema (blunting of septa)	Present	Present
Friability	Common	Uncommon
Spontaneous petechiae	Common	Rare
Superficial to small ulcerations	Occasional	Frequent
Large (> 1 cm) ulceration	Severe disease	Common
Deep, longitudinal ulceration	Rare	Common
Linear ulceration	Rare	Common
Aphthoid ulceration	Absent	Characteristic
Serpiginous ulceration	Rare	Common
Pseudopolyps	Occasional	Occasional
Bridging	Occasional	Occasional
Mucosa surrounding ulcer	Abnormal	Normal

Figure 11.66 Differential diagnosis of ulcerative colitis and Crohn's disease.

a normal rectal appearance favors a diagnosis of Crohn's disease.

A continuous, symmetrical, diffuse pattern of mucosal involvement strongly favors ulcerative colitis. Although there may be some variability in activity, the mucosa should always be abnormal over the involved segment. Occasionally the endoscopic abnormalities may be subtle and consist only of minor loss of shininess. In this case, even with a visible, sharply demarcated, vascular pattern, one is often surprised by the heavy amount of mononuclear infiltration seen at biopsy.

Ulceration seen in a background of diffuse mucosal abnormality is the most important indicator of ulcerative colitis. This acute mucosal inflammation may consist of ery-

thema, friability, or mucopurulent exudate. A patulous or effaced ileocecal valve with a patent opening favors the diagnosis of ulcerative colitis. In contrast, the presence of extensive ulceration around a closed or stenotic ileocecal valve favors the diagnosis of Crohn's disease.

FACTORS FAVORING DIAGNOSIS OF CROHN'S DISEASE

Patchy, discontinuous, and segmental distribution of lesions is a key finding favoring the diagnosis of Crohn's disease. Areas of apparently normal mucosa alternate with ulcerations, or there may be asymmetrical distribution of ulceration within a given segment.

Absence of rectal involvement, which may occur in 30%

Types of Infectious Colitis

Disorder	Similarity to *	
	Ulcerative Colitis	Crohn's Disease
Campylobacter colitis	2	1
Yersinia enterocolitica colitis	1	3
Salmonellosis	3	1
Shigellosis	3	
Tuberculosis	1	3
Mycobacterium avium-intracellulare	1	
Gonorrhea	1	
Syphilis	2	1
Amebiasis	2	2
Schistosomiasis	2	2
Vibrio parahaemolyticus	1	
Cytomegalovirus colitis	3	1
LVG-Chlamydia proctitis	1	3
Non-LVG Chlamydia proctitis	2	
Herpes simplex		1
Antibiotic-associated colitis	2	

*Similarity ranked from 1 to 3, 3 being most similar.

Figure 11.67 Types of infectious colitis.

of cases of colonic involvement, strongly favors Crohn's disease. When the rectum is involved in Crohn's disease, it is usually in the rectosigmoid or perianal areas.

Ulcers set in relatively normal mucosa with a preserved vascular pattern or at least without evidence of acute inflammation strongly suggest Crohn's disease. Deep, extensive ulceration seems to be more characteristic of Crohn's disease. The adjacent mucosa may appear cobblestoned, heaped-up, nodular, and perhaps slightly pink, but it is not friable. Ulceration, stenosis, or distortion of the ileocecal valve along with a predominantly right-sided involvement strongly favors the diagnosis of Crohn's disease.

BIOPSY

Colonoscopic biopsies of abnormal and normal mucosa are always advisable to supplement the visual impression differentiating ulcerative colitis and Crohn's disease. Colonoscopic biopsies are usually taken with a standard #7 French forceps with round cups or oval jaws, with or without a central spike. Such biopsies are usually small and superficial, and contain only the mucosa and fragments of the muscularis mucosae, with an occasional small bit of submucosa. Biopsy forceps with larger cups are available for use with large-channel colonoscopes.

Nonspecific histologic findings include mucosal ulceration, fibrinous purulent exudate, infiltration by inflammatory cells, crypt abscesses, and lymphoid aggregates. In general, the biopsy finding of multiple basal crypt abscesses in the presence of epithelial cells, with a diminished mucus content and a continuous pattern of activity, favors a diagnosis of ulcerative colitis. The most important histologic feature of Crohn's disease is the presence of focal granulomas or microgranulomas. Other criteria include discontinuity of the inflammatory infiltrate, disproportionate infiltration and transmural extension of the inflammatory infiltrate, marked lymphoid hyperplasia, fissuring, ulceration, and lymphangiectasia. The histologic diagnosis of Crohn's disease varies substantially depending on the number of biopsies and the number of sections examined. However it should be possible to obtain granulomas in at least 30% of cases.

ACUTE SELF-LIMITED COLITIS VS. IDIOPATHIC INFLAMMATORY BOWEL DISEASE

When a patient presents with acute bloody diarrhea, one must consider the possibility that this is the onset of inflammatory bowel disease, either ulcerative colitis or Crohn's disease. On the other hand this may be an episode of acute self-limited colitis. This is not a simple differential diagnosis when the patient first presents. In time the acute self-limited colitis disappears, with gradual resolution over a few weeks. Idiopathic inflammatory bowel disease may also resolve in a period of weeks but the course is usually one of recurrent episodes.

Biopsies of the rectal mucosa may assist in the differential diagnosis between the self-limited colitis and idiopathic inflammatory bowel disease. In the self-limited colitis, the histology appears fairly normal with normal crypt architecture, scattered polymorphs, and few mononuclear cells. Crypt abscesses, if they occur, are superficial, and the main location of the inflammation is the upper half of the mucosa. In idiopathic inflammatory bowel disease the crypts are abnormal with distortion of the crypt architecture and abnormal branching of the crypts. The infiltrate is often predominantly mononuclear. Granulomas may be seen as may lymphoid aggregates. There may be crypt atrophy. In a portion of patients (approximately 1 in 5) biopsy may not distinguish the self-limited type from inflammatory bowel disease.

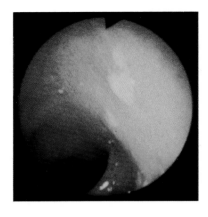

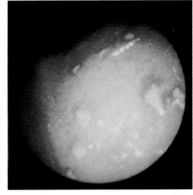

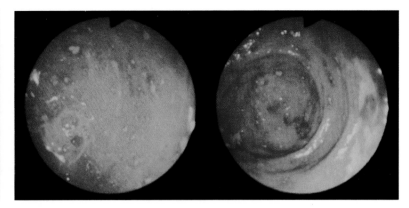

Figure 11.68 Campylobacter colitis. A zone of edema and erythema includes a superficial ulcer with exudate resembling Crohn's disease.

Figure 11.69 Several discrete, small ulcers with pronounced erythematous rims are set in a background of abnormal mucosa in this case of Campylobacter colitis, mimicking ulcerative colitis.

Figure 11.70 Yersiniosis of the terminal ileum, with small aphthoid-like erosions and ulceration.

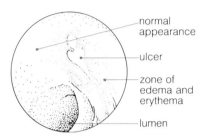

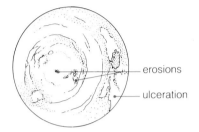

OTHER INFLAMMATORY BOWEL DISORDERS

INFECTIOUS COLITIS

Acute and chronic infectious diseases involving the colon may mimic features of idiopathic inflammatory bowel disease to the point where they cannot be endoscopically differentiated. Thus, endoscopy should not be used as the prime diagnostic modality in infectious colitis, but only when problems of differential diagnosis occur. There are many different organisms which cause colitis; they vary in the degree to which the presenting features mimic ulcerative colitis or Crohn's disease (Fig. 11.67).

Campylobacter fetus, subspecies *jejuni*, is recognized as the etiologic agent in episodes of acute watery diarrhea and acute mucoid bloody diarrhea in otherwise healthy individuals. The endoscopic findings may vary. Occasionally zones of edema, patchy erythema, and friability with some scattered ulcers alternate with areas of relatively normal mucosa, which gives the appearance of Crohn's disease (Fig. 11.68). Also, the presence of tiny aphthoid-like erosions is increasingly recognized. In other patients, erythema, hyperemia, edema, friability, and some superficial ulceration may create an endoscopic appearance similar to ulcerative colitis (Fig. 11.69). Deep ulceration is unusual, although large, shaggy ulcers with markedly friable mucosa at the margins have been observed. In some patients, abundant mucopurulent exudate rather than ulceration may be noted.

Although the rectum is usually involved, occasionally only the more proximal areas of the colon are affected. All these abnormalities disappear in time. On biopsy, the lamina propria contains a variety of inflammatory cells, most of which are polymorphonuclear leukocytes and crypt abscesses but little crypt distortion.

Yersinia enterocolitica may cause acute and chronic diarrhea and colitis. The characteristic endoscopic feature is that of multiple, small, shallow or punched-out aphthoid-like erosions or small ulcers, surrounded by a small zone of erythema and normal-looking adjacent mucosa. The lesions in yersiniosis tend to be small and uniform, although occasionally larger ulcers may develop (Fig. 11.70). The lesions observed in Yersinia colitis almost always have a segmental or patchy distribution. Quite regularly, the lesions may be confined to the terminal ileum, cecum, and ascending colon, but in about 50% of patients the entire colon including the rectum may be involved. Because of the appearance of the lesions and the distribution, yersiniosis may mimic Crohn's disease. Much less commonly, *Yersinia enterocolitica* colitis may be associated with more uniformly edematous, erythematous, and friable mucosa, compatible with the appearance of ulcerative colitis.

Salmonellosis may involve the small or large bowel. Involvement is preferentially on the right side but may include the entire colon; rectal-sparing is common. The endoscopic findings vary from relatively minor abnormalities such as mucosal edema, hyperemia, and loss of vascular pattern to severe pancolitis with diffuse edematous and erythematous mucosa, granularity, friability, and petechial hemorrhages

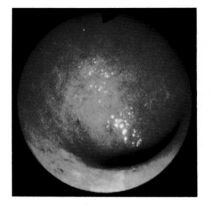

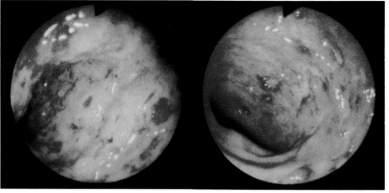

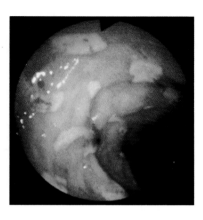

Figure 11.71 Salmonella colitis can mimic ulcerative colitis.

Figure 11.72 *Left,* Severe *Shigella flexneri* colitis with extensive, coalescent, superficial ulceration involves nearly the entire bowel circumference. Increased erythema of the remaining mucosa contrasts with the extensive mucosal necrotic slough. *Right,* Appearance after 2 weeks of antibiotic therapy shows marked improvement.

Figure 11.73 Tuberculosis with ulceration in the cecal area.

similar to ulcerative colitis (Fig. 11.71). Discrete ulcers are usually seen only in the more proximal colon. In severe cases, the markedly edematous mucosa may be covered by a greenish, necrotic slough, similar to antibiotic-associated colitis. Occasionally, multiple, regularly distributed, pustular lymph follicles may be present, suggestive of small Crohn's-like ulcers. This finding, together with the predominant right-sided involvement and the presence of skip areas, may occasionally create an appearance resembling Crohn's disease. Rapid reversal, however, over a 3 to 4 week period is an important finding in favoring the bacterial etiology of the colitis.

Shigellosis may be responsible for severe colitis. In general, the endoscopic appearance may be indistinguishable from idiopathic ulcerative colitis. The severity of the endoscopic abnormalities may vary from intense mucosal erythema and hyperemia with adherent mucus to pronounced hyperemia, minor friability, and superficial ulceration on a background of erythematous mucosa (Fig. 11.72). Although the mucosa may have a magenta hue, the striking friability seen in ulcerative colitis is usually absent. In very severe forms, ulceration may spread and coalesce to involve large segments of the entire circumference. Occasionally in shigellosis, the lesions may be patchy and consist of focal areas of erythema and granularity with some scattered aphthoid erosions or superficial ulcers, usually confined to the rectosigmoid region; this appearance is more suggestive of Crohn's disease.

Tuberculosis has a predilection for the ileocecal area rich in lymphatic tissue. The overall endoscopic appearance of colonic tuberculosis is indistinguishable from that of Crohn's disease, with ulcers, strictures, and skip lesions (Fig. 11.73). The ileocecal valve may show thickened, nodular, and ulcerated patches (Fig. 11.74). Sometimes the valve is gaping, surrounded by heaped-up and ulcerated folds. The cecum and ascending colon may be narrowed and contracted; focal stenotic areas may be deeply ulcerated. The transverse colon may also be involved with ulceration and, at times, irregular stricturing. Shorter segments are involved than in Crohn's disease. The mucosa may be focally erythematous and edematous with superficial and deep ulceration, often with raised, indurated margins. As in Crohn's disease, ulcers are surrounded by normal-looking mucosa. In addition, cobblestoning, segmental involvement, and linear ulceration are seen. At times, a hypertrophic, ulcerated, flaky mass resembling a carcinoma may be discernible, especially in the cecal area. A rare presentation is that of a pancolitis with either diffuse or segmental edema, erythema, friability, and ulceration. The rectum is commonly spared. Strictures, mass lesions, and fistulas may also be noted.

Chronic infection with *Mycobacterium avium-intracellulare* may occur in immunocompromised patients and is responsible for pseudo-Whipple's disease of the rectocolon. Large segments of the circumference of the bowel show a whitish hue caused by the massive accumulation of lipid-filled macrophages, packed with mycobacteria (Fig. 11.75).

The endoscopic features of gonorrhea are nonspecific and include edema, erythema, friability, and—rarely—ulceration. Usually only the 3 to 5 cm immediatley above the anus is involved, with abundant purulent material present in the anal canal. Diagnosis is made by Gram's stain and culture of this material. Several pathogens may be cultured simultaneously, further complicating endoscopic interpretation (Fig. 11.76).

The endoscopic presentation of anorectal syphilis includes solitary or multiple anal and rectal ulcers surrounded by friable and slightly edematous mucosa. At times, thickened, hyperplastic, fibrotic, anorectal masses or condylomas may be seen, which are easily mistaken for anal fissures, cryptitis, fistula, or even cancer.

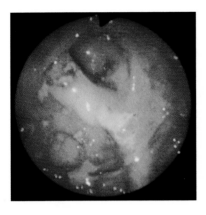

Figure 11.74 In this case of tuberculosis, the diseased ileocecal valve did not allow intubation of the strictured terminal ileum. Ulcerations of the mucosa are similar to those found in Crohn's disease.

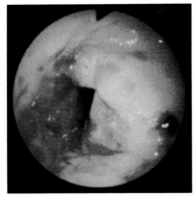

Figure 11.75 Pseudo-Whipple's disease due to *Mycobacterium aviumintracellulare* in an AIDS patient. Characteristic whitish discoloration contrasts with the reddish zones representing uninvolved mucosa.

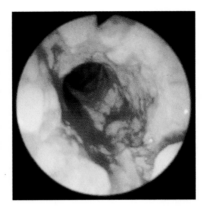

Figure 11.76 Proctitis caused by gonorrhea, Chlamydia, and beta-hemolytic streptococci. Appearance 7 days after ampicillin therapy still shows erythema and ulcerations.

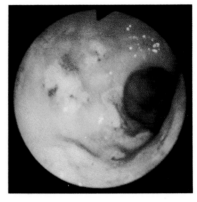

Figure 11.77 Discrete ulcers with slightly undermined edges are depicted in this view of amebiasis.

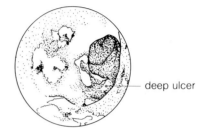

deep ulcer

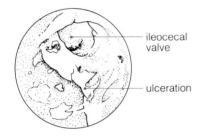

ileocecal valve

ulceration

Amebiasis caused by *Entamoeba histolytica* has a predilection for the cecal and rectosigmoid area. The endoscopic features of amebic colitis are variable. Especially during acute stages of the disease, the mucosa of the rectum and sigmoid may show diffuse edema, erythema and friability, granularity, and abundant mucopurulent exudate together with scattered ulcerations. This appearance is indistinguishable from that of acute ulcerative colitis. Smears made from the exudate reveal trophozoites, as do biopsies from the ulcerations.

More classical is the appearance reflecting chronic mucosal involvement. Ulcerations a few millimeters in diameter with slightly undermined edges are seen in areas where the mucosa is otherwise normal or minimally abnormal with blurring of the vascular pattern (Fig. 11.77). The ulcers may be covered by a yellow-white exudate and may, at times, resemble aphthoid-type erosions or small ulcers seen in Crohn's disease (Fig. 11.78). Occasionally the ulcers may be deep, punched-out, and surrounded by an intense erythematous halo. Inflammatory pseudopolyps may then be seen, often adjacent to ulcers. Rarely, involvement in amebiasis is limited to the cecal area. Endoscopy may reveal cecal erosions, ulcerations, or mass lesions (amebomas) with superficial ulceration.

The colonic complications of schistosomiasis are related to the deposition of schistosomal eggs in the terminal venules within colonic mucosa. *Schistosoma japonicum* involves primarily the cecum and ascending colon, *Schistosoma mansoni* the descending colon, and *Schistosoma haematobium* the bladder and rectum. The colonic features include edema,

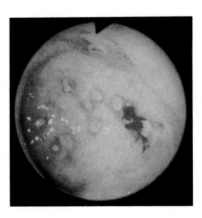

Figure 11.78 Amebiasis of the rectosigmoid junction. Small superficial ulcerations are covered with whitish exudate and surrounded by an erythematous rim. Mucosa adjacent to the ulcers is unremarkable except for some blurring of the vascular pattern. Smearing of the ulcers may cause mild bleeding because of hyperemia at the edges.

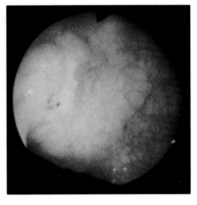

Figure 11.79 Schistosomiasis at the rectosigmoid junction. A shallow ulceration is surrounded by slightly raised, edematous mucosa.

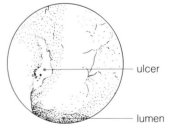

ulcer

lumen

marked hyperemia, friability, punctate hemorrhages, granularity, and focal shallow ulcerations, closely resembling ulcerative colitis (Fig. 11.79). In addition, there may be mucosal thickening and luminal narrowing. A further similarity with ulcerative colitis is the appearance of multiple inflam-

11.21

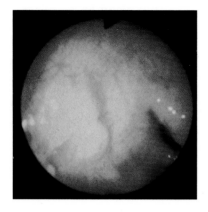

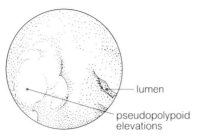
lumen

pseudopolypoid
elevations

Figure 11.80 Pseudopolypoid elevations in schistosomiasis contain degenerating ova.

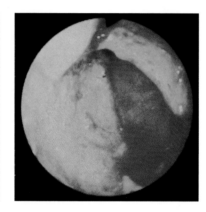

Figure 11.81 Views of lymphogranuloma venerium-type *Chlamydia trachomatis* infection show detail of an ulcer across the distal valve of Houston.

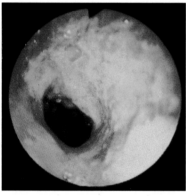

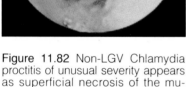

Figure 11.82 Non-LGV Chlamydia proctitis of unusual severity appears as superficial necrosis of the mucosa in the anal canal.

Figure 11.83 This view of herpes proctitis in an AIDS patient shows confluent, nearly circumferential ulceration of anal canal and distal rectum.

matory pseudopolyps largely in the rectum and sigmoid (Fig. 11.80). These polypoid lesions are composed of degenerating ova and surrounding granulomatous inflammatory reaction. Their characteristic feature is central ulceration or the presence of abundant amounts of exudate.

Vibrio parahaemolyticus is usually associated with explosive watery diarrhea and shows striking inflammatory changes in the terminal ileum. Unusually, mucoid bloody diarrhea is noted and at endoscopy, a patchy, erythematous, friable mucosa without ulceration may be observed.

Cytomegalovirus (CMV) infection may present as isolated, large, punched-out ulcers predominantly on the right side in renal transplant patients. In AIDS patients, multiple smaller ulcers may be seen, usually right-sided but occasionally throughout the colon. CMV may also present as multiple discrete zones of intense erythema. There may be thickening of the folds and the mucosal vascular pattern may be blurred or lost, presenting an appearance similar to ulcerative colitis.

Lymphogranuloma venerium-type (LGV) Chlamydia proctitis is a problem in the homosexual population. The rectum and sigmoid are most often involved, with abnormalities that usually do not extend beyond the sigmoid colon. Endoscopically, there is patchy or diffuse edema. The mucosa is erythematous, friable, and granular; skip lesions may be seen. Ulcerations are occasionally noted, with a predilection for the valves of Houston (Fig. 11.81). In more chronic disease, strictures may occur, usually within a few centimeters of the anus. Also, fistula formation may occur which may mimic Crohn's disease.

The abnormalities in non-LGV Chlamydia proctitis are usually milder and consist of erythema, edema with minimal friability, and—rarely—ulceration. In a few patients there may be superficial necrosis of the epithelium (Fig. 11.82).

Herpes simplex virus (HSV) of the anorectal area is an increasingly common diagnosis, especially among homosexuals. At endoscopy, one usually finds patchy or diffuse edema, erythema, and friability, and a variable number of erosions or ulcerations in the anorectal area. Occasionally ulcers coalesce, leading to denudation of nearly the whole circumference of the anorectal canal (Fig. 11.83). Infrequently, small vesicles may be seen in the rectum. HSV intranuclear inclusions and herpes multinucleated cells may be identified in biopsies.

ANTIBIOTIC-ASSOCIATED COLITIS

Certain antibiotics predispose to development of diarrhea, most often without evidence of previous inflammation or *Clostridium difficile* infection. Sometimes, however, this organism emerges with antibiotic use, elaborating a cytotoxin which causes focal necrosis of the epithelium along with an acute inflammatory exudate. If pseudomembranous plaques form over the area of superficial ulceration, the term pseudomembranous colitis is used. This disorder is identified by the presence of sharply demarcated, elevated yellow-white plaques that vary in size from pinhead to several centimeters (Fig. 11.84). The surrounding mucosa may look normal or appear edematous, friable, and covered with mu-

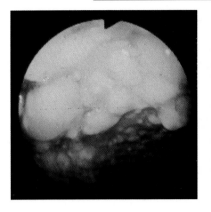

Figure 11.84 After clindamycin therapy, *Clostridium difficile* overgrowth leads to this severe form of pseudomembranous colitis. Raised, strongly adherent, yellow plaques are characteristic features.

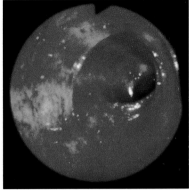

Figure 11.85 Hemorrhagic right-sided colitis after penicillin therapy.

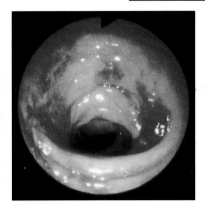

Figure 11.86 Acute phase of ischemic damage involving the sigmoid colon. Patchy erythema contrasts with paler mucosa.

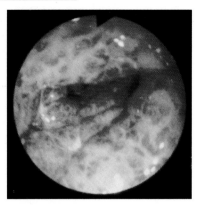

Figure 11.87 Acute phase of ischemic damage. There is severe luminal narrowing because of marked swelling and muscle contraction. Ecchymotic spots are evidence of submucosal bleeding.

copurulent exudate. The mucosa may bleed when the plaques are removed. In severe cases the plaques coalesce, and edema, erythema, and friability with punctate hemorrhages may be seen. Rarely, there is extensive sloughing of necrotic mucosa.

Generally, the involvement is distal or left-sided, but it may be universal, especially if plaques are large. In up to a third of affected patients, the endoscopic changes are seen only above the rectosigmoid area. After treatment with vancomycin, the pseudomembranes usually disappear rapidly.

In up to one-third of cases, only edema and erythema are seen and no obvious pseudomembranes are present. This form of antibiotic-associated colitis has become a major clinical consideration in the differential diagnosis of inflammatory bowel diseases. This is particularly true if the condition presents without raised, whitish plaques attached to the mucosal surface and if the rectum is not involved.

A peculiar, transient, right-sided hemorrhagic colitis is occasionally seen after antibiotic therapy, especially after penicillin and ampicillin, and less often after amoxicillin, erythromycin, and clindamycin. Such patients usually present with bloody diarrhea of acute onset. Edema, friability, and mucosal hemorrhage, sometimes with scattered erosions, are usually located in the hepatic flexure and ascending colon (Fig. 11.85). The affected area may be well-demarcated. Follow-up colonoscopies 7 to 14 days after the initial examination usually demonstrate complete clearing of the hemorrhagic mucosal changes.

ISCHEMIC DAMAGE OF THE COLON

Ischemic colitis caused by inadequate tissue perfusion is being diagnosed with increased frequency, especially in elderly patients. Mesenteric ischemia is most often associated with low cardiac output noted with cardiogenic shock or severe intravascular volume depletion. Less often the ischemia may be secondary to occlusion of the superior or inferior mesenteric artery. Primary venous obstruction is rare. In a substantial percentage of patients, inadequate tissue perfusion is caused by distal colonic obstruction from carcinoma or diverticular disease.

The pathologic changes evoked by ischemia range from submucosal edema to infarction. Between these two extremes are gradations of tissue damage with resulting diverse clinical courses and endoscopic appearances. In mild ischemia, morphologic changes regress and disappear, whereas severe ischemia may result in irreparable damage with gangrene, perforation, or persistent nonresolving colitis.

The most severe form of ischemic damage is transmural gangrene. Patients with severe abdominal pain, high fever, and evidence of peritoneal irritation likely have gangrenous infarction and should not undergo endoscopy because of the risk of perforation. In the rare instance when endoscopy is performed, the whitish-gray or purple-black discoloration characteristic of gangrenous mucosa is evident.

Less severe forms of ischemic damage usually correspond to the clinical variant of transient ischemic colitis. Endoscopy may be useful in this less severe form of ischemia. Three stages have been arbitrarily defined. The acute stage is characterized initially by patchy areas of edematous hyperemia adjacent to paler areas (Fig. 11.86). These pale areas are due to intense vasoconstriction of mucosal blood vessels. Over 24 hours, the erythematous areas may coalesce. At this point, there is usually evidence of submucosal bleeding with petechiae or hemorrhages (Fig. 11.87), or even large submucosal hemorrhagic bluish blebs. In addition, the interhaustral folds may be thickened because of edema and submucosal hemorrhage, creating the characteristic thumbprinting appearance noted radiographically (Fig. 11.88).

11.23

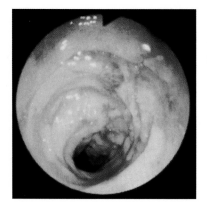

Figure 11.88 Early ischemic damage. Erythema, swelling, and intramural bleeding are evident. This can result in macropseudopolypoid swelling which corresponds with thumbprinting. Superficial necrosis is also noted.

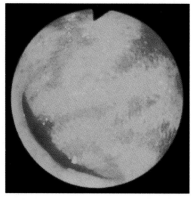

Figure 11.89 Resolving phase after an episode of acute ischemic damage of the sigmoid colon which did not progress to epithelial necrosis.

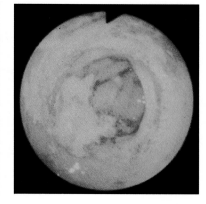

Figure 11.90 Subacute or ulcerative stage of ischemic damage 7 days after an aortic bifurcation prosthesis.

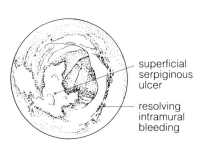

superficial serpiginous ulcer

resolving intramural bleeding

A large serpiginous ulcer and remnants of resolving intramural hemorrhage are evident.

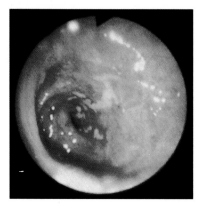

Figure 11.91 Ischemic stricture has a central, longitudinal ulceration.

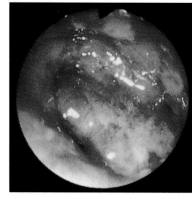

Figure 11.92 Endoscopic findings of ischemic colitis 2 days after onset of sudden hematochezia in a patient with diverticular disease show markedly swollen, hemorrhagic mucosa with early patchy, superficial, epithelial necrosis.

Spots of superficial mucosal necrosis ranging from 2 to 4 mm develop. The overall appearance of this acute stage resembles ulcerative colitis and usually lasts about 3 days (Fig. 11.89).

The subacute stage lasts from the third to the seventh day and is characterized by ulceration. The ulcers may be linear, elongated, and serpiginous or trough-like (Fig. 11.90). Sometimes they are longitudinal, resembling those in Crohn's disease (Fig. 11.91). A more extensive superficial form of ulceration may also be found (Fig. 11.92). The necrotic, ulcerative lesions are sometimes covered initially by a dirty, yellowish-gray, strongly adherent exudate and slough. In some cases, acute inflammatory exudate appears as the predominant lesion, mimicking the pseudomembranous patches in antibiotic-associated diarrhea. The involved segment is usually demarcated at both ends, but occasionally erythema and tiny ulcerations may be separated from the major involved segment by a few centimeters. This

ulcerative stage of ischemic damage is similar to idiopathic inflammatory bowel diseases, especially Crohn's disease. However, the unisegmental distribution of the disease, the predilection for the splenic flexure area or descending colon, the absence of perianal disease, and the histology of biopsies suggest the ischemic nature of the damage.

The chronic state, lasting 2 weeks to 3 months, is characterized by gradual resolution and healing. The edema slowly disappears, the ulcer craters become whitish and clean, devoid of all debris and necrotic material, and gradual reepithelialization of the denuded surfaces occurs. Healing usually takes 6 weeks, but may take as long as 3 months. Colonoscopy at that time may show either normal mucosa or residual granularity; sometimes a crisscross pattern of scarring may be visible. A smooth stricture may develop with slight mucosal pinkness, loss of normal vascularity, and scarring as the only visible abnormalities.

Most peculiar is the nonresolving form of ischemic damage. After 3 months, extensive superficial ulceration remains, leading to chronic blood loss and excessive intestinal loss of protein.

ENDOSCOPIC GUIDELINES

The differential diagnosis of ischemic damage is not simple. It includes carcinoma, inflammatory bowel disease, and diverticulitis. Endoscopy may be helpful in the differential diagnosis and to help to determine the extent of the mucosa affected. This endoscopic information may be useful because at surgery it may be difficult to determine the extent of the ischemic segment. However, one should note that endoscopy in patients with colonic ischemia may be associated with an increased risk of complications. The wall may be ischemic and potentially weakened, increasing the risk of perforation with the endoscope tip. Distension of the colon with gas during colonoscopy may further compromise the blood supply to the wall, worsen the ischemic injury, and increase the chance of a perforation.

The topographical distribution of the lesions of ischemic damage is important in diagnosis. In patients who have had

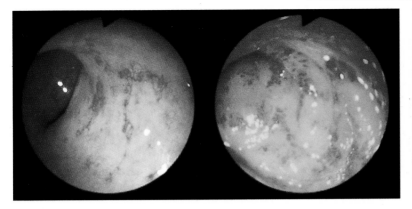
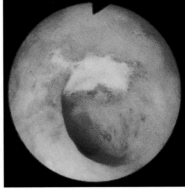
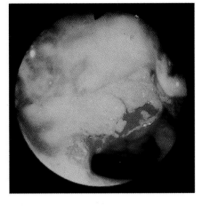

Figure 11.93 Chronic radiation damage at the rectosigmoid junction. Tiny telangiectatic vessels are superimposed on pale and opaque mucosa. The opaque appearance may be caused by fibrosis.

Figure 11.94 Chronic radiation-induced ulcer at the rectosigmoid junction.

Figure 11.95 Huge radiation-induced ulceration in the supra-anal area.

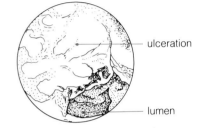

ulceration

lumen

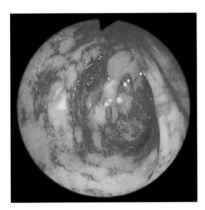
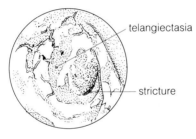

telangiectasia

stricture

Figure 11.96 Radiation-induced stricture at the rectosigmoid junction could not be passed with the colonoscope. Telangiectasia is abundant.

abdominal vascular surgery, preferential sites of involvement are the rectosigmoid area or the left colon, especially around the region of the splenic flexure. This corresponds to the watershed area between the vascular territory of the mesenteric superior and inferior arteries. Rectal involvement is unusual, which is a useful differential point. Moreover, ischemic damage always involves a single segment of the gut with sharp demarcations at the proximal and distal border of the infarcted segment. Therefore, the major endoscopic criteria favoring a diagnosis of ischemia rather than inflammatory bowel disease are:

1. Lack of rectal involvement
2. Presence of petechiae and ecchymoses, and evidence of submucosal edema and hemorrhage
3. Occurrence of unisegmental disease
4. Rapid resolution

Although the outcome of colonic ischemia depends on many factors, the initial response to ischemic damage is the same regardless of the severity. It is therefore impossible to predict the progression and outcome of the ischemic process from the initial clinical or endoscopic evaluation.

RADIATION-RELATED COLITIS

Radiation damage of the rectosigmoid area is common, especially in patients treated for cancer of the cervix. Usually the proximal and distal sigmoid and the intra- and supra-anal area are involved. These are the intestinal segments in close proximity to the cervix and most affected by the radiation treatment.

Radiation damage may present in an acute or chronic form. The acute form is seen during radiation treatment and up to 6 weeks thereafter. Endoscopy may reveal edematous, dusky mucosa with diffuse erythema similar to ulcerative colitis. Severe damage may lead to friability and mucosal ulceration. Delayed effects are seen 6 to 12 months after radiotherapy. Fibrosis and edema of the submucosa may cause the mucosa to appear opaque or pale. Endarteritis causes fibrosis and neovascularization seen as telangiectatic mucosal vessels (Fig. 11.93). Such vessels are excessively fragile and may bleed profusely upon slight touch with the endoscope.

In addition to these changes, acute mucosal inflammation may also be noted, with erythema, friability, and granularity. Ulcerations may appear, especially around the rectosigmoid junction (Fig. 11.94), or into and just proximal to the anal canal (Fig. 11.95). Another common abnormality is the development of a stricture at the rectosigmoid junction (Fig. 11.96). Strictures tend to be associated with either pale

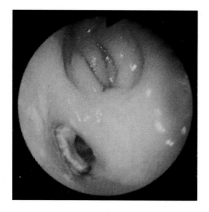

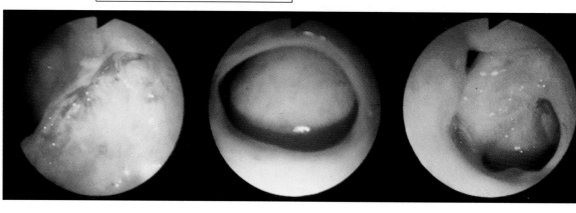

Figure 11.97 Radiation-induced colocolonic fistula narrows the sigmoid lumen.

Figure 11.98 Development of radiation-induced rectovaginal fistula. *Left,* Large radiation-induced ulcer

appears near an impending fistula. *Center,* Wide rectovaginal fistula

developed a few months later. *Right,* Another rectovaginal fistula.

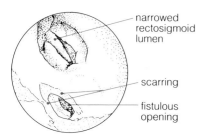

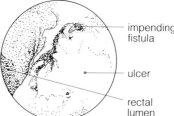

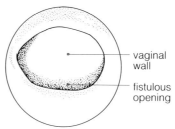

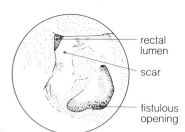

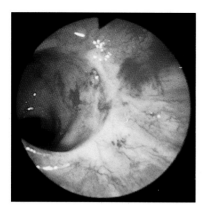

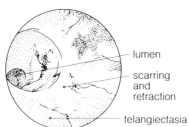

Figure 11.99 Healing stage of an indolent, radiation-induced supra-anal ulcer.

mucosa or with telangiectasias. Strictures may be relatively short but may also extend over a distance, especially in the sigmoid colon, sometimes impeding passage of the endoscope.

A dreadful complication is the development of a fistula either in the sigmoid colon (Fig. 11.97), or in the perianal area, resulting in a rectovaginal connection or fistula (Fig. 11.98). Some caution that biopsy should not be obtained from the anterior rectal wall in a female patient with radiation proctitis because of the risk of development of a rectovaginal fistula.

Radiation-related colitis is extremely difficult to treat. Sometimes ulcers remain for a long time or progress to fistulization. Only occasionally does healing occur with retraction of ulcers (Fig. 11.99).

BYPASS COLITIS

A nonspecific colitis has been observed in colostomy patients with an excluded rectum or rectosigmoid. Also termed divergence or disuse colitis, the most characteristic findings are distorted or absent mucosal vascular pattern, erythema and friability, mucosal granularity, and petechial hemorrhages (Fig. 11.100). Occasionally ulcerations and polypoid excrescences may develop. Such changes are almost exclusively in the distal 2 to 3 cm of the rectum, but may involve the entire excluded segment. Sometimes multiple, small lesions resembling aphthoid erosions, caused by enlarged lymphoid follicles, are seen with red, raised margins and central areas of yellow-white exudate with normal intervening mucosa (Fig. 11.101).

Bypass colitis is indistinguishable from ulcerative colitis endoscopically and histologically. Little is known about the pathogenesis of this entity, which may have important diagnostic and therapeutic implications in colostomy patients. This form of colitis resolves upon reanastomosis.

RARE COLITIS PRESENTATIONS

BEHCET'S DISEASE
Behçet's disease is a rare illness which may present with ulceration of the intestinal tract. Other features include ulcers of the genital area and mouth as well as characteristic associations of eye, joint, and cutaneous lesions. The endoscopic finding is discrete, punched-out ulceration on a mucosal background which either appears normal or shows nonspecific erythema or granularity (Fig. 11.102). The lo-

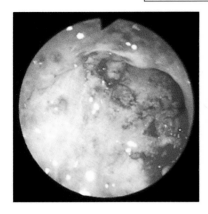 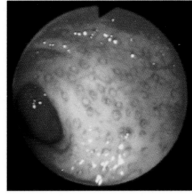 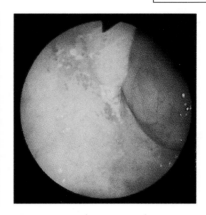 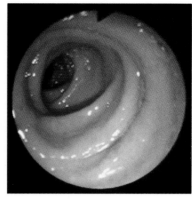

Figure 11.100 Bypass colitis with loss of vascular pattern, erythema, and friability.

Figure 11.101 Bypass colitis with enlarged lymphoid follicles mimics aphthoid-like erosions.

Figure 11.102 Colonic ulceration in a patient with Behçet's disease.

Figure 11.103 Collagenous colitis. Slight opalescence and blurring of the vascular pattern is seen.

cation may be predominantly right-sided or involve the colon diffusely, but rectal involvement is variable. The appearance is suggestive of the aphthoid erosions or small ulcers in Crohn's disease. Even histologically, the two diseases are difficult to differentiate.

NEUTROPENIC COLITIS
Neutropenic colitis is a rare, poorly understood entity characterized by diffuse inflammatory changes of the colonic mucosa. Neutropenic colitis affects predominantly the right colon. The endoscopic abnormalities are mainly characterized by edema, erythema, and friability.

COLLAGENOUS COLITIS
Collagenous colitis is a rare abnormality responsible for chronic diarrhea. The endoscopic abnormalities, if any, are usually rather subtle, characterized by mild opalescence and blurring of the vascular pattern (Fig. 11.103).

11.27

12

Colon III: Diverticular Disease, Vascular Malformations, and Other Colonic Abnormalities

In this chapter we will discuss several common colonic abnormalities including diverticular disease and its complications, vascular malformations, lower gastrointestinal bleeding, and a variety of other colonic abnormalities.

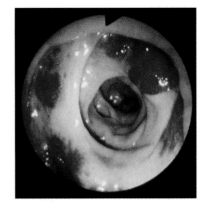

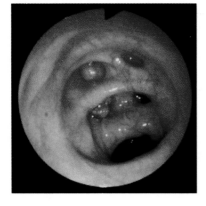 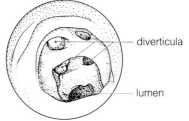

Figure 12.1 Several diverticular out-pouchings are located between thickened haustral folds. The oval-shaped lumen is eccentric.

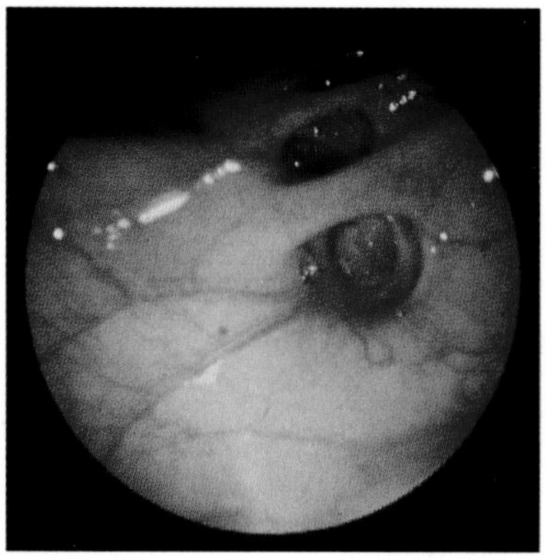

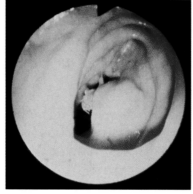

Figure 12.2 The relationship between vessels and diverticular outpouchings is obvious in this view.

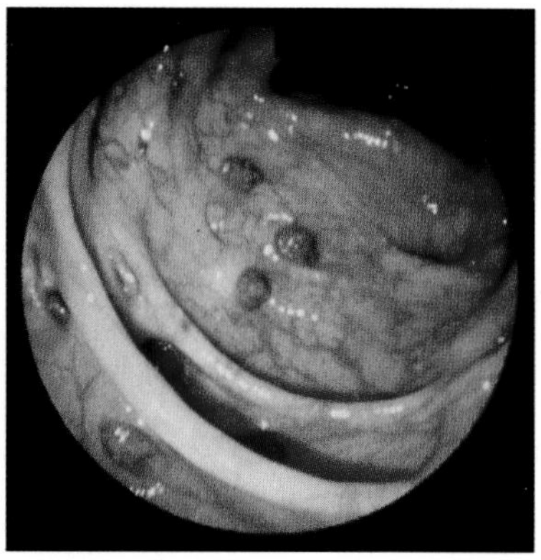

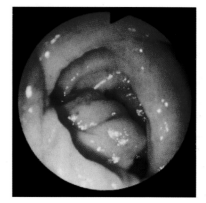

Figure 12.3 Diverticulosis of the entire colon in a young patient. Numerous diverticula in the ascending colon are shown; fecal impaction is evident.

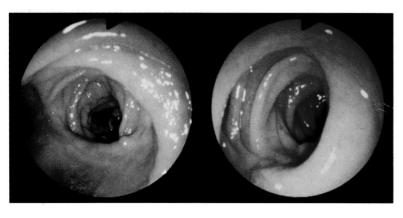

Figure 12.4 Examples of luminal distortion in diverticular disease due to marked muscle thickening and retraction, and twisting of folds.

Figure 12.5 Inverted diverticulum in the sigmoid colon.

Figure 12.6 Prolapsing redundant large folds may result from diverticular disease.

DIVERTICULAR DISEASE

Diverticular disease is an increasingly common clinical problem in the aging population of industrialized countries. It ranks with polyps as one of the most common abnormalities seen during colonoscopy. The muscular hypertrophy and corresponding elastosis are the most striking features. While some patients have no symptoms, others experience cramping or altered bowel habits. Sometimes symptoms are related to complications of the disease, such as diverticulitis, abscess formation, or fistulization.

Colonoscopy is generally not helpful in the evaluation of patients with acute diverticulitis. However, it may be indicated for diagnosis in diverticular disease in the following settings: ambiguous X-ray findings, especially to exclude carcinoma; colonic bleeding; obstructed flow of barium; and after a diverting colostomy for obstruction or perforation to differentiate among polyp, cancer, and inflammation.

Colonoscopy in diverticular disease requires special tech-

niques since the marked muscular hypertrophy causes shortening of the interhaustral segments and marked distortion of the luminal direction. Each fold distorting the lumen must be examined individually. Clues regarding the correct luminal direction may be obtained by observing the arcuate highlights on diverticular folds. However, these may also incorrectly lead the inexperienced endoscopist into a diverticulum.

ENDOSCOPIC APPEARANCE

In general, diverticular orifices are best viewed during the introduction phase of the colonoscopic exam. They represent focal weakness in the wall, usually in the area of penetrating blood vessels (Figs. 12.1 and 12.2). Although the sigmoid is the most common site, diverticular outpouchings may occur throughout the colon (Fig. 12.3). They are seen as small, circular, 2 to 5 mm openings in the central portion of the short haustral segment, situated between large, thick-

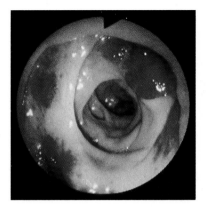

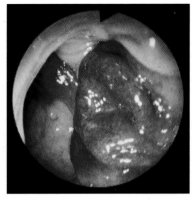

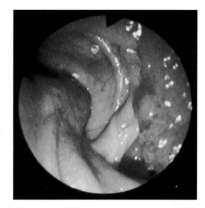

Figure 12.7 In this patient, severe diverticular disease caused strikingly hyperemic patches due to marked congestion.

Figure 12.8 Prolapsing polypoid-appearing folds with striking erythema in severe diverticular disease.

Figure 12.9 Prolapsing redundant folds with slightly elevated red round patches are scattered over the sigmoid colon.

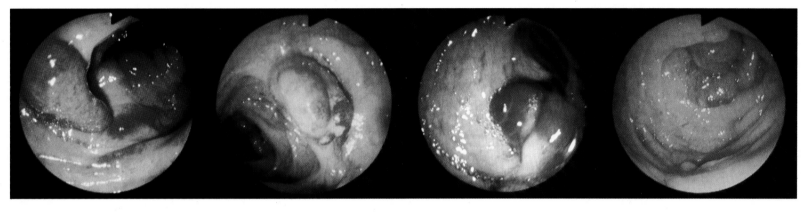

Figure 12.10 Examples of polyp-simulating structures due to redundant mucosal invagination in diverticular disease. Note the patches of striking erythema; however, these lesions are formed of normal mucosa. In the far right view, the redundant mucosa seems to obstruct the lumen.

ened folds. Shortening of the teniae leads to the characteristic concertina-like corrugation of the circular muscle. Occasionally there are two or more diverticula per segment but usually there is only one.

Even in a well-cleaned colon after gut lavage, diverticular openings may be impacted with stool or barium (see Fig. 12.3). Such small fecal pellets within the diverticula may fall into the lumen and obscure endoscopic vision.

A novice endoscopist may confuse the opening of a diverticulum with the lumen, especially when multiple diverticula are associated with prominent haustral folds. There are some helpful clues to help the colonoscopist find the correct luminal axis. Diverticular openings occur between haustral folds, while the lumen is seen at the point where folds converge. Usually the lumen is at an angle with respect to the axis of the colonoscope. A diverticular orifice always appears round when seen closeup, whereas the colonic lumen is usually distorted and slitlike. If there is any doubt, the operator should withdraw and reestablish the general direction of the lumen rather than proceed blindly. The concern is that one might enter and perforate a large diverticulum.

In uncomplicated diverticular disease, the mucosa is smooth and glistening and has a normal vascular pattern. Occasionally, prediverticular disease may be encountered in the form of muscle thickening and retraction, without evidence of diverticular outpouchings (Fig. 12.4). Upon careful inspection of the mucosa, minute outpouchings between the thickened muscle bands are occasionally seen. An inverted diverticulum is a rare finding (Fig. 12.5).

Stretching and compression of redundant mucosal folds is likely to occur in severe diverticular disease because of the underlying motility disorder, excessive cramping, and abnormal contraction (Fig. 12.6). With excessive cramping, patchy areas of markedly hyperemic and even hemorrhagic mucosa may develop (Fig. 12.7), or slightly elevated patches may seem to prolapse and gradually develop into polypoid excrescences (Fig. 12.8). Such polypoid structures are usually bright red hemispheres about 1 cm high, scattered irregularly between diverticula exclusively in the narrow sigmoid segment (Fig. 12.9). These red patches or polypoid lesions may explain minor recurrent bleeding.

In diverticular disease the colonic mucosa may prolapse back and forth through an area of diverticular narrowing. This erythematous lesion may appear similar to an adenoma (Fig. 12.10), but with careful inspection it will become ap-

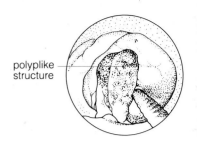

polyplike structure

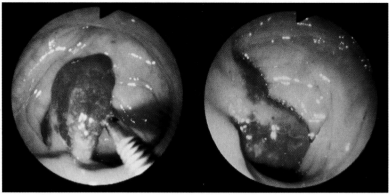

Figure 12.11 *Left,* Markedly congested polyp-simulating structure due to repetitive intraluminal mucosal invagination shows a pedicle-like base. *Right,* A better view of the broad implantation of the polypoid structure.

parent that the red lesion is pliable, moves easily, and has no pedicle (Fig. 12.11). Furthermore, the absence of any lobulation or nodularity, which are common features in larger adenomas, also points to either a fold or a submucosal polypoid lesion. The gradual decrease in the intensity of the erythema from the top to the wide base, merging into normal mucosa, suggests the correct diagnosis. When inspected in detail, the overall texture of the mucosa covering the polypoid structures is identical to that of the surrounding mucosa.

ACUTE DIVERTICULITIS

The development of acute inflammation in and around the diverticula-bearing segment is a major complication of diverticular disease. Pressure on the diverticular outpouchings due to fecaliths or other impacted material leads to necrosis of the mucosal lining; intramural invasion of bacteria produces inflammation and abscess.

The dominant endoscopic features of acute diverticulitis include marked narrowing of the lumen due to excessive spasm, and swelling of the haustral folds (Fig. 12.12). In addition, there is patchy or diffuse erythema of the swollen, contracted folds (Fig. 12.13). Occasionally, purulent material exudes from the mouth of the inflamed diverticula or streams along the colonic wall (Fig. 12.14). The inflamed segment may be narrowed to a tiny orifice, which may not be negotiable with a standard or small-caliber colonoscope. It should be stressed that endoscopic evidence of acute inflammation does not exclude an underlying carcinoma until the area in question has been intubated and examined. After resolution of the acute episode of inflammation, the erythema, luminal narrowing, and edematous swelling of the folds may disappear entirely and the appearance may return to normal (Fig. 12.15).

DIVERTICULAR STRICTURE AND MALIGNANCY

The colonic narrowing in diverticular disease is largely caused by thickening of the muscle layers, and is especially apparent in the increased thickness of the haustral folds. Additional compromise of the lumen can result from a superimposed colic-pericolic inflammatory mass or colic and pericolic fibrosis. Because of the tortuosity of the sigmoid colon, it is often not possible to determine radiologically whether obstruction is secondary to inflammation or to carcinoma. If necessary, a small-caliber colonoscope can usually be inserted to the point of obstruction.

In diverticulitis, the lumen may narrow abruptly, although the overlying mucosa is still intact and the folds themselves appear symmetrical and regular. By contrast, a malignant stricture obliterates and distorts parts of the involved folds. An irregular appearance and a hard consistency of the folds forming the entrance to the narrowed zone are both suggestive of malignancy (Fig. 12.16).

Malignancy is likely when an intraluminal, bulky tumor mass is noted within the narrowed zone. Therefore, all possible effort should be made to pass the obstructed segment with a small-caliber colonoscope. If only markedly inflamed but otherwise intact nonsuspicious mucosa is seen, then the chance of underlying malignancy is remote. If, on the other hand, even a small focus of abnormal suspicious tissue is encountered, then there is a strong chance of malignancy. Multiple biopsies should be obtained from any exophytic growth or excessively necrotic-appearing area. Biopsies taken from the concentric folds encircling the narrowed lumen or even from within the strictured area are usually negative.

If the obstructed segment cannot be passed, no conclusion can be reached regarding the presence or absence of malignancy, and surgical exploration is mandatory. If it cannot be determined at surgery whether the mass is neoplastic or inflammatory, a diversion of the fecal stream is often created with a distal mucous fistula. After several weeks or months, the narrowed area can be reexamined colonoscopically, with

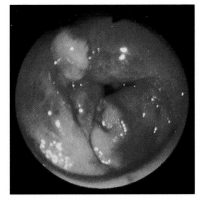

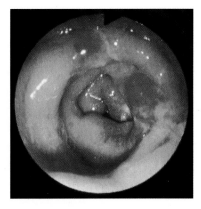

Figure 12.12 Diffuse swelling obliterates the lumen in full-blown diverticulitis. Erythema and focal purulent exudate are also discernible.

Figure 12.13 Acute diverticulitis is characterized by marked swelling and muscle contraction which obliterates the lumen. Intense erythema appears in patches along the folds.

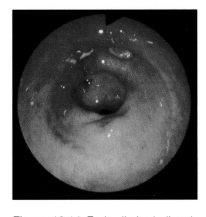

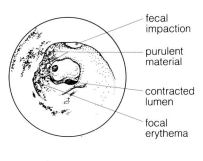

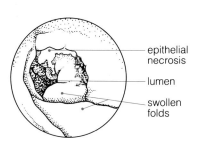

Figure 12.14 Early, limited diverticulitis displays purulent material exuding from the diverticulum. Note the erythema of the adjacent mucosa.

Figure 12.15 Resolution phase of acute diverticulitis exhibits resolving inflammation and reopening of the lumen. Epithelial destruction is present, and patchy areas of erythema are still visible.

biopsies if appropriate, to determine if the inflammatory changes have resolved suggesting diverticulitis, or to determine if malignancy is present. This information will guide decisions regarding further surgical therapy.

VASCULAR MALFORMATIONS

ANGIODYSPLASIA

Angiodysplasia is a microvascular abnormality of the mucosa and submucosa of the colon which may rupture or ulcerate and cause lower intestinal bleeding. It is a common cause of chronic, intermittent, or acute colonic bleeding.

The pathophysiology of the formation of angiodysplastic lesions is not known. Speculations have included the relative obstruction of the small veins passing through the muscularis externa by hypertrophied muscle. This obstruction gradually backs up until the capillaries are dilated and abnormal arteriovenous connections are formed.

Most angiodysplastic lesions occur in the large-diameter cecum and right colon, rarely in the ileum. The greater

Diverticular Stricture and Malignancy

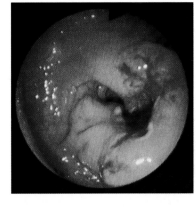

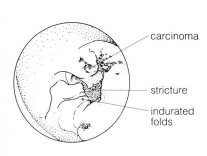

Figure 12.16 Stenosing sigmoid carcinoma with submucosal spread of tumor. The folds at the entrance to the strictured area were firm and indurated in appearance. An Nd-YAG laser had been used earlier to reopen the stenosis.

amount of tension within the bowel wall in these sections contributes to the partial obstruction of the submucosal veins. Angiodysplasia is also encountered in patients with aortic valve disease. Less commonly, angiodysplastic lesions of the colon have been seen in younger people, spreading

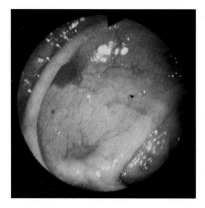

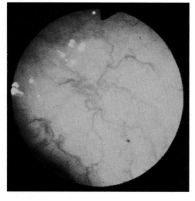

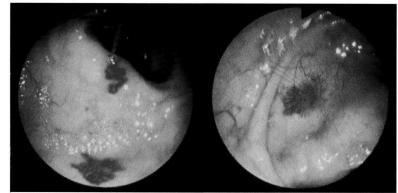

Figure 12.17 Spectrum of congenital angiodysplastic lesions spread throughout the colon in a young patient.

Figure 12.18 Early angiodysplastic lesions are seen as slightly dilated, tortuous vessels.

Figure 12.19 Differently shaped angiodysplastic lesions show distinctly irregular margins. A red capillary tuft

(right) has individually recognizable ectatic vessels.

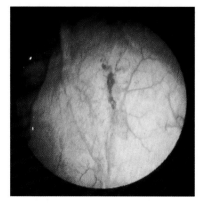

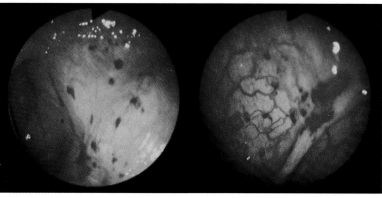

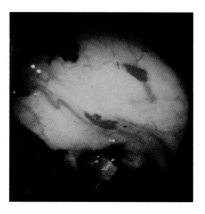

Figure 12.20 A linear angiodysplasia is connected to a pinhead-sized ectasia by capillaries.

Figure 12.21 A larger angiodysplasia and multiple small angiodysplasias

are apparently interconnected in these views.

Figure 12.22 Multiple angiodysplasias with characteristic bluish draining veins.

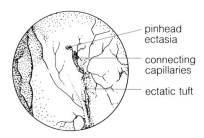

pinhead
ectasia

connecting
capillaries

ectatic tuft

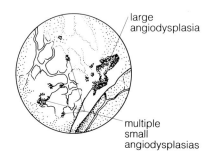

large
angiodysplasia

multiple
small
angiodysplasias

out over the colon and the small bowel (Fig. 12.17). It is possible that congenital abnormalities of the colonic microcirculation lead to the development of this disease in adult life, in conjunction with increased blood pressure and colonic motor disorders.

Angiodysplasia has a variable appearance in the mucosa of the colon. Some of the lesions are large and may seem raised with an irregular border. The smaller lesions appear as bright red spots, often just a few millimeters in diameter. Various shapes are described including linear, flat, and raised (Figs. 12.18 to 12.20). The larger lesions may appear superficially eroded and may be responsible for GI hemorrhage. The lesions may occur singly or they may appear in groups. Lesions of several variable sizes may be noted (Fig. 12.21). These lesions can be located anywhere in the GI tract and colon. Typically, the right colon and cecum are involved.

The degree of distortion of the adjacent vascular architecture varies with each stage in the evolution of the ectasias. In addition to the reddish vascular clusters or tufts, sometimes bluish draining veins may be seen (Fig. 12.22). The vascular clusters have been compared to the petals of a flower, with the bluish draining veins representing the stem.

Angiodysplastic lesions should not be confused with iatrogenic mucosal injury. The irregular margins of angiodysplastic lesions allow them to be distinguished from colonoscope-induced intramucosal hemorrhage (Fig. 12.23). These areas of mucosal trauma often occur at sharply angulated segments such as the descending-sigmoid junction. Angiodysplasia should not be confused with telangiectasia seen in radiation colitis. A rare cause of vascular malformation which may mimic angiodysplasia is that produced after repetitive trauma of the rectal wall during manual evacuation of feces (Fig. 12.24).

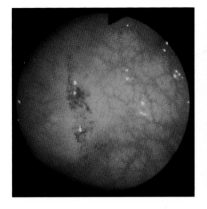

Figure 12.23 Intramucosal bleeding spots in the splenic flexure were induced by the colonoscope.

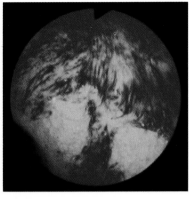

Figure 12.24 Bizarre vascular malformation of the rectal wall occurred after repetitive trauma due to manual evacuation of stool.

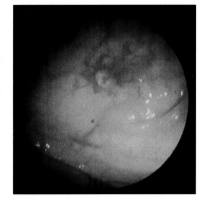

Figure 12.25 This angiodysplastic lesion was treated with one Nd-YAG laser shot, resulting in blanching.

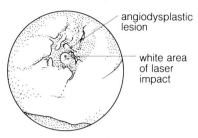

Hemangioma

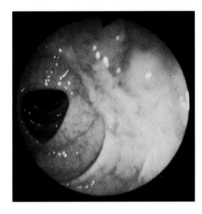

Figure 12.26 Partial treatment with a single Nd-YAG laser application leaves traces of a large cavernous hemangioma.

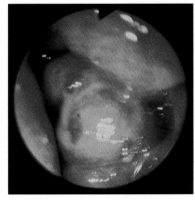

Figure 12.27 A larger rectal hemangioma presents as a polypoid mass which could be confused with a polyp, malignancy, or internal hemorrhoid.

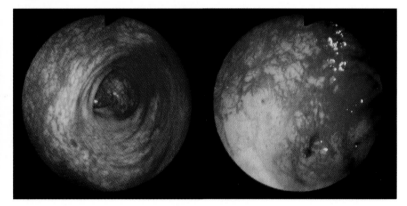

Figure 12.28 *Left,* Various aspects of diffuse hemangioma involving the rectum and sigmoid colon. *Right,* A closeup view shows coalescence of diffuse hemangioma and slight protrusion of the vascular anomaly.

The usual therapy for angiodysplastic lesions is eradication with laser energy or with electrocoagulation using a diathermic or hot-biopsy forceps (Fig. 12.25). In performing a hot biopsy of a vascular ectasia in the cecum, the mucosa should be lifted or "tented" off the underlying submucosa to avoid transmural burns. Such therapy is especially useful in elderly patients and in patients with complicated medical illnesses who are high operative risks. For younger patients with very extensive lesions, some advocate surgical resection.

HEMANGIOMA

Hemangiomas of the large bowel arise from submucosal vascular plexuses, usually of the rectum and distal colon. When they create a masslike deformity, they are usually referred to as cavernous hemangiomas. When they are smaller, they are referred to as the capillary type. They may be responsible for chronic or intermittent bleeding; if so, they may be treated with photocoagulation (Fig. 12.26).

Sizable cavernous hemangiomas are usually recognized endoscopically as ill-defined polypoid masses; distinct ul-

ceration is not ordinarily present. These lesions may bleed heavily if biopsied; therefore, most do not biopsy a lesion if they think that it is a hemangioma. The color is typical of a hemangioma, with a dark blue or dark red appearance. Some are strawberrylike lesions with a deep blue to dull red or port-wine coloration (Fig. 12.27).

Hemangiomas may also present as infiltrating vascular lesions involving large segments of the rectum and sigmoid. Such flat or minimally elevated diffuse lesions are often poorly defined and of a bluish color (Fig. 12.28).

RARE VASCULAR ABNORMALITIES

Other vascular lesions may be encountered in the colon. Varicose veins may occur in patients with portal hypertension. These tend to occur in the rectum and the distal sigmoid colon. The color may appear normal or the varices may have a bluish appearance. These veins tend to run in a longitudinal fashion and are often tortuous, typical of varicose veins elsewhere in the GI tract. One must be careful that these are not mistaken for a polyp. An endoscopic

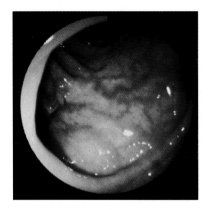

Figure 12.29 Early varices in the sigmoid colon.

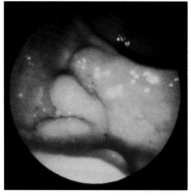

Figure 12.30 Large varix of the sigmoid colon runs perpendicularly to haustral folds.

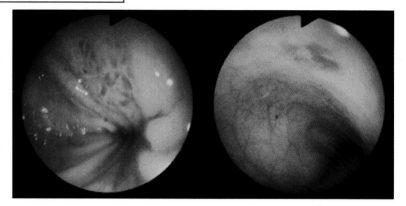

Figure 12.31 Henoch-Schönlein vasculitis appears as multiple petechiae *(left)* or as a central purpura within an area of blanching adjacent to normal vasculature *(right)*.

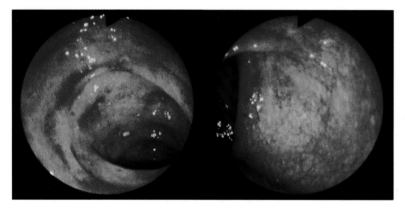

Figure 12.32 Vasculitic changes involving the colon are mainly characterized by focal erythema *(left)* and, occasionally, by discrete intramural bleeding *(right)*.

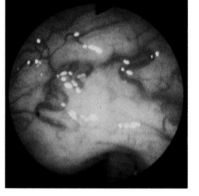

Figure 12.33 Bizarre vascular malformation.

Doppler device might be useful to detect venous flow in what otherwise appears to be a polyp. Careful visual inspection at colonoscopy usually reveals that the varices are part of a venous system (Figs. 12.29 and 12.30).

Evidence of vasculitis may also be found in Henoch-Schönlein syndrome. These patients may present with evidence of GI hemorrhage, and at colonoscopy there may be evidence of vascular injury of the wall with petechiae (Fig. 12.31). In polyarteritis nodosa the changes may include ulceration and erythema (Fig. 12.32).

Vascular malformations consisting of excessively tortuous, protuberant, bizarrely developed vascular structures are occasionally encountered in the colon. Such abnormalities, which may be responsible for chronic blood loss, are difficult to classify at present (Fig. 12.33).

DIAGNOSIS OF COLONIC BLEEDING

Bleeding from the colon is a frequent problem, especially in the elderly population. Colonic bleeding is most often chronic and intermittent, although occasionally bleeding may be massive. A scala of lesions may be responsible for colonic bleeding, as listed in Figure 12.34.

Hemorrhoids and anal fissures should be easily ruled out by appropriate endoscopic examination. Many feel that the best way to examine for the presence of internal hemorrhoids is to perform the toilet test. The patient is asked to sit on a toilet and gently bear down, causing internal hemorrhoids and rectal prolapse to protrude from the anal verge. The anus can be carefully and conveniently inspected indirectly by using a mirror. This may be the only method of seeing large, bleeding, internal hemorrhoids which may be difficult to appreciate by other diagnostic approaches.

Diverticular disease can cause either acute or chronic intermittent colonic bleeding. Stretching and distortion of the vessel walls through increased intraluminal pressure is thought to weaken the vessels and to predispose to rupture into the diverticulum. Localization of the bleeding site to the left colon in a patient with diverticular disease and no other distinguishable lesions strongly suggests a diverticular origin. However, one must remember that right-sided diverticula can also bleed. The diagnosis is often one of exclusion since a single bleeding diverticulum is only rarely identified. If there is any doubt, colonoscopy should be repeated soon after the bleeding ceases. Diverticular bleeding may be so brisk that the lumen is obscured. Occasionally, blood may be seen welling up from the bleeding diverticulum, resulting in copious amounts of blood filling up the distal colon.

Causes of Rectal Bleeding

Hemorrhoids

Anal fissures

Diverticular disease

Idiopathic inflammatory bowel disease

    Ulcerative colitis

    Crohn's disease

Radiation colitis

Ischemic colitis

Infectious colitis

Vascular malformations (angiodysplasia/varices)

Colonic polyps

Colorectal cancer

Distal small bowel lesions

Upper gastrointestinal lesions

Idiopathic ulcerations

Figure 12.34 Causes of rectal bleeding.

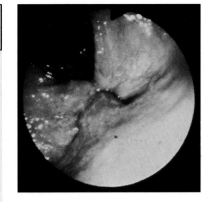
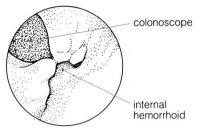

Figure 12.35 An internal hemorrhoid is seen after retroflexing the colonoscope.

Inflammatory bowel disease is occasionally detected during colonoscopy performed for chronic or intermittent bleeding. Ulcerative colitis is usually associated with severe inflammation and diffuse, continuous bleeding from the inflamed mucosal surface. In Crohn's disease, focal deep ulceration involving major vessels causes the brisk bleeding. Infectious colitis and radiation damage rarely cause major bleeding.

Occasionally, ischemic damage of the colon may produce bleeding, typically in the splenic flexure area, descending colon, and sigmoid colon. Marked mucosal friability with spontaneous bleeding is seen in conjunction with extensive intramural hemorrhage, as evidenced by the presence of petechiae and ecchymoses.

Vascular malformations, especially angiodysplasia, are increasingly recognized as a cause of intermittent brisk or chronic low-grade bleeding. The visible angiodysplasia is only a manifestation of a diffusely deranged mucosal and submucosal vascular network.

Neoplasms in the form of adenomatous polyps or colorectal cancer are the most common lesions identified at colonoscopy in patients with colonic bleeding. The adenomatous polyps which bleed tend to be large, causing the polyps to be repeatedly traumatized. Twisting and bending leads to fracture of the stalk and vascular obstruction, leading to congestion and hemorrhage. In addition, the surface of a polyp which has bled becomes fragile. Bleeding also occurs after autoamputation.

When a patient notes red blood streaking the stool, a polypoid carcinoma of the sigmoid colon may be encountered. Other cancers detected because of bleeding, especially in the right colon, are usually large, centrally ulcerated masses. Distal small bowel lesions may be a cause of colonic bleeding, especially in patients whose detectable angiodysplastic lesions of the colon have been adequately treated endoscopically.

The possibility of an upper GI bleeding site should always be considered in patients passing large amounts of red blood per rectum. If an upper GI site is suspected, it is worthwhile to first pass an endoscope into the stomach and duodenum to see if there is evidence of active bleeding and to determine the bleeding site.

A careful history usually offers considerable information about the source of the bleeding. Red blood on toilet tissue or unrelated to defecation is often due to hemorrhoids or fissures external to the sphincter muscles. Dripping red blood following defecation is also usually hemorrhoidal. When a stripe of blood is seen on the stool, or flecks of blood are mixed with the stool, the lesion usually lies above the rectum in the area of the sigmoid colon and is of more significance. Bleeding proximal to the descending colon is mixed with the stool and may not be grossly visible, but may be detected by fecal occult blood testing.

For any patient with hematochezia, an anorectal sigmoidoscopic examination should be performed first to look for anal or rectal pathology. Blood attributed to hemorrhoids may be related to a low-lying carcinoma or polyp. Although a rigid anoscope is the standard technique, the flexible sigmoidoscope can be retroflexed in the rectal ampulla to examine the hemorrhoidal ring (Fig. 12.35). If no lesion is obvious, it may be necessary to perform a total

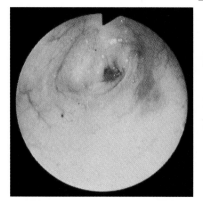

Figure 12.36 Endometriosis of the sigmoid colon causes luminal narrowing. A reddish area is evident.

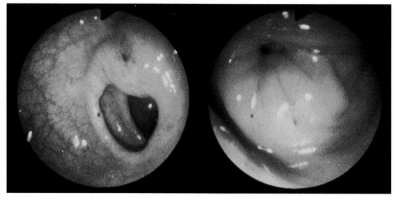

Figure 12.37 Views of luminal narrowing due to endometrial masses.

Intramural bleeding *(left)* is often seen.

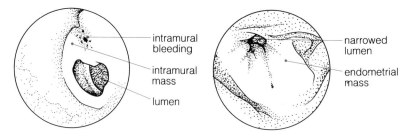

intramural bleeding
intramural mass
lumen

narrowed lumen
endometrial mass

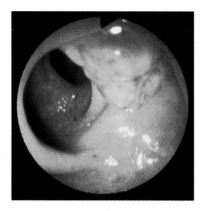

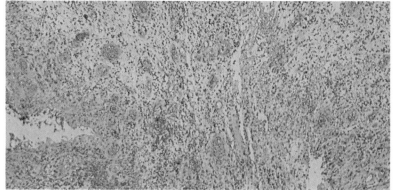

Figure 12.38 *Left,* Polypoid lesion at the rectosigmoid junction consisting

of granulation tissue is caused by chronic suppurative inflammation of

the left adnexa. *Right,* Histology of the granulation polyp.

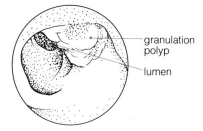

granulation polyp
lumen

colonoscopy. If certain lesions are found in the sigmoid colon, it may still be necessary to perform a total colonoscopy. For example, if the lesion detected is an adenomatous polyp, colonoscopy is indicated to detect a synchronous polyp or carcinoma above the low-lying lesion.

To identify a bleeding site, blood must be seen actively trickling or spurting. Presence of blood in the vicinity of an apparent vascular ectasia or diverticulum is not convincing evidence. On the other hand, rapid bleeding usually overwhelms the cleaning capacity of the colonoscope.

The role of colonoscopy in cases of massive, dramatic bleeding is debatable. Large amounts of blood and clots may make it difficult to examine the colon. Nevertheless, for some patients with massive bleeding, colonoscopy has been reported as having a high diagnostic yield.

Colonoscopy is most valuable for patients with intermittent or moderate bleeding. With moderate bleeding, the blood acts as a cathartic to clean the bowel and minimal preparation is necessary. However, blood clots should be evacuated from the rectum by enema before starting the

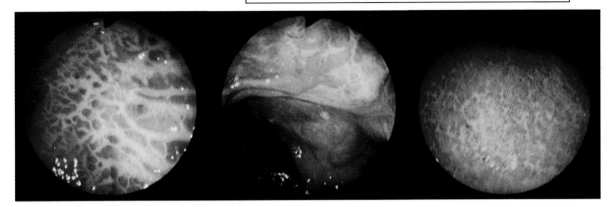

Figure 12.39 Different appearances of pseudomelanosis of the colon. Discoloration ranges from brown to black.

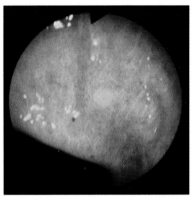

Figure 12.40 Small unstained adenoma stands out in pseudomelanosis.

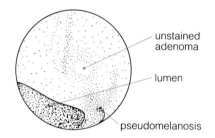

examination, to prevent blockage of the instrument suction channel during the examination. If there is a pool of blood, the patient can be repositioned so that the blood forms a layer at the bottom of the endoscopic field of vision, and the instrument can then be advanced over it. By maintaining an almost constant spray of water, the image can be kept clear as the insertion proceeds.

The goal of colonoscopy in chronic, more occult bleeding is to define accurately the bleeding source, to provide effective therapy whenever possible, and to help guide the surgical approach.

Some of the causes of colonic bleeding are amenable to endoscopic treatment. Polyps may be removed easily and safely. Telangiectases may be treated, either with laser coagulation or electrocoagulation. Rebleeding, however, is not uncommon with angiodysplasias due to the widespread nature of the vascular abnormality.

OTHER COLONIC ABNORMALITIES

ABNORMALITIES OF GENITAL ORIGIN

Because of its proximity to the uterus, the sigmoid colon may become involved with endometriosis. Abrupt, severe narrowing is the characteristic finding. The mucosa at the mouth of the narrowed zone appears intact except for some swelling and a glassy appearance (Figs. 12.36 and 12.37). The obstructing mass is of firm consistency. When examined at the time of the menstrual period, reddish spots or reddish flecks may be observed surrounded by somewhat irregular granular mucosa.

Extrinsic compression of the sigmoid by an enlarged fibroid uterus or enlarged ovary may distort the lumen and create an asymmetrical, stricture-like appearance. If the fold pattern remains intact and there is no evidence of significant diverticular disease, the examiner should suspect extrinsic compression.

Other suppurative inflammation of the adnexa may occasionally lead to fistulization into the sigmoid colon and the formation of a granulation polyp (Fig. 12.38). Usually the sigmoid colon is markedly fixed to the adnexal mass, which makes polypectomy difficult. The histologic nature of the polyp suggests the correct pathology.

PSEUDOMELANOSIS COLI AND CATHARTIC COLON

Pseudomelanosis coli is caused by the accumulation of a brownish-black lipofuscin pigment in the lysosomes of the subepithelial macrophages, resulting from the ingestion of anthraquinone laxatives. Depending upon the mode of administration of anthraquinone-containing laxatives, the lesions may be distributed throughout the colon or limited to the rectosigmoid area.

The striking feature at endoscopy is the mucosal coloration, which varies from slightly gray to anthracite or completely black. This discoloration may be seen in patches or streaks (Fig. 12.39). Characteristically, there is a sharp demarcation at the ileocecal valve between the normal-colored small intestine and the pigmented colonic mucosa. When adenomatous polyps are present in pseudomelanosis coli, they characteristically lack the blackish pigment and stand out as whitish excrescences against the dark background (Fig. 12.40). Upon cessation of the anthraquinone laxative,

12.11

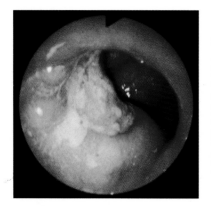

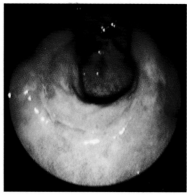

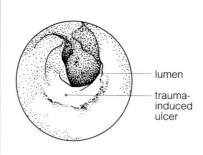

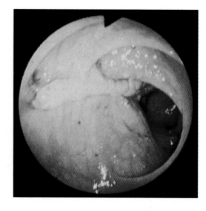

Figure 12.41 A solitary ulcer of the rectum may be caused by repetitive injury to a small area.

Figure 12.42 Chronic trauma induced an indolent solitary ulcer of the anterior wall in a homosexual patient.

Figure 12.43 Longitudinal laceration of the upper rectum is due to forceful insertion of an enema cannula.

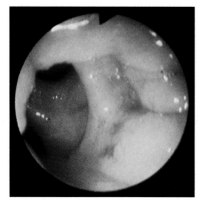

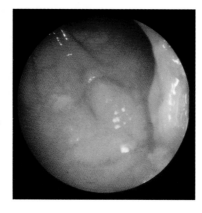

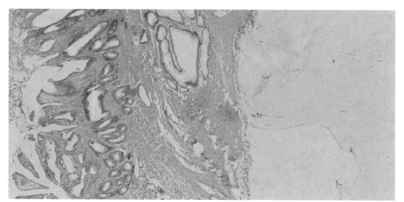

Figure 12.44 Colitis cystica profunda. *Left,* The thickened area in the distal rectum characterizes the disorder. *Center,* Here the lesion simulates a tumor. *Right,* Corresponding biopsy shows mucin-filled submucosal cysts.

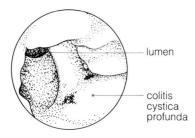

the coloration gradually disappears over several months. Inflammatory changes of the mucosa, such as erythema or granularity, are usually not present in a pseudomelanotic colon.

COLONIC ULCERS

SOLITARY RECTAL ULCER

The solitary rectal ulcer syndrome is thought to be a consequence of excessive straining which may cause internal prolapse of the mucosa, with stretching and compression eventually leading to ischemia, inflammation, and an anterior rectal wall ulcer (Fig. 12.41). A solitary rectal ulcer must be distinguished from traumatic ulceration, as seen in homosexual males (Fig. 12.42). In some patients, the trauma to the rectal wall is self-induced by digital extraction of fecal material to assist defecation or by repeated manual manipulation with foreign objects. Traumatic ulceration may also occur after intramucosal injection of hypertonic topical laxative solutions or laceration by instruments such as an enema tip (Fig. 12.43). The ulcers themselves are large, with a well-defined edge. Despite the name, solitary ulcers quite often are multiple.

COLITIS CYSTICA PROFUNDA

This syndrome is not well understood. It refers to the finding of mucus retention cysts in the submucosa of the colonic wall. This occurs in the distal colon and rectum, and may be related to the solitary rectal ulcer syndrome. These lesions appear endoscopically as slightly raised mucosa which may feel firm and be superficially eroded. The firm consistency and abnormally deep cysts may simulate carcinoma but this can be differentiated by histologic interpretation of biopsies (Fig. 12.44).

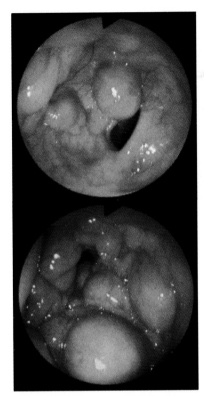

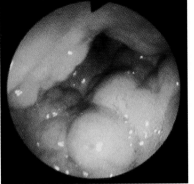

Figure 12.46 Obvious transparent character of cysts in pneumatosis coli.

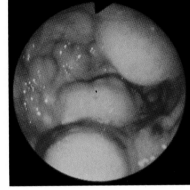

Figure 12.47 Focal tip erythema in pneumatosis coli.

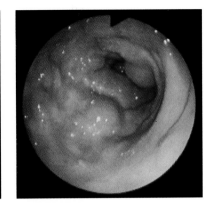

Figure 12.48 Hyperbaric oxygen therapy can cause regression of cysts.

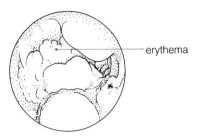

erythema

Figure 12.45 Pneumatosis coli. *Top,* Gas-filled cysts are seen. *Bottom,* Here the cysts seem to occlude the lumen.

PNEUMATOSIS COLI

Pneumatosis coli is characterized by the presence of gas-filled cysts within the mucosa and submucosa of the colon. Usually, only one segment of the colon is involved, especially the sigmoid or descending colon. At endoscopy, clusters of broad-based, smooth, polypoid bulges are seen which may have a peculiar transparency (Figs. 12.45 and 12.46). Quite often there is erythema at the tip of these bulges, presumably secondary to friction (Fig. 12.47). When they are multiple, the cysts may appear to obstruct the lumen, but the endoscope can usually be passed. Some bleeding may occur as a result of breakdown of the hemorrhagic mucosa on the surface of the cysts. When punctured, gas may escape. Such lesions should not be removed with electrocautery snares because the gas within the cysts may be explosive. Upon treatment with pure or hyperbaric oxygen, the cysts may gradually disappear, leaving behind a somewhat thickened, brownish discolored granular mucosa (Fig. 12.48).

HIRSCHSPRUNG'S DISEASE AND STERCORAL ULCERATION

Hirschsprung's disease is a rare indication for colonoscopy. Proper cleansing of the colon in such circumstances is usually extremely difficult. The distal, denervated segment typically has a normal caliber and an unremarkable mucosa (Fig.

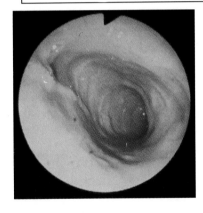

Figure 12.49 Adult Hirschsprung's disease. The distal denervated segment has normal caliber and mucosal appearance.

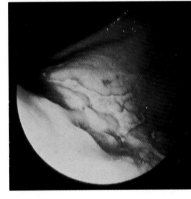

Figure 12.50 Hirschsprung's disease. Widely dilated segment of the colon often shows bizarre stercoral ulceration due to fecal stasis.

12.49). Above the denervated segment is a tremendously dilated colon. Not uncommonly, bizarre-shaped stercoral ulcers are present in the area where the widely dilated colon joins the denervated segment (Fig. 12.50). Stercoral ulcers may develop whenever there is colonic stasis with fecalith or fecaloma formation. Fecaliths are stonelike formations of fecal matter. When they reach a size of 2 cm or more they are termed fecalomas. These firm masses of feces may injure and necrose the mucosal lining.

12.13

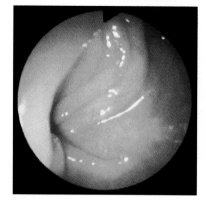 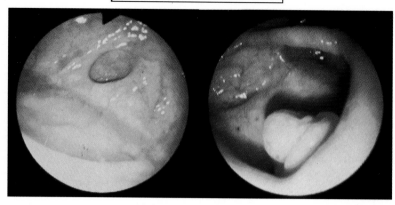

Figure 12.51 Colonic volvulus. The twisting mucosal fold pattern is characteristic.

Figure 12.52 Appendix. *Left,* Normal appearance of opening. *Right,* In a different patient, the root of the appendix protrudes upon the appendiceal contraction.

DEROTATION OF COLONIC VOLVULUS

Colonoscopy is used in the diagnosis and therapy of intermittent volvulus of the sigmoid colon. Usually at the point of obstruction, twisted mucosal folds can be seen (Fig. 12.51). The mucosa usually looks normal, but may have an appearance suggesting a compromised vascular supply with cyanosis. Derotation of the volvulus may occur if the twisted area can be gently entered and liquid stool and gas can be removed through the suction channel of the endoscope.

APPENDIX AND APPENDICEAL LESIONS

The normal appendiceal orifice is a slitlike, semilunar pocket on the posterior medial wall of the cecum. The root may protrude from the opening, especially when the appendix contracts (Fig. 12.52). Fecal material may be present in the appendiceal opening and can be the cause of partial intussusception of the appendiceal structure (Fig. 12.53).

A common abnormality is an inverted appendiceal stump after appendectomy, which may appear as a smooth, oblong mass (Fig. 12.54). Such a masslike deformity can easily be mistaken for an adenomatous polyp, especially if adenomatous polyps are present in the cecal area or if surveillance colonoscopy is performed after previous removal of adenomatous polyps. It is usually covered by normal-appearing mucosa. When in doubt, biopsies should be obtained. Such a lesion should not be removed with a polypectomy snare if there is the slightest suspicion that it might be an inverted appendiceal stump.

It is most unusual to see purulent material exuding from the appendiceal orifice (Fig. 12.55). More often, an appendiceal inflammatory mass compresses the medial or posterior cecal wall with some edema and opalescence of the mucosa and stretching or swelling of the folds (Fig. 12.56).

The appendiceal region and bottom of the cecum have a unique appearance after intussusception of the ileocecal area. This is a very rarely noted lesion. Because of marked venous congestion, there may be impressive petechial or ecchymotic discoloration of the mucosa.

POSTOPERATIVE APPEARANCES

The colonoscopist needs to be aware of the range of appearances after colonic resection and colonic anastomosis.

An anastomosis between the small intestine and colon may be either side-to-end or end-to-end (Fig. 12.57). The overall color and texture of the two segments are sufficiently different to allow easy differentiation of the anastomotic line. This line can also be indicated by differences in the vascular pattern. The anastomosis between the ileum and colon may be regular and smooth or nodular (Fig. 12.58). Ringlike Kerckring's folds are often seen just beyond the anastomosis. Features such as erythema and nodularity of the anastomotic line are not specific and should not be interpreted as evidence of recurrent inflammatory disease by itself.

A colocolonic anastomosis is usually fashioned end-to-end. The anastomotic line may be a thin, perfectly smooth scar (Fig. 12.59). When interrupted sutures are used, the anastomotic site may reveal nodularity (Fig. 12.60). Sometimes the nodular folds may exceed 5 mm, and the overlying mucosa appears erythematous. However, the mucosa is soft and pliant, and tents easily upon biopsy. In case of side-to-end colocolonic anastomosis, the closed end of the anastomosed segment may be inverted, creating a polyp-simulating configuration which may fool the endoscopist and lead to inappropriate removal (Fig. 12.61). When in doubt, the polypoid protuberance should be biopsied to prove its nonneoplastic composition.

If a suture granuloma occurs at the anastomosis, the area is usually erythematous and may be eroded or ulcerated (Fig. 12.62).

A peculiar and poorly understood abnormality is the development of chronic ulceration after ileorectal anastomosis, especially on the ileal side (Fig. 12.63). Such ulcers appear resistant to any form of therapy.

Narrowing of a colonic anastomosis to the point where a colonoscope cannot pass suggests disease at the anastomosis such as inflammation, cancer, or concomitant diverticular disease. The presence of a symmetrical stricture without rigidity, masses, or ulcerations favors the diagnosis

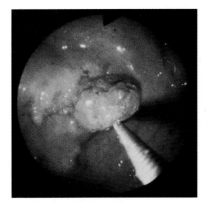

Figure 12.53 Partial spontaneous intussusception of the appendix encrusted with fecal material.

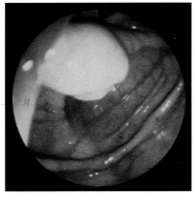

Figure 12.54 An inverted appendiceal stump is a common appearance after appendectomy.

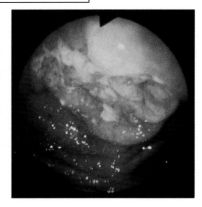

Figure 12.55 Acute appendicitis is presumably responsible for exudate surrounding the appendiceal opening.

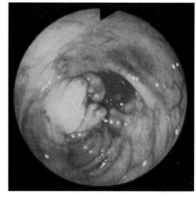

Figure 12.56 Appendiceal inflammation with swollen folds.

Postoperative Appearances

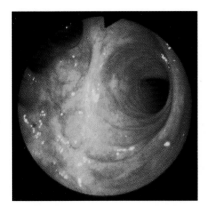

Figure 12.57 Normal end-to-side ileocolonic anastomosis. Note the differences in color and fold pattern between small bowel and colon.

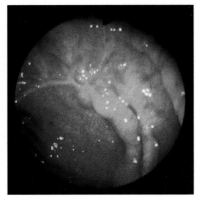

Figure 12.58 Ileocolonic anastomosis shows slight nodularity at the anastomotic line.

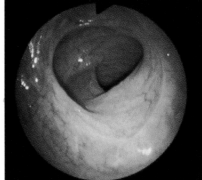

Figure 12.59 Perfectly smooth colocolonic anastomosis. *Left,* Appearing as a fine line of scarring.

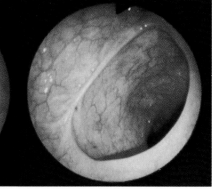

Right, Appearing as a very thin scar fold.

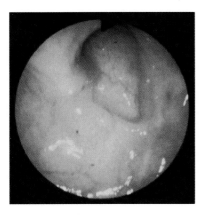

Figure 12.60 Colocolonic anastomosis with some nodularity at the suture line.

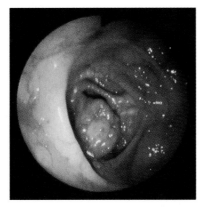

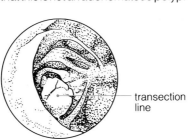

Figure 12.61 Inverted anastomotic line after side-to-end anastomosis. If uncertain, a biopsy will establish that this is not an adenomatous polyp.

transection line

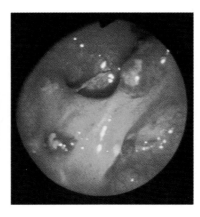

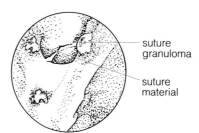

Figure 12.62 Suture granulomas at the anastomotic line with some evidence of inflammation.

suture granuloma

suture material

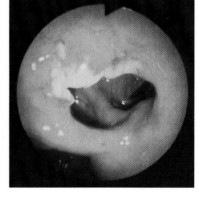

Figure 12.63 Chronic ulceration after ileorectal anastomosis for polyposis coli.

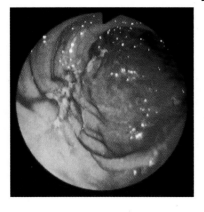

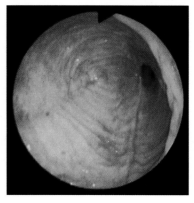

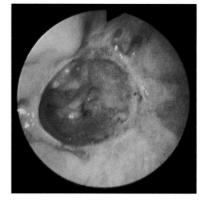

Figure 12.64 Healing stage after creation of a small intestinal pelvic pouch. Lines of ulceration and exudate mark the site of anastomosis between ileal loops.

Figure 12.65 Fully healed ileal pouch has anastomotic lines perpendicular to Kerckring's folds

Figure 12.66 A fully healed ileoanal anastomosis appears as a fine line between squamous and columnar mucosa.

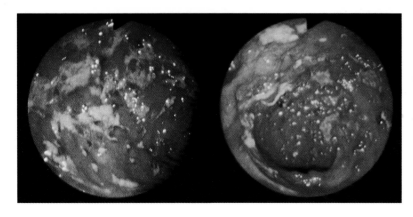

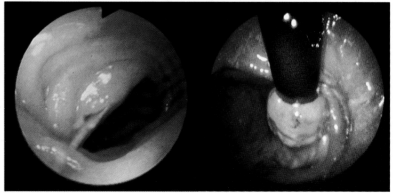

Figure 12.67 *Left,* Severe ulcerating pouchitis, seen after creation of a pelvic pouch with ileoanal anastomosis. *Right,* Here we see that the prepouch ileum was severely inflamed and ulcerated.

Figure 12.68 *Left,* The endoscope is being inserted in the nipple of the Koch pouch. *Right,* The nipple is seen on retroflexion.

of a benign anastomotic stricture rather than recurrent malignancy. Malignancy can never be excluded with certainty, even if biopsy and brush cytology are negative.

Endoscopy can also be useful in the evaluation of a Koch pouch or an ileoanal anastomosis with creation of a pelvic pouch. These types of surgery are usually carried out for ulcerative colitis or familial polyposis coli. During the healing stage after creation of a pouch, superficial ulceration and exudate may mark the lines of anastomosis between the small bowel loops (Fig. 12.64). After complete healing, Kerckring's folds are seen, with the surgical deformity of longitudinally dissecting parallel anastomotic lines (Fig. 12.65). The ileoanal anastomotic line is seen as a fine, whitish rim connecting the anal squamous mucosa to the columnar mucosa of the ileal limb (Fig. 12.66). Inflammation in the pouch and prepouch ileum or in the Koch pouch can presumably develop by overgrowth of anaerobic microorganisms. Pouchitis is characterized by diffuse erythema and occasionally superficial ulceration (Fig. 12.67).

If dysfunction of a Koch pouch is suspected, the nipple can be inspected by inserting a small-caliber endoscope into the pouch and retroflexing the scope (Fig. 12.68). Dysfunction of the nipple may occasionally be due to the presence of adhesions between the nipple and the wall of the pouch. In other instances, the nipple valve may become shorter and patulous due to loosening of the sutures between the invaginated ileum and the mesenteric site of the adjacent small bowel loop.

Colonoscopy is also frequently used for inspecting the defunctionalized limb of the left colon following colostomy. In most instances, the colostomy is performed for sigmoid inflammation or abscess formation, perforation, or other abdominal catastrophes. Usually the colonoscope can be passed into the left limb of a double-barrel colostomy down to and occasionally through the point of obstruction. If the narrowed segment cannot be intubated from above, the colonoscope may be inserted rectally and advanced to the point of obstruction.

Bibliography

GENERAL READINGS

Berk JE: Bockus Gastroenterology, 4th ed. Saunders, Philadelphia, 1985.

Blackstone MO: Endoscopic Interpretation. Raven Press, New York, 1984.

Cotton PB, Williams CB: Practical Gastrointestinal Endoscopy, 2nd ed. Blackwell Scientific, Oxford, 1982.

Silvis SE: Therapeutic Gastrointestinal Endoscopy. Igaku-Shoin, New York, 1985.

Sleisenger MH, Fordtran JS: Gastrointestinal Disease, 3rd ed. Saunders, Philadelphia, 1983.

Suggested Readings

1 THE NORMAL GASTROINTESTINAL TRACT

Becker V, Classen M, et al: Gastroenterologishche Endoskopie. Ferdinand Enke Verlag, Stuttgart, 1979.

Demling L, Elster K, et al: Endoscopy and Biopsy of Esophagus, Stomach and Duodenum. Saunders, Philadelphia, 1982.

Goldberg SM, Gordon PH, et al: Essentials of Anorectal Surgery. Lippincott, Philadelphia, 1980.

Hunt RH, Waye JD: Colonoscopy. Year Book, Chicago, 1981.

Kozarek RA: Evaluation of the larynx, hypopharynx, and nasopharynx at the time of diagnostic upper gastrointestinal endoscopy. Gastrointestinal Endoscopy 31:271, 1985.

Lieberman DA: Common anorectal disorders. Annals of Internal Medicine 101:837, 1984.

Nagasako K: Differential Diagnosis of Colorectal Diseases. Igaku-Shoin, Tokyo, 1982.

Stewart ET, Vennes JA, et al: Atlas of Endoscopic Retrograde Cholangiopancreatography. Mosby, St. Louis, 1977.

2 ESOPHAGUS I: DIVERTICULA, HIATAL HERNIAS, WEBS, RINGS, REFLUX, AND BARRETT'S METAPLASIA

Benjamin SB, Kerr R, et al: Complications of the Angelchik antireflux prosthesis. Annals of Internal Medicine 100:570, 1984.

Bozymski EM, Herlihy KJ, et al: Barrett's esophagus. Annals of Internal Medicine 97:103, 1982.

Brand DL, Eastwood IR, et al: Esophageal symptoms, manometry, and histology before and after antireflux surgery. Gastroenterology 76:1393, 1979.

Brühlmann WF, Zollikofer CL, et al: Intramural pseudodiverticulosis of the esophagus: Report of seven cases and literature review. Gastrointestinal Radiology 6:199, 1981.

Cameron AJ, Ott BJ, et al: The incidence of adenocarcinoma in columnar-lined (Barrett's) esophagus. New England Journal of Medicine 313:857, 1985.

Dumon JF, Meric B, et al: A new method of esophageal dilation using Savary-Gilliard bougies. Gastrointestinal Endoscopy 31:379, 1985.

Eckardt VF, Adami B, et al: The esophagogastric junction in patients with asymptomatic lower esophageal mucosal rings. Gastroenterology 79:426, 1980.

Graham DY, Smith JL: Balloon dilatation of benign and malignant esophageal strictures. Gastrointestinal Endoscopy 31:171, 1985.

Hamilton SR, Hutcheon DF, et al: Adenocarcinoma in Barrett's esophagus after elimination of gastroesophageal reflux. Gastroenterology 86:356, 1984.

Hendrix TR: Schatzki ring, epithelial junction, and hiatal hernia—an unresolved controversy. Gastroenterology 79:584, 1980.

Knuff TE, Benjamin SB, et al: Pharyngoesophageal (Zenker's) diverticulum: A reappraisal. Gastroenterology 82:734, 1982.

Patterson DJ, Graham DY, et al: Natural history of benign esophageal stricture treated by dilatation. Gastroenterology 85:346, 1983.

Pope CE: Pathophysiology and diagnosis of reflux esophagitis. Gastroenterology 70:445, 1976.

Richter JE, Castell DO: Gastroesophageal reflux. Annals of Internal Medicine 97:93, 1982.

Shiflett DW, Gilliam JH, et al: Multiple esophageal webs. Gastroenterology 77:556, 1979.

Spechler SJ, Goyal RK: Barrett's Esophagus. Elsevier, New York, 1985.

Wesdorp ICE, Bartelsman J, et al. Results of conservative treatment of benign esophageal strictures: A follow-up study in 100 patients. Gastroenterology 82:487, 1982.

Wesdorp ICE, Bartelsman J, et al: Effect of long-term treatment with cimetidine and antacids in Barrett's esophagus. Gut 22:724, 1981.

3 ESOPHAGUS II: NEOPLASMS, INFECTIONS, AND INVOLVEMENT IN GRAFT-VERSUS-HOST DISEASE

Den Hartog Jager FCA, Bartelsman JFWM, et al: Palliative treatment of obstructing esophagogastric malignancy by endoscopic positioning of a plastic prosthesis. Gastroenterology 77:1008, 1979.

Faintuch J, Shepard KV, et al: Adenocarcinoma and other unusual variants of esophageal cancer. Seminars in Oncology 11:196, 1984.

Fleischer D, Sivak MJ, et al: Endoscopic Nd:YAG laser therapy as palliation for esophagogastric cancer. Gastroenterology 89:827, 1985.

Franzin G, Musola R, et al: Squamous papillomas of the esophagus. Gastrointestinal Endoscopy 29:104, 1983.

Froelicher P, Miller G: The European experience with esophageal cancer limited to the mucosa and submucosa. Gastrointestinal Endoscopy 32:88, 1986.

Gertler SL, Pressman J, et al: Gastrointestinal cytomegalovirus infection in a homosexual man with severe acquired immunodeficiency syndrome. Gastroenterology 85:1403, 1983.

Graham DY, Schwartz JT, et al: Prospective evaluation of biopsy number in the diagnosis of esophageal and gastric carcinoma. Gastroenterology 82:228, 1982.

Guanrei Y, He H, et al: Endoscopic diagnosis of 115 cases of early esophageal carcinoma. Endoscopy 14:157, 1982.

Howiler, W Goldberg HI: Gastroesophageal involvement in herpes simplex. Gastroenterology, 70:775, 1976.

Kodsi BE, Wichremesinghe PC, et al: Candida esophagitis. Gastroenterology 71:715, 1976.

Lightdale CJ, Winawer SJ: Screening diagnosis and staging of esophageal cancer. Seminars in Oncology 11:101, 1984.

McDonald GB, Sharma P, et al: Esophageal infections in immunosuppressed patients after marrow transplantation. Gastroenterology 88:1111, 1985.

McDonald GB, Shulman HM, et al: Intestinal and hepatic complications of human bone marrow transplantation, Part 1. Gastroenterology 90:460, 770, 1986.

McDonald GB, Sullivan KM, et al: Esophageal abnormalities in chronic graft-versus-host disease in humans. Gastroenterology 80:914, 1981.

Murney RG Jr., Huston JD: Endoscopic evaluation of the esophagogastric polyp and fold. Gastrointestinal Endoscopy 29:294, 1983.

Seremetis MG, Lyons WS, et al: Leiomyomata of the esophagus. Cancer 38:2166, 1976.

4 ESOPHAGUS III: MOTOR DYSFUNCTION, VASCULAR ABNORMALITIES, AND TRAUMA

Brayko CM, Kozarek RA, et al: Bacteremia during esophageal variceal sclerotherapy: Its cause and prevention. Gastrointestinal Endoscopy 31:10, 1985.

Cello JP, Grendell JH, et al: Endoscopic sclerotherapy versus portacaval shunt in patients with severe cirrhosis and variceal hemorrhage. New England Journal of Medicine 311:1589, 1984.

Cohen S: Motor disorders of the esophagus. New England Journal of Medicine, 301:184, 1979.

Collins FJ, Matthews HR, et al: Drug-induced oesophageal injury. British Medical Journal 1:1673, 1979.

de Caestecker JS, Blackwell JN, et al: The esophagus as a cause of recurrent chest pain: Which patients should be investigated and which tests should be used? Lancet 2:1143, 1985.

di Costanzo J, Noirclerc M. et al: New therapeutic approach to corrosive burns of the upper gastrointestinal tract. Gut 21:370, 1980.

Eckardt VF, Grace ND: Gastroesophageal reflux and bleeding esophageal varices. Gastroenterology, 76:39, 1979.

Fleischer D: Endoscopic Nd:YAG laser therapy for active esophageal variceal bleeding. Gastrointestinal Endoscopy 31:4, 1985.

Garcia-Tsao G, Groszmann RJ, et al: Portal pressure, presence of gastroesophageal varices and variceal bleeding. Hepatology 5:419, 1985.

Goldman LP, Weigert JM: Corrosive substance ingestion: A review. American Journal of Gastroenterology 79:85, 1984.

Grobe JL, Kozarek RA, et al: Venography during endoscopic infection sclerotherapy of esophageal varices. Gastrointestinal Endoscopy 30:6, 1984.

Haynes WC, Sanowski RA, et al: Esophageal strictures following endoscopic variceal sclerotherapy: Clinical course and response to dilation therapy. Gastrointestinal Endoscopy 32:202, 1986.

Kikendall JW, Friedman AC, et al: Pill-induced esophageal injury. Digestive Diseases and Sciences 28:174, 1983.

Papazian A. Capron J-P, et al: Mucosal bridges of the upper esophagus after radiotherapy for Hodgkin's disease. Gastroenterology 84:1028, 1983.

Smith JL, Graham DY: Variceal hemorrhage. Gastroenterology 82:968, 1982.

Tucker HJ, Snape WJ, et al: Achalasia secondary to carcinoma: Manometric and clinical features. Annals of Internal Medicine 89:315, 1978.

Turner R, Rittenberg G, et al: Esophageal dysfunction in collagen disease. American Journal of the Medical Sciences 265:191, 1973.

Westaby D, MacDougall BRD, et al: Improved survival following infection sclerotherapy for esophageal varices: Final analysis of a controlled trial. Hepatology 5:827, 1985.

5 STOMACH I: GASTRIC ULCERS, ANATOMIC AND VASCULAR ABNORMALITIES, AND POSTOPERATIVE EVALUATION

Bachman BA, Brady PG: Localized gastric varices: Mimicry leading to endoscopic misinterpretation. Gastrointestinal Endoscopy 30:244, 1984.

Cameron AJ, Higgins JA: Linear gastric erosion. A lesion associated with large diaphragmatic hernia and chronic blood loss anemia. Gastroenterology 91:338, 1986.

Caygill CPJ, Hill MJ, et al: Mortality from gastric cancer following gastric surgery for peptic ulcer. Lancet 1(8487):929, 1986.

Dekker W, Tytgat GN: Diagnostic accuracy of fiberendoscopy in the detection of upper intestinal malignancy. A follow-up analysis. Gastroenterology 73:710, 1977.

Goldman RL: Submucosal arterial malformation ("aneurysm") of the stomach with fatal hemorrhage. Gastroenterology 46:589, 1964.

Graham DY, Schwartz JT: The spectrum of the Mallory-Weiss tear. Medicine 57:307, 1977.

Graham DY, Schwartz JT, et al: Prospective evaluation of biopsy number in the diagnosis of esophageal and gastric carcinoma. Gastroenterology 82:228, 1982.

Gunnlaugsson O: Angiodysplasia of the stomach and duodenum. Gastrointestinal Endoscopy 31:251, 1985.

Hirschowitz BI, Luketic GC: Endoscopy in the post-gastrectomy patient. Gastrointestinal Endoscopy 18:27, 1971.

Klarfeld J, Resnick G: Gastric remnant carcinoma. Cancer 44:1129, 1979.

Ludwig S, Ippoliti A: Objective evaluation of symptomatic alkaline reflux after antrectomy. Digestive Diseases and Sciences 29:824, 1984.

Malagelada J-R, Phillips SF, et al: Postoperative reflux gastritis: Pathophysiology and long-term outcome after Roux-en-Y diversion. Annals of Internal Medicine 103:178, 1985.

Martinez NS, Morlock CG, et al: Heterotopic pancreatic tissue involving the stomach. Annals of Surgery 147:1, 1958.

Nelson RS, Urrea LH, et al: Evaluation of gastric ulcerations. Digestive Diseases 21:389, 1976.

Piper DW, McIntosh JH, et al: Analgesic ingestion and chronic peptic ulcer. Gastroenterology 80:427, 1981.

Shepherd HA, Harvey J, et al: Recurrent retching with gastric mucosal prolapse. Digestive Diseases 29:121, 1984.

Sun DCH, Stempien SJ: Site and size of the ulcer as determinants of outcome. Gastroenterology 61:576, 1971.

Vizcarrondo FJ, Brady PG, et al: Foreign bodies of the upper gastrointestinal tract. Gastrointestinal Endoscopy 29:208, 1983.

Woodard JC, Mainz DL, et al: Afferent-efferent loop intragastric intussusception: Diagnosed by gastroscopy. Gastroenterology 64:120, 1973.

Wortzel E, Ferrer JP, et al: Medical treatment of the postgastrectomy bezoar. American Journal of Gastroenterology 67:565, 1977.

Zuckerman GR, Cornette GL, et al: Upper gastrointestinal bleeding in patients with chronic renal failure. Annals of Internal Medicine 102:588, 1985.

6 STOMACH II: TUMORS AND POLYPS

Appelman HD, Helwig EB: Sarcomas of the stomach. American Journal of Clinical Pathology 67:2, 1977.

Bemvenuti GA, Hattori K, et al: Endoscopic sampling for tissue diagnosis in gastrointestinal malignancy. Gastrointestinal Endoscopy 21:159, 1975.

Blackstone MO: The endoscopic diagnosis of early gastric cancer. Gastrointestinal Endoscopy 30:105, 1984.

Burt RW, Berenson MM, et al: Upper gastrointestinal polyps in Gardner's syndrome. Gastroenterology 86:295, 1984.

Dworkin B, Lightdale CJ, et al: Primary gastric lymphoma. Digestive Diseases and Sciences 27:986, 1982.

Fleischer D, Sivak MV: Endoscopic Nd:YAG laser therapy as palliative treatment for advanced adenocarcinoma of the gastric cardia. Gastroenterology 87:815, 1984.

Friedman SL, Wright TL, et al: Gastrointestinal Kaposi's sarcoma in patients with acquired immunodeficiency syndrome. Gastroenterology 89:102, 1985.

Gordon SJ, Rifkin MD, et al: Endosonographic evaluation of mural abnormalities of the upper gastrointestinal tract. Gastrointestinal Endoscopy 32:193, 1986.

Gray GM, Rosenberg SA, et al: Lymphomas involving the gastrointestinal tract. Gastroenterology 82:143, 1982.

Green PHR, O'Toole KM, et al: Early gastric cancer. Gastroenterology 81:247, 1981.

Harvey RF, Bradshaw MJ, et al: Multifocal gastric carcinoid tumours, achlorhydria, and hypergastrinaemia. Lancet 1:951, 1985.

Iida M, Yao T, et al: Natural history of fundic gland polyposis in patients with familial adenomatosis coli/Gardner's syndrome. Gastroenterology 89:1021, 1985.

Kamiya T, Morishita T, et al: Histoclinical long-standing follow-up study of hyperplastic polyps of the stomach. American Journal of Gastroenterology 75:275, 1981.

Kawai K: Diagnosis of early gastric cancer. Endoscopy 1:23, 1971.

Lanza FL, Graham DY, et al: Endoscopic upper gastrointestinal polypectomy. American Journal of Gastroenterology 75:345, 1981.

Llanos O, Guzman S, et al: Accuracy of the first endoscopic procedure in the differential diagnosis of gastric lesions. Annals of Surgery 195:224, 1982.

Menuck LS, Amberg JR: Metastatic disease involving the stomach. Digestive Diseases 20:903, 1975.

Morrissey JF: Small polypoid lesions of the stomach. Gastrointestinal Endoscopy 28:266, 1982.

Niv Y, Bat L: Gastric polyps—a clinical study. Israel Journal of Medical Sciences 21:841, 1985.

Seifert E, Gail K, et al: Gastric polypectomy: Long-term results (survey of 23 centres in Germany). Endoscopy 15:8, 1983.

Tio TL, Den Hartog Jager FCA, et al: Endoscopic ultrasonography of non-Hodgkin lymphoma of the stomach. Gastroenterology 91:401, 1986.

Yokoyama Y, Yokoyama H, et al: On biopsy of excavated gastric lesions. Stomach and Intestine 9:8, 1974.

7 STOMACH III: GASTRITIS AND UPPER GASTROINTESTINAL BLEEDING

Andre C, Gillon J, et al: Randomised placebo-controlled double-blind trial of two dosages of sodium cromoglycate in treatment of varioliform gastritis: Comparison with cimetidine. Gut 23:348, 1982.

Emmanouilidis A, Nicolopoulou-Stamati P, et al: The histologic pattern of bile gastritis. Gastrointestinal Endoscopy 30:179, 1984.

Fleischer D: Endoscopic therapy of upper gastrointestinal bleeding in humans. Gastroenterology 90:217, 1986.

Fleischer D: Etiology and prevalence of severe persistent upper gastrointestinal bleeding. Gastroenterology 84:538, 1983.

Gad A: Erosion: A correlative endoscopic histopathologic multicenter study. Endoscopy 18:76, 1986.

Griffiths WJ, Neumann DA, et al: The visible vessel as an indicator of uncontrolled or recurrent gastrointestinal hemorrhage. New England Journal of Medicine 300:1411, 1979.

Hirao M, Kobayashi T, et al: Endoscopic local injection of hypertonic saline-epinephrine solution to arrest hemorrhage from the upper gastrointestinal tract. Gastrointestinal Endoscopy 31:313, 1985.

Johnston JH, Sones JQ, et al: Comparison of heater probe and YAG laser in endoscopic treatment of major bleeding from peptic ulcers. Gastrointestinal Endoscopy 31:175, 1985.

Karvonen AL, Lehtola J: Outcome of gastric mucosal erosions. Scandinavian Journal of Gastroenterology 19:228, 1984.

Levine DS, Surawicz CM: Severe intestinal damage following acid ingestion with minimal findings on early endoscopy. Gastrointestinal Endoscopy 30:247, 1984.

O'Brien JD, Day SJ, et al: Controlled trial of small bipolar probe in bleeding peptic ulcers. Lancet 1:464, 1986.

Papp JP: Endoscopic Control of Gastrointestinal Hemorrhage. CRC Press, Boca Raton, 1981.

Poelman JR, Hausman RH, et al: Endoscopy in lye burns of oesophagus and stomach. Endoscopy 9:172, 1977.

Ritchie WP: Alkaline reflux gastritis: A critical reappraisal. Gut 25:975, 1984.

Rutgeerts P, van Gompel F, et al: Long term results of treatment of vascular malformations of the gastrointestinal tract by Neodymium Yag laser photocoagulation. Gut 26:586, 1985.

Sauerbruch T, Schreiber MA, et al: Endoscopy in the diagnosis of gastritis. Diagnostic value of endoscopic criterion in relation to histological diagnosis. Endoscopy 16:101, 1984.

Scharschmidt BF: The natural history of hypertrophic gastropathy (Menetrier's disease). American Journal of Medicine 63:644, 1977.

Shorvon PJ, Leung JWC, et al: Preliminary clinical experience with the heat probe at endoscopy in acute upper gastrointestinal bleeding. Gastrointestinal Endoscopy 31:364, 1985.

Silverstein FE, Gilbert DA, et al: The national ASGE survey on upper gastrointestinal bleeding. Gastrointestinal Endoscopy 27:73, 80, 94, 1981.

Silvoso GR, Ivey KJ, et al: Incidence of gastric lesions in patients with rheumatic disease on chronic aspirin therapy. Annals of Internal Medicine 91:517, 1979.

Soehendra N, Grimm H, et al: Infection of nonvariceal bleeding lesions of the upper gastrointestinal tract. Endoscopy 17:129, 1985.

Storey DW, Bown SG, et al: Endoscopic prediction of recurrent bleeding in peptic ulcers. New England Journal of Medicine 305:915, 1981.

Swain CP, Kirkham JS, et al: Controlled trial of Nd-YAG laser photocoagulation in bleeding peptic ulcers. Lancet 1:1113, 1986.

Swain CP, Storey DW, et al: Nature of the bleeding vessel in recurrently bleeding gastric ulcers. Gastroenterology 90:595, 1986.

Tanaka M, Kimura K, et al: Long-term follow-up for minute gastroduodenal lesions in Crohn's disease. Gastrointestinal Endoscopy 32:206, 1986.

Tytgat GNJ: Endoscopic diagnosis. In Salmon PR (ed.): Gastrointestinal Endoscopy. Advances in Diagnosis and Therapy, vol. I. Chapman and Hall, London, 1984.

Weinstein WM: The diagnosis and classification of gastritis and duodenitis. Journal of Clinical Gastroenterology 3:7, 1981.

8 SMALL BOWEL

Ament ME, Rubin CE: Relation of giardiasis to abnormal intestinal structure and function in gastrointestinal immunodeficiency syndromes. Gastroenterology 62:216, 1972.

Brown P, Salmon PR, et al: The endoscopic, radiological, and surgical findings in chronic duodenal ulceration. Scandinavian Journal of Gastroenterology 13:557, 1978.

Corachan M, Oomen HAPC, et al: Parasitic duodenitis. Transactions of the Royal Society of Tropical Medicine and Hygiene 75:385, 1981.

Frandsen PJ, Jarnum S, et al: Crohn's disease of the duodenum. Scandinavian Journal of Gastroenterology 15:683, 1980.

Greenlaw R, Sheahan DG, et al: Gastroduodenitis: A broader concept of peptic ulcer disease. Digestive Diseases and Sciences 25:660, 1980.

Ikeda K, Murayama H, et al: Massive intestinal bleeding in hemangiomatosis of the duodenum. Endoscopy 12:306, 1980.

Kerremans RP, Lerut J, et al: Primary malignant duodenal tumors. Annals of Surgery 190:179, 1979.

Kozarek RA: Hydrostatic balloon dilation of gastrointestinal stenoses: A national survey. Gastrointestinal Endoscopy 32:15, 1986.

Kreel L, Ellis H: Pyloric stenosis in adults: A clinical and radiological study of 100 consecutive patients. Gut 6:253, 1965.

Laufer I, Mullens JE, et al: The diagnostic accuracy of barium studies of the stomach and duodenum—correlation with endoscopy. Radiology 115:569, 1975.

Lockard OO Jr, Ivey KJ, et al: The prevalence of duodenal lesions in patients with rheumatic diseases on chronic aspirin therapy. Gastrointestinal Endoscopy 26:5, 1980.

Lumsden K, MacLarnon JC, et al: Giant duodenal ulcer. Gut 11:592, 1970.

Mee AS, Burke M, et al: Small bowel biopsy for malabsorption: Comparison of the diagnostic adequacy of endoscopic forceps and capsule biopsy specimens. British Medical Journal 291:769, 1985.

Merrell DE, Mansbach C II, et al: Carcinoid tumors of the duodenum: Endoscopic diagnosis of two cases. Gastrointestinal Endoscopy 31:269, 1985.

Reddy RR, Schuman BM, et al: Duodenal polyps: Diagnosis and management. Journal of Clinical Gastroenterology 3:139, 1981.

Rogers BHG: Hydrostatic dilation of upper gastrointestinal strictures with endoscopic control. Gastrointestinal Endoscopy 31:343, 1985.

Roth RI, Owen RL, et al: Intestinal infection with *Mycobacterium avium* in acquired immune deficiency syndrome (AIDS). Digestive Diseases and Sciences 30:497, 1985.

Solt J, Rauth J, et al: Balloon catheter dilation of postoperative gastric outlet stenosis. Gastrointestinal Endoscopy 30:359, 1984.

Yamase H, Norris M, et al: Pseudomelanosis duodeni: A clinicopathologic entity. Gastrointestinal Endoscopy 31:83, 1985.

Zukerman GR, Mills BA, et al: Nodular duodenitis. Digestive Diseases and Sciences 28:1018, 1983.

9 ENDOSCOPIC RETROGRADE CHOLANGIOPANCREATOGRAPHY AND SPHINCTEROTOMY

Alderson D, Lavelle MI, et al: Endoscopic sphincterotomy before pancreaticoduodenectomy for ampullary carcinoma. British Medical Journal 282:1109, 1981.

Bilbao MK, Dotter CT, et al: Complications of endoscopic retrograde cholangiopancreatography (ERCP). Gastroenterology 70:314, 1976.

Cooperman A, Gelbfish G, et al: Choledochoscopy. Surgical Clinics of North America 62:853, 1982.

Delhaye M, Engelholm L, et al: Pancreas divisum: Congenital anatomic variant or anomaly? Gastroenterology 89:951, 1985.

Guelrud M, Siegel JH: Hypertensive pancreatic duct sphincter as a cause of pancreatitis. Digestive Diseases and Sciences 29:225, 1984.

Hagenmüller F, Soehendra N: Non-surgical biliary drainage. Clinics in Gastroenterology 12:297, 1983.

Huibregtse K, Tytgat GN: Palliative treatment of obstructive jaundice by transpapillary introduction of large bore bile duct endoprosthesis. Gut 23:371, 1982.

Lehman GA, O'Connor KW: Coexistence of annular pancreas and pancreas divisum—ERCP diagnosis. Gastrointestinal Endoscopy 31:25, 1985.

Leung JWC, Del Favero G, et al: Endoscopic biliary prostheses: A comparison of materials. Gastrointestinal Endoscopy 31:93, 1986.

Mueller PR, Ferrucci JT, et al: Biliary stent endoprosthesis: Analysis of complications in 113 patients. Radiology 156:637, 1985.

Nakao NL, Siegel JH, et al: Tumors of the ampulla of Vater: Early diagnosis by intraampullary biopsy during endoscopic cannulation. Gastroenterology 83:459, 1982.

Osnes M, Kahrs T: Endoscopic choledochoduodenostomy for choledocholithiasis through choledochoduodenal fistula. Endoscopy 9:162, 1977.

Phillip J, Koch H, et al: Variations and anomalies of the papilla of Vater, the pancreas and biliary duct system. Endoscopy 6:70, 1974.

Richter JM, Silverstein MD: Suspected obstructive jaundice: A decision analysis of diagnostic strategies. Annals of Internal Medicine 99:46, 1983.

Riemann JF, Seuberth K, et al: Mechanical lithotripsy of common bile duct stones. Gastrointestinal Endoscopy 31:207, 1985.

Siegel JH: Precut papillotomy: A method to improve success of ERCP and papillotomy. Endoscopy 12:130, 1980.

Thomas E, Reddy KR: Cholangitis and pancreatitis due to a juxtapapillary duodenal diverticulum. American Journal of Gastroenterology 77:303, 1982.

Winstanley PA, Ellis WR, et al: Medium term complications of endoscopic biliary sphincterotomy. Gut 26:730, 1985.

Wurbs D, Phillip J, et al: Experiences with the long standing nasobiliary tube in biliary diseases. Endoscopy 12:219, 1980.

10 COLON I: POLYPS AND TUMORS

Avgerinos A, Kalantzis N, et al: Bowel preparation and the risk of explosion during colonoscopic polypectomy. Gut 25:361, 1984.

Brunetaud JM, Mosquet L, et al: Villous adenomas of the rectum. Gastroenterology 89:832, 1985.

Caccese WJ, McKinley MJ, et al: Endoscopic confirmation of colonic endometriosis. Gastrointestinal Endoscopy 30:191, 1984.

Christie JP: Colonoscopic excision of large sessile polyps. American Journal of Gastroenterology 67:430, 1977.

DiPalma JA, Brady CE, et al: Comparison of colon cleansing methods in preparation for colonoscopy. Gastroenterology 86:856, 1984.

Fenoglio CM, Pascal RR: Colorectal adenomas and cancer. Cancer 50:2601, 1982.

Gardner EJ, Burt RW, et al: Gastrointestinal polyposis: Syndromes and genetic mechanisms. Western Journal of Medicine 132:488, 1980.

Green JP, Schaupp WC, et al: Anal carcinoma: Current therapeutic concepts. American Journal of Surgery 140:151, 1980.

Haggitt RC, Glotzbach RE, et al: Prognostic factors in colorectal carcinomas arising in adenomas: Implications for lesions removed by endoscopic polypectomy. Gastroenterology 89:328, 1985.

Love RR, Morrissey JF: Colonoscopy in asymptomatic individuals with a family history of colorectal cancer. Archives of Internal Medicine 144:2209, 1984.

Lynch HT, Albano WA, et al: Surveillance/management of an obligate gene carrier: The cancer family syndrome. Gastroenterology 84:404, 1983.

McGrew W, Dunn GD: Colonic lipomas: Clinical significance and management. Southern Medical Journal 78:877, 1985.

Morson B: The polyp-cancer sequence in the large bowel. Proceedings of the Royal Society of Medicine 67:451, 1974.

Mortensen NJMcC, Eltringham WK, et al: Direct vision brush cytology with colonoscopy: An aid to the accurate diagnosis of colonic strictures. British Journal of Surgery 71:930, 1984.

Pagana TP, Ledesma EJ, et al: The use of colonoscopy in the study of synchronous colorectal neoplasms. Cancer 53:356, 1984.

Shinya H, Wolff WI: Morphology, anatomic distribution and cancer potential of colonic polyps. Annals of Surgery 190:679, 1979.

Sivak MV Jr, Fleischer DE: Colonoscopy with a videoendoscope: Preliminary experience. Gastrointestinal Endoscopy 30:1, 1984.

Tavassolie H, Mir-Madjlessi SH, et al: The endoscopic demonstration of Kaposi's sarcoma of the colon. Gastrointestinal Endoscopy 29:331, 1983.

Varano VJ, Bonanno CA: Colonoscopic findings in *pneumatosis cystoides intestinalis*. American Journal of Gastroenterology 59:353, 1973.

Winawer SJ, Leidner SD, et al: Colonoscopic biopsy and cytology in the diagnosis of colon cancer. Cancer 42:2849, 1978.

Wolff WI, Shinya H: Polypectomy via the fiberoptic colonoscope. New England Journal of Medicine 288:329, 1973.

11 COLON II: INFLAMMATORY AND INFECTIOUS DISORDERS

Bartlett JG, Chang TW, et al: Antibiotic-associated pseudomembranous colitis due to toxin-producing clostridia. New England Journal of Medicine 298:531, 1978.

Bhargava DK, Tandon HD, et al: Diagnosis of ileocecal and colonic tuberculosis by colonoscopy. Gastrointestinal Endoscopy 31:68, 1985.

Coremans G, Rutgeerts P, et al: The value of ileoscopy with biopsy in the diagnosis of intestinal Crohn's disease. Gastrointestinal Endoscopy 30:167, 1984.

den Hartog Jager FCA, van Haastert M, et al: The endoscopic spectrum of late radiation damage of the rectosigmoid colon. Endoscopy 17:214, 1985.

Farmer RG, Whelan G, et al: Long-term follow-up of patients with Crohn's disease. Gastroenterology 88:1818, 1985.

Iida M, Matsui T, et al: Radiographic and endoscopic findings in penicillin-related non-pseudomembranous colitis. Endoscopy 17:64, 1985.

Lambert ME, Schofield PF, et al: Campylobacter colitis. British Medical Journal 1:857, 1979.

Luterman L, Alsumait AR, et al: Colonoscopic features of cecal amebomas. Gastrointestinal Endoscopy 31:204, 1985.

Maratka Z, Nedbal J, et al: Incidence of colorectal cancer in proctocolitis: A retrospective study of 959 cases over 40 years. Gut 26:43, 1985.

Novak JM, Collins JT, et al: Effects of radiation on the human gastrointestinal tract. Journal of Clinical Gastroenterology 1:9, 1979.

Quinn TC, Corey L, et al: The etiology of anorectal infections in homosexual men. American Journal of Medicine 71:395, 1981.

Reeders JWAJ, Tytgat GNJ, et al: Ischaemic Colitis. Martinus Nijhoff Publishers, Boston, 1984.

Rosenstock E, Farmer RG, et al: Surveillance for colonic carcinoma in ulcerative colitis. Gastroenterology 89:1342, 1985.

Surawicz CM, Belic L: Rectal biopsy helps to distinguish acute self-limited colitis from idiopathic inflammatory bowel disease. Gastroenterology 86:104, 1984.

Teague RH, Read AE: Polyposis in ulcerative colitis. Gut 16:792, 1975.

Tedesco FJ, Hardin RD, et al: Infectious colitis endoscopically simulating inflammatory bowel disease: A prospective evaluation. Gastrointestinal Endoscopy 29:195, 1983.

Watier A, Devroede G, et al: Small erythematous mucosal plaques: An endoscopic sign of Crohn's disease. Gut 21:835, 1980.

Waye JD: Endoscopy in inflammatory bowel disease. Clinics in Gastroenterology 9:279, 1980.

Wolff BG, Culp CE, et al: Anorectal Crohn's disease. Disease of the Colon and Rectum 28:709, 1985.

12 COLON III: DIVERTICULAR DISEASE, VASCULAR MALFORMATIONS, AND OTHER COLONIC ABNORMALITIES

Almy TP, Howell DA: Diverticular disease of the colon. New England Journal of Medicine 302:324, 1980.

Boushey HA, Warnock DG, et al: Diagnosis and management of lower gastrointestinal tract hemorrhage. Western Journal of Medicine 143:80, 1985.

Franzin G, Fratton A, et al: Polypoid lesions associated with diverticular disease of the sigmoid colon. Gastrointestinal Endoscopy 31:196, 1985.

Gekas P, Schuster MM: Stercoral perforation of the colon: Case report and review of the literature. Gastroenterology 80:1054, 1981.

Mahoney, TJ, Bubrick MP, et al: Nonspecific ulcers of the colon. Diseases of the Colon and Rectum 21:623, 1978.

Mathus-Vliegen EMH, Tytgat GNJ: Polyp-simulating mucosal prolapse syndrome in (pre-) diverticular disease. Endoscopy 18:84, 1986.

Meyer CT, Troncale FJ, et al: Arteriovenous malformations of the bowel. Medicine 60:36, 1981.

Shah NC, Ostrov AH, et al: Benign ulcers of the colon. Gastrointestinal Endoscopy 32:102, 1986.

Tedesco FJ, Gottfried EB, et al: Prospective evaluation of hospitalized patients with nonactive lower intestinal bleeding—timing and role of barium enema and colonoscopy. Gastrointestinal Endoscopy 30:281, 1984.

Tedesco FJ, Sumner HW, et al: Colitis cystica profunda. American Journal of Gastroenterology 65:339, 1976.

Wittoesch JH, Jackman RJ, et al: Melanosis coli: General review and a study of 887 cases. Diseases of the Colon and Rectum 1:172, 1958.

Wolff WI, Grossman MB, et al: Angiodysplasia of the colon: Diagnosis and treatment. Gastroenterology 72:329, 1977.

Index

Note: Numbers in **bold** refer to Figure numbers.